Glioblastoma - Current Evidence

Edited by Amit Agrawal and Daulat Singh Kunwar

Published in London, United Kingdom

Glioblastoma - Current Evidence
http://dx.doi.org/10.5772/intechopen.100846
Edited by Amit Agrawal and Daulat Singh Kunwar

Contributors
Robert A. Newman, Yuchen Du, Peiying Yang, Xiao-Nan Li, Bertil Rolf Ragnar Persson, Leif G. Salford, Peter Siesjö, Gunnar Skagerberg, Anna Rydelius, Catharina Blennow, Åsa Lilja, Susanne Strömblad, Edward Visse, Bengt Widegren, Tariq D. Al-Saadi, Roberto J. Diaz, Lee Roy Morgan, Branko S. Jursic, Marcus Ware, Roy S. Weiner, Atit Silsirivanit, Maria Angeles Vaz, Maria Villamayor, Juan M. Sepúlveda, Maria Vieito, Sonia Del Barco Berrón, Raquel Luque, Bhabani Sankar Satpathy, Binapani Barik, Ladi Alik Kumar, Sangram Biswal, Meenakshi Tiwari, Lokendra Kumar Sharma, Ajit Kumar Saxena, Raphael Bastianon Santiago, Mauricio Mandel, Hamid Borghei-Razavi, Surabhi Ranjan, Badih Adada, Bhavika Gupta, Assad Ali, James M. Angelastro, Nicole M. Yost, Frank Y. Shan, Dachun Zhao, Carlos A. Tirado, Ekokobe Fonkem, Yi-lu Zhang, Dong-xia Feng, Jason H. Huang, Amit Agrawal, Daulat Singh Kunwar, Ved Prakash Maurya, Balachandar Deivasigamani, Rakesh Mishra

First published in London, United Kingdom, 2023 by IntechOpen
IntechOpen is the global imprint of INTECHOPEN LIMITED, registered in England and Wales, registration number: 11086078, 5 Princes Gate Court, London, SW7 2QJ, United Kingdom

British Library Cataloguing-in-Publication Data
A catalogue record for this book is available from the British Library

Additional hard and PDF copies can be obtained from orders@intechopen.com

Glioblastoma - Current Evidence
Edited by Amit Agrawal and Daulat Singh Kunwar
p. cm.
Print ISBN 978-1-80356-128-8
Online ISBN 978-1-80356-129-5
eBook (PDF) ISBN 978-1-80356-130-1

For EU product safety concerns:
IN TECH d.o.o., Prolaz Marije Krucifikse Kozulić 3, 51000 Rijeka, Croatia,
info@intechopen.com or visit our website at intechopen.com.

Meet the editors

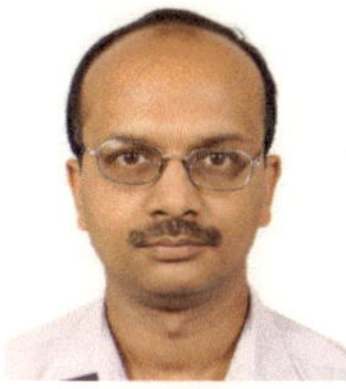

Dr. Amit Agrawal completed his MCh in Neurosurgery at the National Institute of Mental Health and Neurosciences, Bangalore, India, and is now a member of many field-related societies including the World Federation of Neurological Societies, Congress of Neurological Societies, American Association of Neurological Surgeons, International Stroke Society, World Association of Medical Editors, Indian Society of Neuro-oncology, and World Endoscopic Spine Society.

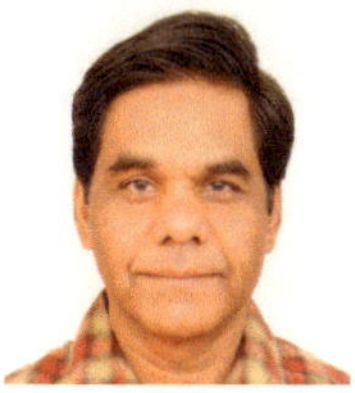

Dr. Daulat Singh obtained his MD from Gandhi Medical College, India. He has vast experience in managing oncology clinical practice. He worked closely to establish the Radiation Oncology Department, including helping to install a dual-energy linear accelerator, as well as the tele-radiation therapy and chemotherapy unit at Government Doon Medical College, India.

Contents

Preface

Glioblastoma multiforme (GBM) has a complex pathogenesis and mutates and alters several key cellular pathways involving cell proliferation, cell migration, and tumor vessel angiogenesis. GBM is known for its rapidly progressive nature. It is a debilitating disease associated with limited response to therapies, poor outcomes, and a very short median overall survival. The diagnosis and management of glioblastomas require multimodal strategies and a multidisciplinary approach. Treatment may involve surgical resection, radiation therapy, and chemotherapy. Significant advances have been made to understand the pathology of GBM, particularly molecular mechanisms and targets for immunotherapy. Recent advances in genetic testing have improved our understanding of the glioblastoma category of brain tumors and have helped us decide on management and follow-up strategies. This book discusses the management of glioblastoma, isocitrate dehydrogenases (IDH)-mutated gliomas, evolving molecular diagnosis strategies, management of lesions involving the corpus callosum, glycan and glycosylation as potential targets for designing therapies, systemic treatment in glioblastoma, the potential utility of lipid-based nano-drug carriers, the role of cancer stem cells and cardiac glycosides in disease evaluation and treatment, management of glioblastoma in the elderly, research related to immunization with autologous IFN-D, and the use of canine glioma as a model for human glioblastoma. This book is a useful resource for understanding and exploring current advances in GBM treatment, including the identification of the molecular characteristics that determine the malignant phenotype, which t may further help to develop effective management strategies including immunotherapy.

Amit Agrawal
Professor,
Department of Neurosurgery,
All India Institute of Medical Sciences,
Bhopal, India

Daulat Singh Kunwar
Department of Radiotherapy and Clinical Oncology,
Government Doon Medical College,
Dehradun, India

Section 1

Glioblastoma

Chapter 1

Glioblastoma in Elderly Population

Raphael Bastianon Santiago, Hamid Borghei-Razavi, Mauricio Mandel, Bhavika Gupta, Asad Ali, Badih Adada and Surabhi Ranjan

Abstract

Glioblastoma (GBM) is the third most common primary intracranial tumor and the commonest primary malignant brain tumor in adults. The peak incidence is between 65 and 84 years old. The incidence of GBM increases starkly with age—from 1.3/100,000 between the ages of 35–44 to 15.3/100,000 between the ages of 75–84 years. Elderly patients with GBM have increased comorbidities, lower functional status, aggressive tumor biology, and an overall worse outcome as compared with their younger counterparts. Age is an independent and powerful prognosticator of GBM outcomes, even if the performance status is controlled. Elderly patients with GBM represent a vulnerable heterogeneous cohort. Surgical resection in elderly patients offers a better outcome and improved quality of life as compared with biopsy alone and nowadays can be safely tolerated by elderly patients in specialized centers. The standard of care treatment of glioblastoma based on the Stupp's protocol excluded patients over the age of 70. Thus, the standard of care treatment in elderly patients with GBM remains controversial. Selected elderly patients with excellent performance status may be treated with Stupp's protocol. Elderly patients with lower functional status may be treated with a hypofractionated treatment regimen with concomitant and adjuvant temozolomide. Frail patients with MGMT methylated tumor can be treated with temozolomide monotherapy alone. It is also not unreasonable to treat elderly frail patients with MGMT unmethylated GBM with hypofractionated RT alone. Thus, treatment of elderly patients with GBM needs a multidisciplinary approach based on the extent of the tumor, MGMT methylation status, performance status, and even the social situation unique to the elderly patient. This chapter seeks to bring a comprehensive and updated review on the treatment of glioblastoma in the elderly population.

Keywords: glioblastoma, high-grade glioma, elderly, geriatric, hypofractionated, aged, frail, temozolomide, chemoradiation, tumor-treating field

1. Introduction

Glioblastoma (WHO grade 4) is the third most common primary intracranial tumor and the most common primary malignant brain tumors in adults [1]. While death rates for many common cancers are declining due to prevention (e.g. tobacco control policies) [2], cancer screening [3], and immunotherapy (i.e. lung cancer, melanoma) [4, 5] and other advances in chemotherapeutics, the prognosis for patients with glioblastoma remains dismal with an overall survival of 12–18 months. The standard of care treatment for glioblastoma is maximum safe resection, followed by combined radiotherapy and temozolomide chemotherapy, and then monthly temozolomide for 6 months [6]. In 2011, a medical device called tumor-treating field was approved to deliver low frequency electromagnetic field locally to the tumor site and was found to further improve the median overall survival by 4.9 months [7].

Though glioblastoma can affect people at any age, it preferentially occurs in older individuals, with a peak incidence between 65 and 84 years old. The 2021 WHO classification of the central nervous system tumors has mandated that the term glioblastoma be used to indicate only IDH wildtype (WT) astrocytoma, WHO grade 4, and *not* IDH-mutant astrocytoma, WHO grade 4 [8]. IDH-WT glioblastoma occurs de novo and its prognosis is much worse than IDH-mutant astrocytoma, WHO grade 4. IDH-mutant astrocytoma, WHO grade 4 were previously also called secondary glioblastoma, and were found in younger patients. The reality is that IDH-wildtype glioblastoma is mostly a disease of the elderly. Yet, there continues to be a lack of clarity and unresolved challenges in treatment of elderly glioblastoma patients leading to a stark contrast in survival outcomes of the elderly (median overall survival of 4 months) vs. non-elderly glioblastoma population (median overall survival 15 months) [9].

What are some unique challenges faced by elderly glioblastoma patients? Elderly patients whose initial symptoms are confusion, memory loss, fatigue or depression are often diagnosed late and have a longer lead time to radiological and pathological diagnosis as compared to patients who present with seizures [10, 11]. Stroke and transient ischemic attacks are common in the elderly population and many glioblastomas are initially misdiagnosed as sub-acute infarcts. This delay in precious lead times often results in a larger tumor size and a worse neurological state at the time of surgery and initiation of treatment. It is well known that patients who undergo resection or de-bulking over a biopsy have better survival outcomes. Yet, elderly GBM patients are more likely to get biopsy over resection due to their frailty, neurological symptom burden, co-morbidities, large tumor size and lower surgical risk tolerance by surgical team and patient families. Therefore, by the time the elderly patient is radiographically and pathologically diagnosed, their condition may have declined too far to be able to tolerate the standard 6 weeks of combined chemoradiotherapy. Their treatment is usually tailored to either hypofractionated chemoradiotherapy, hypofractionated radiotherapy (HFRT) alone or temozolomide alone [12] Even if they are able to get the standard of care 6 weeks concurrent chemoradiation and adjuvant temozolomide, the treatment toxicity is much higher as compared to the non-elderly GBMs [13] and often necessitate treatment discontinuation. The next issue is the uniqueness of tumor biology in elderly glioblastoma. Is it possible that the tumor itself is more aggressive than their non-elderly counterpart? Is the aged brain parenchyma more conducive to tumor growth? Does aging decrease systemic immune-surveillance in the elderly? Further, complex socio-economic factors come in play in regard to treatment access to the elderly. Patients often live by themselves, in assisted living facilities or nursing homes. The treatment of glioblastoma is fully outpatient, thus making it vital that a full-time caregiver be available so that the patient can access the healthcare system. This is often not the case for elderly patients, and it is a not uncommon for them to be diagnosed with GBM and be transitioned to hospice care at the time of initial hospitalization.

In the following book chapter, we closely examine each of the above issues and present the most up-to-date evidence on the unique aspects of glioblastoma in the elderly.

2. Epidemiology

The incidence of primary brain tumors increases with age [14]. Glioblastoma is the most common malignant brain tumor in the aging population and accounts for 58% of all gliomas in the elderly [15]. The definition of elderly itself is a contested topic. Some researchers consider age 65+ or even 60+ as elderly, while in general most will agree that the population over 70 is elderly. The incidence rate of glioblastoma progressively increases as we grow older—from 1.3/100,000 between the ages of 35–44, 3.6/100,000 between the ages of 45–54, 8.1/100,000 between the ages of 55–64 to the dramatically higher rate of 13/100,000 between the ages of 65–74 and 15.3/100,000 between 75 and 84 years of age [1]. According to a recent study, non-Hispanic whites make up the majority of that population, and males were 1.62 times more likely to be affected than females. The study also concluded that the incidence of glioblastoma remained stable in the past couple of years [16]. Incidence rates for glioblastomas were highest in supratentorial regions and lowest in extra-cranial regions like the spinal cord [1].

3. Signs and symptoms

In a study on 339 elderly GBM patient over the age 70, the most common presenting symptoms were confusion (38%), hemiparesis (35%), speech disturbance (34%) and seizure (29%) [17]. Another study on 189 elderly GBM patients found that patients most commonly presented with global symptoms of cognitive dysfunction, headache, dizziness and fatigue (66%), followed by loss of neurological function (58%), headache (33%) and seizure (32%) [11]. This study also found if behavioral change, memory impairment and confusion were the presenting symptoms, elderly patients had the shortest overall survival because these symptoms were misinterpreted as normal aging by patients' families and even their healthcare teams. Patients who present with seizures had a significantly longer survival and tend to be younger [11, 18].

4. Prognostic factors

Age alone is a prognostic factor in GBM [19–21], as elderly patients usually have increased incidence of comorbidities, lower functional status [22, 23] and a unique tumor biology as compared to younger population [21]. In elderly patients with GBM, age and performance status form a complex interplay. The most common performance status assessment tool for primary brain tumors is the Karnofsky Performance Scale (KPS) [24]. A patient with a KPS of 70% is self-caring but is unable to carry on normal activity or do active work. Interestingly, a large study of over 48,000 patients with GBM over the age of 60, found that that even when performance status is good ($KPS \geq 70$), overall survival is poorer with advancing age—15.2 months (age 60–69) vs. 9.6 months (age 70–79) vs. 6.8 months ($age \geq 80$) [25]. A poor $KPS < 70$ has also been associated with a poorer overall survival as patients with a lower KPS usually cannot tolerate a more aggressive treatment (i.e., radical resection followed by chemotherapy and radiotherapy) [26].

5. Tumor biology

There are molecular, epigenetic, and genomic biomarkers unique to elderly GBMs which are associated with a worse prognosis [19–21, 26]. Elderly GBMs usually lack the isocitrate dehydrogenase (IDH) mutation, which is usually found in younger glioblastoma patients (currently, reclassified as IDH-mutant astrocytoma, WHO grade 4) and is associated with an improved prognosis [12, 27]. It is well established that methylation of DNA repair O(6)methylguanine-DNA methyltransferase (MGMT) is related to response to alkylating agents, and the lack of promoter methylation in this elderly group leads to a poor response to chemotherapy [12, 27, 28]. Fukai et al. in a cohort of 212 patients found that *TERT* promoter mutation, copy number alterations such as *PTEN* deletion and *CDK4* amplification/gain, and co-amplification of *MDM2* and *CDK4* were more frequent in the older group (>70 years old) [20]. There was also a higher triple overlapping of *PTEN*, *CDKN2A* and *EGFR* in the older group, which is positively associated with tumor invasiveness and resistance to therapy [29–31].

As the central nervous system ages, markers of cellular senescence come to the fore [32–34]. One may assume that the senescent cells are growth-arrested and are the polar opposite of oncogenic cells which divide uncontrollably. However, these senescent cells release pro-inflammatory factors called secretory associated senescent phenotype (SASP) which exacerbate cancer. SASP factors such are TGF-beta, IL-6, IL-8, VEGF, matrix metalloprotein-2 (MMP-2) and MMP-9 play a role in diseases such as cancer, neuroinflammation and neurodegeneration [14, 35].

6. Preoperative assessment

Age alone, even in octogenarian and nonagenarian, should not be the criterion to exclude surgical resection [36–41]. A comprehensive assessment using risk prediction tools for outcomes after a GBM resection in elderly patients is recommended. Patient's performance status is commonly evaluated using KPS (100 = normal to 0 = dead) [24] or the ECOG scale (0 = fully active to 5 = dead) [36] A KPS value lower than 70 is associated with a poor prognosis [21, 38, 39] and is commonly used as a cut-off for patient enrollment for newly diagnosed glioblastoma trials. A more comprehensive appraisal using *Comprehensive Geriatric Assessment* (CGA) which takes in account an older patient's functional status, comorbid medical conditions, cognition, psychological state, social support, nutritional status, and a review of the patient's medications has demonstrated prognostic and predictive role for treatment eligibility [21, 42–44]. CGA is interdisciplinary and multidimensional evaluation that includes eight major criteria (**Figure 1**) to formulate a better plan to anticipate and address challenges in management of geriatric patients. Lombardi et al. in a retrospective study of 133 patients found a prognostic significance for CGA in elderly patients with GBM [43]. Cloney et al. applying *The Canadian Study on Health and Aging Modified Frailty Index (CSHA-mFI)* found that frailer patients, independently of age, KPS or cardiovascular risk, were less likely to undergo surgery, had a longer inpatient stay, had more post-operative complications

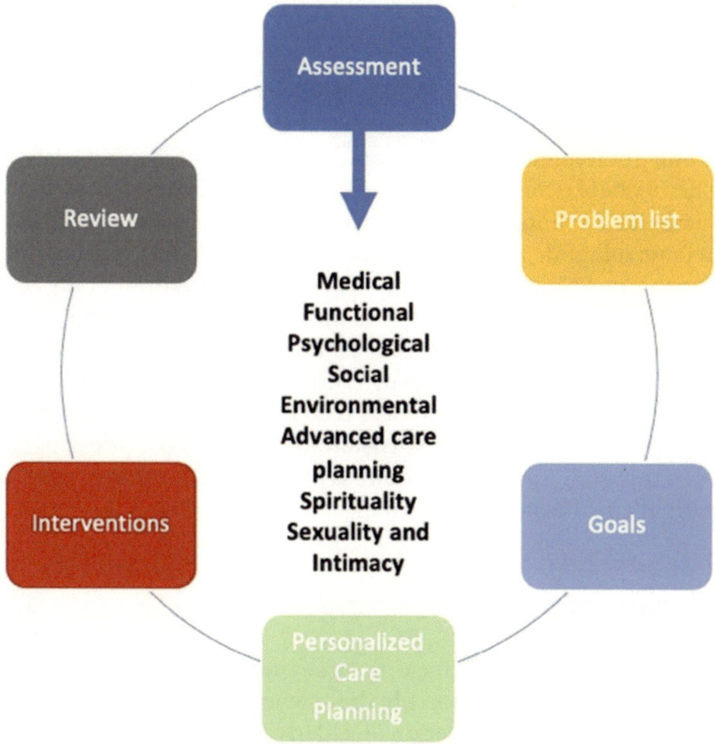
Assessment
Problem list
Goals
Personalized Care Planning
Interventions
Review
Medical
Functional
Psychological
Social
Environmental
Advanced care planning
Spirituality
Sexuality and Intimacy

Figure 1.
Comprehensive geriatric assessment consisting in eight general topics: medical, functional, social, environmental, advanced care, spirituality and sexuality and intimacy. CGA has been advocated for elderly patients with cancer by The International Society of Geriatric Oncology.

and a shorter overall survival [45]. Thus, in this heterogeneous group a complete and thorough assessment should be performed. While CGA is mainstream in the practice of geriatric oncology, its use is not prevalent in assessment of elderly GBM patients and needs to be encouraged.

7. Treatment overview

A radical total resection followed by combined temozolomide and standard fractionated radiotherapy (SFRT), followed by adjuvant temozolomide for six cycles, is the standard first line of treatment of glioblastoma. This treatment is based on the EORTC/NCIC study on in which 573 patients after biopsy or resection were treated with 6 weeks of focal radiotherapy (total 60 Gy in 30 fractions) vs. radiotherapy plus continuous daily temozolomide (75 mg/m^2 of body-surface area per day, 7 days per week from the first to the last day of radiotherapy), followed by six cycles of adjuvant temozolomide (150–200 mg/m^2 for 5 days during each 28-day cycle) [6]. This seminal study found that the median survival in the radiotherapy only group was 12.1 months and was significantly improved to 14.6 months in the combined radiotherapy and chemotherapy group. It is noteworthy that this study excluded patients above the age of 70. Interestingly this study found that in patients >60 years, median survival was 11.8 months with radiotherapy alone vs. 10.9 months with combination therapy. However, this was an exploratory analysis, and no firm conclusion could be drawn from this subset.

The best treatment approach for elderly glioblastoma patients remains controversial [46]. Due to patient's lower KPS, higher prevalence of risk factors, and the question of ability to tolerate combined standard of care 60Gy chemoradiotherapy, studies on elderly glioblastoma have focused on making the treatment regimens tolerable to patients. Patients with a poor performance status (i.e., KPS < 70) can benefit from temozolomide monotherapy (especially if *MGMT* promoter methylated) or radiotherapy alone [27, 28, 46–50]. The specific dose of radiotherapy adopted is usually different from standard protocol, as the standard radiotherapy dose of 60 Gy can be difficult to tolerate, especially when combined with temozolomide [28]. In this context, hypofractioned radiotherapy (HFRT) has shown not inferior to SFTR with less side effects [51]. Another important factor to consider is that drugs for symptomatic management such as corticosteroids and antiepileptic drugs as they are less tolerated in this group [47]. Thus, there is a need to tailor the therapy for each individual patient's profile in this age group.

8. Surgical treatment

Some authors have questioned if age alone should be the criterion to decide whether elderly GBM patients, especially those who are 80+, should undergo a surgical resection. The surgical question on elderly GBM patients is two-pronged. First, can the elderly tolerate a major brain surgery or biopsy similar to their non-elderly counterparts? And second, does resection as opposed to biopsy only, confer a survival benefit in elderly patients similar to non-elderly patients? The hesitation for craniotomies on elderly GBM patients, hinges on the fact that octogenarians have an increased incidence of comorbidities and lower functional status, and therefore may not be good candidates for a major surgery [52]. The higher prevalence of metabolic, neurologic, cardiac comorbidities and a loss of reserve capacity seen in this age-group is associated with a lengthier hospitalization [53].

The first question on the safety and tolerance of brain surgery in elderly is answered by several retrospective studies. In a retrospective cohort study of 741 patients with surgically assessable brain tumors, of whom 570 patients were between the ages of 60 and 79 (senior) and 83 were aged 80 or above (elderly), pre- and post-operative change to modified Rankin score, surgical complications, length of stay, and 30-days readmission were performed [36]. No statistical significance was found comparing the elderly patients with their counterparts of senior and young (20–29 years) (surgical complication rates of 6, 7.2 and 4.5% respectively). Post-operative complications such as neurological deficits, infection, DVTs are similar to those described in younger patients [10, 54, 55]. Thus, it appears that surgical resection in elderly can be safely performed in specialized centers without overt risk as compared to the non-elderly population.

The second question on the benefit of surgical resection as opposed to biopsy stems from the fact that elderly GBMs inherently have a more aggressive biology [19, 21, 35] and that the survival benefit from a radical resection seen in younger GBM patients may not translate to elderly GBM patients. This answer was explored by Chaichana et al. in a retrospective study comparing biopsy in 40 elderly GBM (65 years and older) patients to resection in 40 matched elderly GBM patients [56].

Overall survival in the resection group (5.7 months) was significantly greater than the biopsy group (4 months). Surgical resection offers a better outcome and is associated with an improved quality of life [57, 58] than biopsy in elderly with GBM [26, 59–62]. Gross total resection (GTR) is related to longer survival time, progression free survival and improved functional recovery without increased morbidity or mortality, when compared to subtotal resection [10, 63, 64].

9. Post-operative assessment

Length of stay (LOS) has been shown to be longer in the elderly who undergo surgery. There is a positive correlation with LOS and delirium in aged patient [65, 66]. In a study highlighting the incidence of delirium in the elderly, it was found that patients with advanced age had a higher rate of post-operative delirium (POD) and post-operative cognitive dysfunction (POCD) [67, 68]. A possible approach to dealing with POD in the elderly is to optimize pharmacologic intervention. Antipsychotic regimen and use of dexmedetomidine may reduce post-operative delirium and are possible options for pharmacologic interventions to reduce LOS [69–71]. Other factors that could influence the LOS difference between elder and younger groups are mechanical factors such as early ambulation and the use of physical therapy. Chiu et al. found that additional factors such as geriatric consultation, care giver education, and music therapy can also play an important role in decreasing LOS [72].

10. Radiotherapy

The importance of SFRT in the treatment of glioblastoma has been established more than a decade ago [6]. The time to initiate radiation treatment is between 3 and 6 weeks after surgery [6, 73]. The standard course of 60Gy divided in 30 fractions is widely used in management of glioblastoma, although it is associated with a higher incidence of radionecrosis [74], and may not be well-tolerated in elderly population [12]. Hypofractionated radiotherapy has been shown to be non-inferior to standard radiotherapy in elderly patients. A randomized phase III trial by the Nordic Clinical Brain Tumor Study Group, enrolled patients over 60 years of age in three arms—temozolomide only, standard course of radiotherapy (60 Gy, 30 fractions) or hypofractionated radiotherapy HFRT) (34 Gy, 10 fractions) [12]. There was no cut-off for performance status so that real-world scenario could be replicated. For patients aged 70 and older, outcomes were worse in the standard radiotherapy group. For temozolomide vs. hypofractionated radiotherapy, median survival was similar. Only 72% of patients in the standard radiotherapy group could complete their treatment as opposed to 94% patients in the hypofractionated group. If elderly patients had difficulty tolerating 6 weeks of radiation only, then it may be extrapolated that tolerance would be much worse if they were to receive the combined 6 weeks radiation plus concomitant temozolomide. However, this may not apply to fitter elderly patients with KPS 70 or more. A randomized trial of 695 patients testing tumor-treating fields (TTF) after standard chemoradiotherapy and adjuvant temozolomide included 134 patients aged 65 or older and KPS of 70 or higher [7]. In this group of relatively fit elderly patients, the median overall survival was 13.7 months in the adjuvant temozolomide group vs. 17.4 months in the adjuvant temozolomide plus TTF group. Though this study did not discuss the tolerability of standard chemoradiation in the elderly population, the median survival of over 12 months in the each of the elderly group suggests that elderly patients with a good KPS can in fact tolerate standard 6 weeks of chemoradiation.

HFRT schedules were developed in an effort to improve treatment tolerability and decrease the daily burden of radiotherapy treatment for elderly. In a pre-temozolomide era prospective study on 100 GBM patients, 60 years and older were treated with either HFRT (40 Gy in 15 fractions) vs. standard radiotherapy (60 Gy in 30 fractions) [75]. Overall survival was similar in HFRT group (5.6 months) as compared to the standard radiotherapy group (5.1 months). The Nordic study showed a longer survival in patients over 70 years when treated with temozolomide or HFRT as compared to standard radiotherapy [12]. Based on these studies, it appears that HFRT is at least non-inferior to standard radiotherapy in elderly patients. A small phase III prospective study on elderly and/or frail in which patients were randomized to either a very short-course RT (25 Gy in five fractions delivered over 1 week) or commonly used HFRT (40 Gy in 15 fractions delivered over 3 weeks) [51], and showed an overall survival of 7.9 months in the 1 week radiotherapy group and 6.4 months in the 3 weeks radiotherapy group. However, the 1-week short course radiotherapy for GBM is controversial, and not commonly utilized in mainstream practice.

11. Chemotherapy

The alkylating agent temozolomide is the drug of choice for glioblastoma. Traditional treatment protocol that combines temozolomide (75 mg/m^2/day) with standard RT/HFRT after surgical resection followed by 200 mg/m^2 for 5 days with cycles repeated every 28 days for up to six cycles is the choice for patients with a good KPS ($\geq$70) [21, 76]. Elderly glioblastoma patients who have a good KPS and reasonably controlled co-morbidities can be treated with the standard combined chemoradiation and adjuvant chemotherapy [7, 77]. No prospective study on elderly patients so far has compared standard chemoradiotherapy with hypofractionated chemoradiotherapy.

However, for fragile elderly patients who cannot tolerate the standard treatment, the use of temozolomide alone is non-inferior to standard radiation alone. A phase III randomized trial in patients older than 65 tested with dense temozolomide regimen to 6 weeks standard radiotherapy and found that temozolomide alone was non-inferior to radiotherapy alone [50]. This study also confirmed the role of MGMT as a predictive biomarker for chemotherapy monotherapy in these patients. The most common side effects described in this population are fatigue and thrombocytopenia [13]. Malmström et al., in the Nordic trial that included a arm of temozolomide found an overall survival (OS) significantly longer specially in patients above 70 years old with MGMT promoter methylated (9.7 vs. 6.8 months, compared to non- methylated). A phase III randomized trial of patients 65 years or older tested HFRT alone (40 Gy in 15 fractions) vs. HFRT concurrent with temozolomide, followed by adjuvant temozolomide [78]. The median overall survival was longer in the combined group than with radiotherapy alone (9.3 vs. 7.6 months). The benefit with combined treatment was much greater in the MGMT methylated GBMs. A non-significant survival benefit was also found in the MGMT unmethylated GBM patients. For MGMT unmethylated elderly GBM patients, RT only should be favored over temozolomide monotherapy [50].

Bevacizumab is not recommended for people with newly diagnosed glioblastoma due to high rates of adverse events and no improvement in overall survival [79–81]. In select cases, bevacizumab may be cautiously used to treat tumor-related edema and to avoid the side-effects of steroids.

12. Tumor-treating field

Tumor-treating field (TTF) is a device which is worn locally over the patient's shaved scalp and is FDA approved for treatment of glioblastoma. It delivers low-intensity alternating electric field to the tumor and thus has an anti-mitotic effect on glioblastoma. A phase III randomized clinical trial showed that the overall survival was significantly longer in the chemoradiotherapy + adjuvant temozolomide + TTF group (20.9 months) as compared to chemoradiotherapy + adjuvant temozolomide group (16 months) [7]. This study enrolled 695 patients with glioblastoma over the age of 18 and included 134 patients aged 65 or older. Patients 65 years or older had significantly increased survival on addition of TTF vs. temozolomide alone (HR, 0.51; 95% CI, 0.33–0.77). Device side-effects are mild as compared to chemotherapy or radiation and usually consist of mild to moderate skin toxicity underneath the transducer arrays. TTF is a local therapy and needs to be worn daily for long-term, optimally for over 18 h a day. Elderly patients will often require lifestyle modification and caregiver support when using it. It can be an attractive antineoplastic therapy for elderly as it does not have systemic side-effects.

13. Conclusion

GBM is the GBM is the most common primary brain tumor in the elderly population. It has been shown that GBM has a unique more aggressive biology in aged patients. Molecular patterns have not been thoroughly elucidated yet and many of these factors are thought to have a negative impact to the prognosis in these patients. If well-tolerated, surgical treatment should aim at gross total resection, and comprehensive pre-operative assessment is recommended. An active post-operative care can reduce the length of stay in these patients and consequently, the risk of post-operative complications and the incidence of delirium. Selected elderly patients with good performance status and well-controlled co-morbidities may receive standard 6 weeks of combined chemoradiotherapy, adjuvant temozolomide and TTF or HFRT combined with temozolomide. In patients with unmethylated tumors and poor KPS patients, HFRT alone has been commonly indicated. Chemotherapy alone is an option for patients with a low performance status and whose tumor is hypermethylated. Elderly patients with GBM represent a special and vulnerable group. Treatment in the elderly and very elderly patients with glioblastoma requires an individualized plan with a multi-disciplinary team. Patient's age, KPS, MGMT status, patient's wishes, and even social factors should guide the overall treatment plan.

Author details

Raphael Bastianon Santiago[1], Hamid Borghei-Razavi[1*], Mauricio Mandel[1], Bhavika Gupta[2], Asad Ali[3], Badih Adada[1] and Surabhi Ranjan[1]

1 Department of Neurosurgery, Cleveland Clinic Florida, United States

2 School of Medicine, St George's University, Grenada

3 Dr. Kiran C. Patel College of College of Osteopathic Medicine, NOVA Southeastern University, United States

*Address all correspondence to: borgheh2@ccf.org

References

[1] Ostrom QT et al. CBTRUS statistical report: Primary brain and other central nervous system tumors diagnosed in the United States in 2013-2017. Neuro-Oncology. 2020;**22**(12 Suppl. 2):iv1-iv96

[2] Jeon J et al. Smoking and lung cancer mortality in the United States from 2015 to 2065: A comparative modeling approach. Annals of Internal Medicine. 2018;**169**(10):684-693

[3] Coleman C. Early detection and screening for breast cancer. Seminars in Oncology Nursing. 2017;**33**(2):141-155

[4] Siegel RL et al. Cancer statistics, 2022. CA: A Cancer Journal for Clinicians. 2022;**72**(1):7-33

[5] Luke JJ et al. Targeted agents and immunotherapies: Optimizing outcomes in melanoma. Nature Reviews Clinical Oncology. 2017;**14**(8):463-482

[6] Stupp R et al. Radiotherapy plus concomitant and adjuvant temozolomide for glioblastoma. The New England Journal of Medicine. 2005;**352**(10):987-996

[7] Stupp R et al. Effect of tumor-treating fields plus maintenance temozolomide vs maintenance temozolomide alone on survival in patients with glioblastoma: A randomized clinical trial. JAMA. 2017;**318**(23):2306-2316

[8] Louis DN et al. The 2021 WHO classification of tumors of the central nervous system: A summary. Neuro-Oncology. 2021;**23**(8):1231-1251

[9] Jordan JT et al. Glioblastoma care in the elderly. Cancer. 2016;**122**(2):189-197

[10] Tanaka S et al. Presentation, management, and outcome of newly diagnosed glioblastoma in elderly patients. Journal of Neurosurgery. 2013;**118**(4):786-798

[11] Bruhn H et al. Initial cognitive impairment predicts shorter survival of patients with glioblastoma. Acta Neurologica Scandinavica. 2022;**145**(1):94-101

[12] Malmström A et al. Temozolomide versus standard 6-week radiotherapy versus hypofractionated radiotherapy in patients older than 60 years with glioblastoma: The Nordic randomised, phase 3 trial. The Lancet Oncology. 2012;**13**(9):916-926

[13] Wasilewski A, Alam A, Mohile N. Chemotherapy toxicities and geriatric syndromes in older patients with malignant gliomas. Journal of Geriatric Oncology. 2021;**12**(1):134-138

[14] Berben L et al. Cancer and aging: Two tightly interconnected biological processes. Cancers (Basel). 2021;**13**(6):1400

[15] Nayak L, Iwamoto FM. Primary brain tumors in the elderly. Current Neurology and Neuroscience Reports. 2010;**10**(4):252-258

[16] Chen B et al. Recent incidence trend of elderly patients with glioblastoma in the United States, 2000-2017. BMC Cancer. 2021;**21**(1):54

[17] Lorimer CF et al. Challenges to treating older glioblastoma patients: The influence of clinical and tumour characteristics on survival outcomes. Clinical Oncology (Royal College of Radiologists). 2017;**29**(11):739-747

[18] Lu VM et al. Quantifying the prognostic significance in glioblastoma of seizure history at initial presentation:

A systematic review and meta-analysis. Clinical Neurology and Neurosurgery. 2018;**164**:75-80

[19] Bozdag S et al. Age-specific signatures of glioblastoma at the genomic, genetic, and epigenetic levels. PLoS One. 2013 Apr 29;**8**(4):e62982

[20] Fukai J et al. Molecular characteristics and clinical outcomes of elderly patients with IDH-wildtype glioblastomas: Comparative study of older and younger cases in Kansai Network cohort. Brain Tumor Pathology. 2020;**37**(2):50-59

[21] Bruno F et al. Glioblastoma in the elderly: Review of molecular and therapeutic aspects. Biomedicine. 2022;**10**(3):644

[22] Ewen EF Jr, Keating HJ 3rd. Alternatives to major surgery in the high-risk elderly. Clinics in Geriatric Medicine. 1990;**6**(3):481-492

[23] Sudlow A et al. Outcomes of surgery in patients aged ≥90 years in the general surgical setting. Annals of the Royal College of Surgeons of England. 2018;**100**(3):172-177

[24] Mor V et al. The Karnofsky performance status scale: An examination of its reliability and validity in a research setting. Cancer. 1984;**53**(9):2002-2007

[25] Al Feghali KA et al. Real-world evaluation of the impact of radiotherapy and chemotherapy in elderly patients with glioblastoma based on age and performance status. Neuro-Oncology Practice. 2021;**8**(2):199-208

[26] Álvarez de Eulate-Beramendi S et al. Prognostic factors and survival study in high-grade glioma in the elderly. British Journal of Neurosurgery. 2016;**30**(3):330-336

[27] Wick W et al. MGMT testing-the challenges for biomarker-based glioma treatment. Nature Reviews Neurology. 2014;**10**(7):372-385

[28] Brandes AA et al. Temozolomide concomitant and adjuvant to radiotherapy in elderly patients with glioblastoma: Correlation with MGMT promoter methylation status. Cancer. 2009;**115**(15):3512-3518

[29] Saadeh FS, Mahfouz R, Assi HI. EGFR as a clinical marker in glioblastomas and other gliomas. The International Journal of Biological Markers. 2018;**33**(1):22-32

[30] Hatanpaa KJ et al. Epidermal growth factor receptor in glioma: Signal transduction, neuropathology, imaging, and radioresistance. Neoplasia. 2010;**12**(9):675-684

[31] Chakravarti A et al. The epidermal growth factor receptor pathway mediates resistance to sequential administration of radiation and chemotherapy in primary human glioblastoma cells in a RAS-dependent manner. Cancer Research. 2002;**62**(15):4307-4315

[32] Ladomersky E et al. The coincidence between increasing age, immunosuppression, and the incidence of patients with glioblastoma. Frontiers in Pharmacology. 2019;**10**:200

[33] Lian J et al. Immunosenescence: A key player in cancer development. Journal of Hematology & Oncology. 2020;**13**(1):151

[34] Huff WX et al. The evolving role of CD8(+)CD28(−) immunosenescent T cells in cancer immunology. International Journal of Molecular Sciences. 2019;**20**(11):2810

[35] Kim M et al. Glioblastoma as an age-related neurological disorder in

adults. Neuro-Oncology Advances. 2021;**3**(1):vdab125

[36] Eichberg DG et al. Brain tumor surgery is safe in octogenarians and nonagenarians: A single-surgeon 741 patient series. World Neurosurgery. 2019;**132**:e185-e192

[37] Poon MT et al. Outcome of elderly patients undergoing intracranial meningioma resection—A systematic review and meta-analysis. British Journal of Neurosurgery. 2014;**28**(3):303-309

[38] Osawa T et al. Elderly patients aged over 75 years with glioblastoma: Preoperative status and surgical strategies. Interdisciplinary Neurosurgery. 2021;**25**:101127

[39] Barbagallo GMV et al. High grade glioma treatment in elderly people: Is it different than in younger patients? Analysis of surgical management guided by an intraoperative multimodal approach and its impact on clinical outcome. Frontiers in Oncology. 2021;**10**:631255

[40] Dobran M et al. Surgical treatment and outcome in patients over 80 years old with intracranial meningioma. Clinical Neurology and Neurosurgery. 2018;**167**:173-176

[41] D'Andrea G et al. Thirty-seven cases of intracranial meningiomas in the ninth decade of life: Our experience and review of the literature. Neurosurgery. 2005;**56**(5):956-961 discussion 956-61

[42] Repetto L et al. Comprehensive geriatric assessment adds information to Eastern cooperative oncology group performance status in elderly cancer patients: An Italian group for geriatric oncology study. Journal of Clinical Oncology. 2002;**20**(2):494-502

[43] Lombardi G et al. Validation of the comprehensive geriatric assessment as a predictor of mortality in elderly glioblastoma patients. Cancers (Basel). 2019;**11**(10):1509

[44] Cohen-Inbar O. Geriatric brain tumor management part II: Glioblastoma multiforme. Journal of Clinical Neuroscience. 2019;**67**:1-4

[45] Cloney M et al. Frailty in geriatric glioblastoma patients: A predictor of operative morbidity and outcome. World Neurosurgery. 2016;**89**:362-367

[46] Zarnett OJ et al. Treatment of elderly patients with glioblastoma: A systematic evidence-based analysis. JAMA Neurology. 2015;**72**(5):589-596

[47] Laigle-Donadey F. Glioblastoma in the elderly. Geriatrie et Psychologie Neuropsychiatrie du Vieillissement. 2019;**17**(2):173-178

[48] Ducray F et al. Complete response after one cycle of temozolomide in an elderly patient with glioblastoma and poor performance status. Journal of Neuro-Oncology. 2008;**88**(2):185-188

[49] Wick A et al. Superiority of temozolomide over radiotherapy for elderly patients with RTK II methylation class, MGMT promoter methylated malignant astrocytoma. Neuro-Oncology. 2020;**22**(8):1162-1172

[50] Wick W et al. Temozolomide chemotherapy alone versus radiotherapy alone for malignant astrocytoma in the elderly: The NOA-08 randomised, phase 3 trial. The Lancet Oncology. 2012;**13**(7):707-715

[51] Roa W et al. International atomic energy agency randomized phase III study of radiation therapy in elderly and/or frail patients with newly

diagnosed glioblastoma multiforme. Journal of Clinical Oncology. 2015;**33**(35):4145-4150

[52] St-Louis E et al. The outcomes of the elderly in acute care general surgery. European Journal of Trauma and Emergency Surgery. 2016;**42**(1):107-113

[53] Martins S, Fernandes L. Delirium in elderly people: A Review. Frontiers in Neurology. 2012;**3**:101

[54] D'Amico RS et al. The safety of surgery in elderly patients with primary and recurrent glioblastoma. World Neurosurgery. 2015;**84**(4):913-919

[55] Johans SJ et al. Identification of preoperative and intraoperative risk factors for complications in the elderly undergoing elective craniotomy. World Neurosurgery. 2017;**107**:216-225

[56] Chaichana KL et al. Supratentorial glioblastoma multiforme: The role of surgical resection versus biopsy among older patients. Annals of Surgical Oncology. 2011;**18**(1):239-245

[57] Minniti G, Lombardi G, Paolini S. Glioblastoma in elderly patients: Current management and future perspectives. Cancers (Basel). 2019;**11**(3):336

[58] Halani SH, Babu R, Adamson DC. Management of glioblastoma multiforme in elderly patients: A review of the literature. World Neurosurgery. 2017;**105**:53-62

[59] Almenawer SA et al. Biopsy versus partial versus gross total resection in older patients with high-grade glioma: A systematic review and meta-analysis. Neuro-Oncology. 2015;**17**(6):868-881

[60] Uzuka T et al. Treatment outcomes in glioblastoma patients aged 76 years or older: A multicenter retrospective cohort study. Journal of Neuro-Oncology. 2014;**116**(2):299-306

[61] Noorbakhsh A et al. Gross-total resection outcomes in an elderly population with glioblastoma: A SEER-based analysis. Journal of Neurosurgery. 2014;**120**(1):31-39

[62] Sanai N et al. An extent of resection threshold for newly diagnosed glioblastomas. Journal of Neurosurgery. 2011;**115**(1):3-8

[63] Han Q et al. Gross total vs. subtotal resection on survival outcomes in elderly patients with high-grade glioma: A systematic review and meta-analysis. Front Oncologia. 2020;**10**:151

[64] Oszvald Á et al. Glioblastoma therapy in the elderly and the importance of the extent of resection regardless of age: Clinical article. Journal of Neurosurgery. 2012;**116**(2):357-364

[65] Cristelo D et al. Quality of recovery in elderly patients with postoperative delirium. Saudi Journal of Anaesthesia. 2019;**13**(4):285-289

[66] Janssen TL et al. Prevention of postoperative delirium in elderly patients planned for elective surgery: Systematic review and meta-analysis. Clinical Interventions in Aging. 2019;**14**:1095-1117

[67] Gleason LJ et al. Effect of delirium and other major complications on outcomes after elective surgery in older adults. JAMA Surgery. 2015;**150**(12):1134-1140

[68] Bhaskar SB, Bajwa SJ. From pre-operative comorbidities to post-operative cognitive dysfunction: The challenging face of geriatric anaesthesia. Indian Journal of Anaesthesia. 2014;**58**(3):248-250

[69] Larsen KA et al. Administration of olanzapine to prevent postoperative delirium in elderly joint-replacement patients: A randomized, controlled trial. Psychosomatics. 2010;**51**(5):409-418

[70] Su X et al. Dexmedetomidine for prevention of delirium in elderly patients after non-cardiac surgery: A randomised, double-blind, placebo-controlled trial. Lancet. 2016;**388**(10054):1893-1902

[71] Tremblay P, Gold S. Prevention of post-operative delirium in the elderly using pharmacological agents. Canadian Geriatrics Journal. 2016;**19**(3):113-126

[72] Chiu L et al. Quality of life in patients with primary and metastatic brain cancer as reported in the literature using the EORTC QLQ-BN20 and QLQ-C30. Expert Review of Pharmacoeconomics & Outcomes Research. 2012;**12**(6):831-837

[73] Sulman EP et al. Radiation therapy for glioblastoma: American society of clinical oncology clinical practice guideline endorsement of the American society for radiation oncology guideline. Journal of Clinical Oncology. 2017;**35**(3):361-369

[74] Azoulay M et al. New hypofractionation radiation strategies for glioblastoma. Current Oncology Reports. 2017;**19**(9):58

[75] Roa W et al. Abbreviated course of radiation therapy in older patients with glioblastoma multiforme: A prospective randomized clinical trial. Journal of Clinical Oncology. 2004;**22**(9):1583-1588

[76] Chahal M, Thiessen B, Mariano C. Treatment of older adult patients with glioblastoma: Moving towards the inclusion of a comprehensive geriatric assessment for guiding management. Current Oncology. 2022;**29**(1):360-376

[77] Hanna C et al. Treatment of newly diagnosed glioblastoma in the elderly: A network meta-analysis. Cochrane Database of Systematic Reviews. 2020;**3**(3):Cd013261

[78] Perry JR et al. Short-course radiation plus temozolomide in elderly patients with glioblastoma. The New England Journal of Medicine. 2017;**376**(11):1027-1037

[79] Mohile NA et al. Therapy for diffuse astrocytic and oligodendroglial tumors in adults: ASCO-SNO guideline. Journal of Clinical Oncology. 2022;**40**(4):403-426

[80] Barrascout E, Lamuraglia M. Glioblastoma and bevacizumab in elderly patients: Monocentric study. Journal of Oncology Pharmacy Practice. 2021;**27**(4):842-846

[81] Wirsching HG et al. Bevacizumab plus hypofractionated radiotherapy versus radiotherapy alone in elderly patients with glioblastoma: The randomized, open-label, phase II ARTE trial. Annals of Oncology. 2018;**29**(6):1423-1430

Chapter 2

Glioblastomas: Molecular Diagnosis and Pathology

Frank Y. Shan, Dachun Zhao, Carlos A. Tirado, Ekokobe Fonkem, Yi-lu Zhang, Dong-xia Feng and Jason H. Huang

Abstract

Glioblastoma (GBM) is a fatal human brain tumor of grade IV/4 by WHO classification, with a very poor prognosis. At the molecular level and clinical, GBM has at least two types, primary and secondary. Each has a different tumorigenesis and clinical presentation. In this chapter, some major molecular biomarkers and diagnostic hallmarks of GBM will be reviewed and discussed.

Keywords: epigenetic, biomarker

1. Introduction

Glial tissue in the human brain includes astrocytes, oligodendrocytes, microglia, and ependymal cells, and each cell type has its own function. Like oligodendrocytes, proving the myelin sheath covering the axons, making the signal transporting faster. While the ependymal cells cover the surface of ventricles. When a specific mutation happens, each glial cell may produce its own glioma (glial neoplasm), the terminology of the glioma will follow the origin of the glial cells. Like oligodendrocyte-original glioma named as oligodendroglioma. Each glioma has different grading, which indicates the tumors' malignancy as well as the clinical behavior. Such as adult's astrocytomas have three grades, from grade 2 to grade 4, the highest grade, (CNS WHO grade 4) astrocytoma also called glioblastoma (GBM). GBM is the most common malignant brain tumor and accounts for 46% of primary malignant brain tumors, which occurs in older patients with a mean age of 64 years old. The most common location of GBM is in the supratentorial region (frontal, temporal, parietal, and occipital lobes), with the highest incidence in frontal lobe, rarely occurs in the cerebellum and spinal cord. GBMs show on MRI scan an enhancing lesion, after administration of contract agent, heterogenic enhancing, or ring-enhancing mass lesion will be presented (**Figure 1**) GBM is a malignant neoplasm, by current treatment including surgery, chemo, and radiation therapy, most patients with GBM have only about 15 months of survival time due to the aggressive nature of this tumor and some other reasons.

Annual age-adjusted incidence rates for GBM have increased in recent years to 3–6 cases per 100,000 people, as the reports from the USA, Canada, UK, and Australia [1].

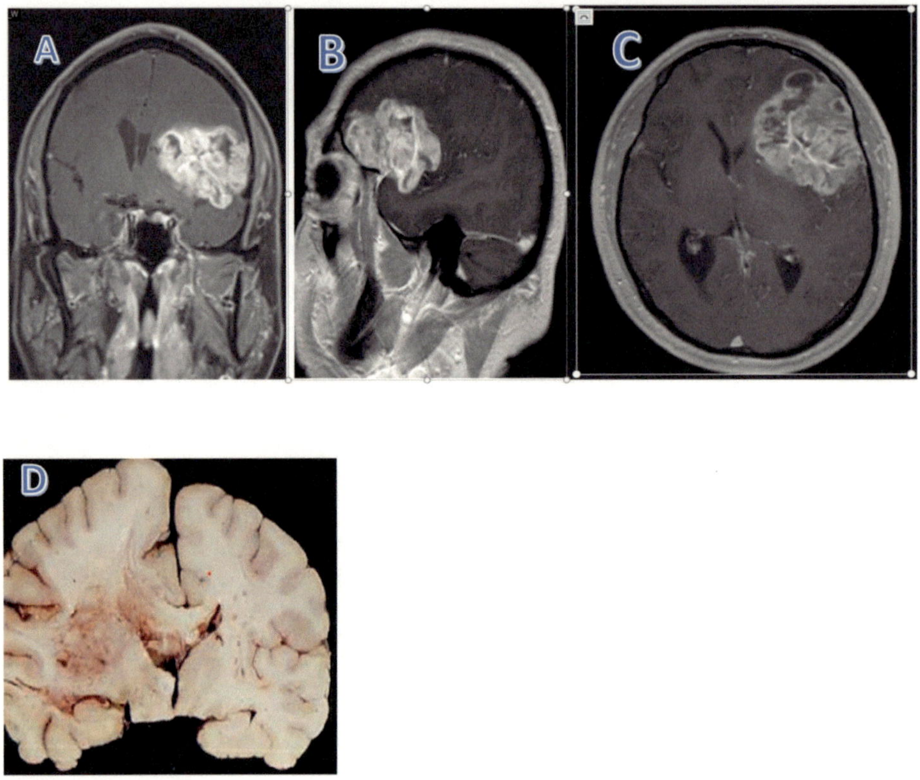

Figure 1.
On this patient, the left parietal heterogenic enhancing mass lesion is most likely a GBM (MRI scan, A. coronal, B. sagittal, and C. axial). An autopsy gross picture of a GBM on the right hemisphere with focal invasion into corpus callosum (D).

In the last two decades, the research discovered that GBMs have two different subtypes by their distinct genetic alteration, each subtype has its own clinical behavior and molecular background. This review will briefly cover this knowledge of the current understanding of GBMs, and include some diagnostic and brief molecular information about this malignant brain neoplasm.

1.1 Migration and metastasis of GBM

Biologically, astrocytomas, no matter low or high grade, are characterized by their infiltrating growth. For example, GBM usually deeply infiltrates the white matter of the brain and sometimes goes to cross the corpus callosum and makes a terrible butterfly pattern in MRI scan **(Figure 2A)**. This nature of infiltrating growth makes the astrocytoma one of the most challenging tumors for surgical resection, since no distinctive clear surgical margin can be archived without damaging the brain function during the tumor resection surgery by neurosurgeons.

Due to the aggressive infiltration of the gliomas, migration of tumor cells is not a surprise. For example, if a mass of GBM occurs in one side of the brain, it may try to cross the corpus coliseum into the other half of the brain to make a so-called "Butterfly" sign on MRI scan (bi-hemisphere GBMs) **(Figure 2A)**. which is an almost an unresectable feature for neurosurgeons.

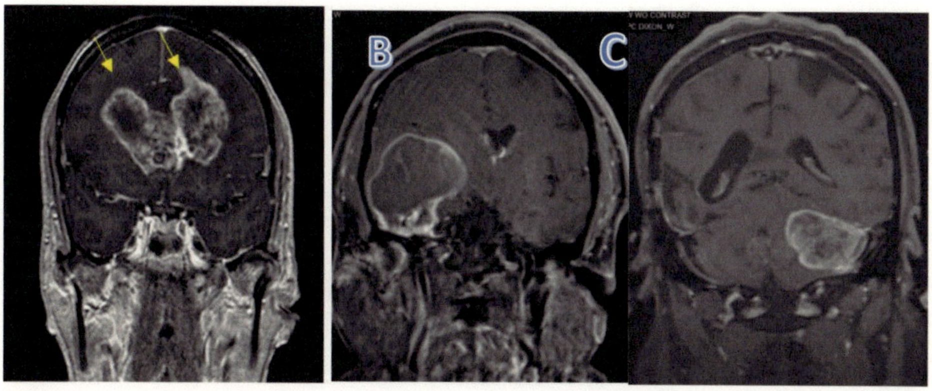

Figure 2.
A 52-year-old male with newly diagnosed GBM showed a butterfly sign on MRI scan (A). (see yellow arrows). A patient with right temporal GBM (B) and surgically resected successfully, but years later another nodule with the feature of GBM (C) in the left cerebellum, suggesting an intracranial metastasis.

A few decades ago, a chemotherapy agent called Gliadel wafer (Azurity pharmaceutical, Atlanta, GA, USA) went into the market, which contains carmastatin, and is implanted in the brain along the walls and floor of the cavity created after a GBM has been surgically removed. The residual tumor cells felt the threat from the Gliade and started to run away from it. Some tumor cells run through the unhealed surgical wound and form a subcutaneous nodule, with biopsy confirmed, it was GBM. Some surgeons did not like it since it delayed the wound healing, it actually caused by tumor cells running through the surgical wound. In addition, the chemotherapy agent might have some effect on the inhibition of tissue recovery (healing process).

The metastasis of GBM is very rare and only reported as case reports [2]. However, (**Figure 2B** and **C**) showed a patient with right temporal GBM, successfully surgical removed; but sometime later, another enhancing nodule showed up on his left cerebellum, suggesting an intracerebral metastatic GBM from the right temporal lobe to left cerebellum.

2. Histopathology of glioblastomas

2.1 Macroscopy

GBMs are often showing signs of elevated intracranial pressure due to the mass effect, while surprisingly large at the time of presentation, and can occupy much of a lobe. Most GBMs of the cerebral hemispheres are clearly intraparenchymal with an epicenter in the white matter (**Figure 1D**). Those records in the pathology application form by neurosurgeon's description of a specimen during surgery always include poorly delineated, the cut surface is variable in color, with peripheral grayish tumor masses and central areas of yellowish necrosis. After formalin fixation, GBMs are fragmented and soft, gray to pink rim with peripheral brain tissue. Necrotic or hemorrhagic tissue may also border adjacent brain structures without an intermediate zone of macroscopically detectable tumor tissue. Some of the tumor's present macroscopic cysts, contain a turbid fluid, and constitute liquefied necrotic tumor tissue (**Figure 3**).

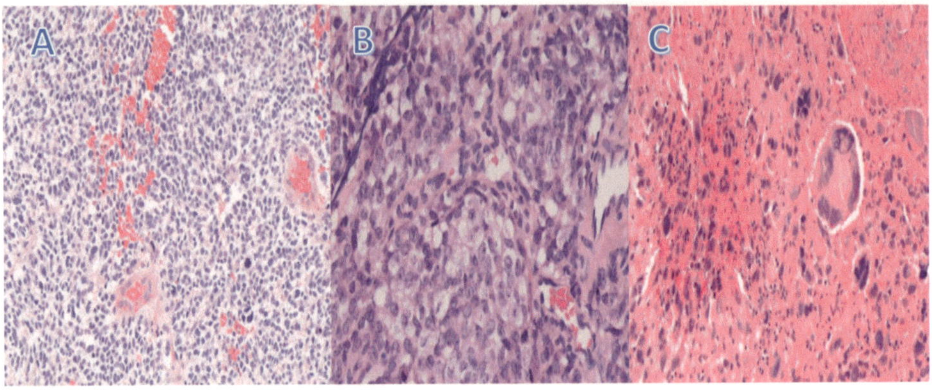

Figure 3.
Small cell glioblastomas are remarkably uniform in both cell size and distribution. Although the cells are often a bit elongated rather than round, the overall appearance resembles that of lung or other primary small cell carcinomas (A, x200). Epithelioid glioblastomas with plump cytoplasm and sharp cell borders simulate metastatic carcinoma or melanoma. It is difficult to distinguish in some cases, especially intraoperation. BRAF v600E is a marker of characteristic expression in epithelioid glioblastoma, and other immunohistochemistry markers such as HMB45, Melan-a may usually resolve the issue (B, x200). Giant cell glioblastoma is consist predominantly of pleomorphism, multinucleation of large or giant cells, atypical mitoses may be numerous. Sometimes microvascular proliferation is absent (C, x200).

2.2 Cell proliferation

The main cellular feature of malignant glial cells is local tissue invasion that typically occurs along deep white matter tracts. Most GBMs exhibit nuclear atypia, greater cellularity, multiple mitotic figures, and a high degree of nuclear pleomorphism. The neoplastic cells are marked pleomorphism, enlarged hyperchromatic nuclei with clumped chromatin, which is an important histological feature to differentiate astrocytic tumors from oligodendrogliomas. Significant variation in cellularity is often seen in different parts of the tumor and can lead to misdiagnosis if the specimens are obtained by stereotactic needle biopsy [3]. Although most of the cases show readily visible mitoses, the distribution is very unevenly in the same tumor. When pathologists use the Ki-67 proliferation index to evaluate it, different regions could range from 5% to over 70% within a GBM.

2.3 Microvascular proliferation

Since the grading system had been set up at the World Health Organization (WHO) classification of tumors of the central nervous system, microvascular proliferation is the major histological feature of high-grade gliomas, especially at GBMs. The morphology manifests as multilayered small-caliber blood vessels to indicate that they grow rapidly. In some cases, endothelial and smooth muscle cell overgrowth in an organoid structure, so-called "Glomeruloid shape" [4]. In addition to glomeruloid appearance, some remarkably proliferated vessels may be accompanied by necrosis and mitoses [5]. During the intraoperative frozen section, the presence of microvascular proliferation within a hypercellular glial neoplasm is a reliable histological feature to support the diagnosis of a high-grade tumor. As the evidence given by different researches, a number of mechanisms, which include perinecrotic hypoxia, stimulate the growth factor expression, lead to new angiogenesis [6].

2.4 Necrosis

Necrosis is another important histological character in GBM apart from microvascular proliferation. Necrosis in GBM can take on a variety of morphologies, from single tumor cell necrosis to extensive diffuse necrosis, which can be seen under light microscopy. The typical necrosis is the so-called "Pseudopalisading" [7], whereby tumor cells are arranged radially in a picket fence-like distribution around a central area of necrosis. Evidence from other studies suggests that exclusion of microvascular proliferation results in markedly increased of vascular permeability, often with a decrease in microthrombosis. Thrombosis leads to the infarction of surrounding tissues [8]. The relationship between thrombosis and necrosis is much stronger in IDH-wildtype glioblastoma than in IDH-mutant high-grade astrocytomas [9].

2.5 Cytology

The cytologic appearance of GBM is extremely variable and pleomorphic. The background of the smear may be fibrillary, or necrotic, which is helpful to make the diagnosis at intraoperative frozen section. Some cases show an appearance essentially similar to that of low-grade astrocytoma, especially when the surgeon sends a peripheral part of the tumor. Pathologic mitosis, single-cell necrosis, and gradual thinning to dense cell distribution suggest that it is possible to see the boundary region of the tumor. For small cell glioblastoma or very poorly differentiated tumors, cytological features will show up similar to lymphomas or embryonal tumors, at that time spectrum of progressive dedifferentiation, we may find that all intermediate possible aspects, such as cellular anaplastic changes, vascular proliferative changes, and necrotic phenomena add up and combine each other.

2.6 Histological patterns of glioblastoma

GBM is a highly variable morphologic tumor, as the old term "glioblastoma multiforme" mentioned, forming the pivot of the tumor is fusiform, atypia, and pleomorphic cells, but low-grade neoplastic astrocytes are often detectable, more or less. Cellular pleomorphism includes small, undifferentiated, giant, epithelioid, spindled, gemistocytic, lipidized, and sarcomatoid cells. Some tumors may present one kind of pattern dominantly; these can be established in different subtypes of GBMs.

Three main subtypes of GBM are giant cell glioblastoma, epithelioid glioblastoma, and gliosarcoma, each of them has been described in Individual chapters at the World Health Organization (WHO) classification of tumors of the central nervous system since 2016 [10–14]. In addition to these subtypes, there are several patterns that are characterized by predominant cell type that can be observed in GBM.

Giant cell glioblastoma is histologically characterized by numerous large, bizarre giant cells, which have multiple nuclei and atypical mitosis, small fusiform syncytial cells, and a reticulin background [15]. The giant cells are often extremely bizarre, sometime it can be larger than 0.5 mm in diameter. The pleomorphism shows not only the size of cells, but also multiple nuclei, cytoplasmic inclusions, palisading, and large ischemic necrosis. Giant cell glioblastomas are frequently rich in reticulin, tend to well-circumscribed structure on MRI, and may be diagnosis as a metastasis tumor. The intraoperative consultation of these lesions will be misguided by clinical information, especially when the giant cells spread over carcinoma or melanoma-like pattern. The perivascular accumulation of tumor cells with the formation of a pseudorossettes-like pattern, which is detected in the frozen slides as a typical feature in GBM may be useful for differential diagnosis. Not the same as Non-CNS tumors, most giant cells indicate a poor prognosis, the giant cell subtype of GBM is slightly better in prognosis than that of other ordinary GBM by some studies [16, 17].

Epithelioid glioblastomas are dominated by a relatively uniform population of discohesive rounded epithelioid cells with eccentric nuclei and abundant eosinophilic cytoplasm, distinct cell membrane, paucity of cytoplasmic processes, and laterally positioned nucleus. Tumor cells can display features of squamous or adenomatous epithelial cells, and are immunoreactive to cytokeratin by IHC stain, when it contains keratin pearls or typical glandular structures that will mimic metastatic carcinoma [18, 19]. Rosenthal fibers and eosinophilic granular bodies are not features in this type of tumor and the necrosis is usually showing zonal type compared with ordinary GBM. The pleomorphic xanthoastrocytoma and epithelioid GBM are BRAF p.V600E positive tumors and they will share similar histology, molecular tests will be more important for differential diagnoses [20].

Gliosarcomas are a special subtype of GBM with the biphasic component, which can either present glial or spindled sarcomata's morphology. The glial part of the mixture is astrocytic, showing features about GBM, and the mesenchymal part of the tumor is most manifesting as spindled fibroblast-like sarcoma. Sometimes the glial component includes epithelial differentiation, such as glandular, adenoid, and squamous formation. The mesenchymal component may be variable, like bone, cartilage, osteoid-chondroid tissue, smooth, and striated muscle, and even lipomatous features could be seen in the tumor [21– 23].

Stains can be useful to distinguish different components of the tumor for the sarcomatous part is rich in collagen and reticulin, which can be seen in the well-developed intensely staining network around spindle cells, and the glial component is seen as reticulin-free nests, which are immunoreactive for GFAP (**Figure 4B**) [24].

GBM is one of the most morphologically heterogeneous tumors, there are several histological patterns that can be detected if a particular cellular morphology predominates besides three main subtypes. Gemistocytic regions in GBMs are similar to other astrocytic neoplasms, which reveal the distinctive cells with large eosinophilic, plump to slightly angulated cytoplasm, and eccentric nuclei. Perivascular lymphocytic infiltrates appear to be more common in this variant. Oligodendrocyte-like cells with uniform round nuclei and variable perinuclear haloes may be seen in some GBMs, including a chichen wire-like capillary network and microcalcifications, suggestive of a presence of low-grade glioma, like secondary GBM. Previous studies suggest that such tumors have a better prognosis than ordinary GBMs, but since evidence from molecular tests prompts that like the outdated name oligoastrocytomas often referred as "mixed glioma" with two components, GBMs with oligodendroglial cells are molecularly heterogeneous. Since 2016, only IDH-wild-type tumor with this pattern is classified as GBM based on the WHO classification [25]. Small cells with highly monomorphic, round to oval, hyperchromatic nuclei, and minimal discernible cytoplasm, which is similar to the small cell neuroendocrine tumor of other organs can be a predominant feature of GBM, as referred as "small cell GBM", which is with a very poor prognosis [26]. The mitotic activity is vibrant and the Ki-67 index proliferation index is very high in this component. Granular cells which is large, periodic acid Schiff positive cytoplasm can be observed in some cases, occasionally, GBM may be composed of granular cells dominantly. Some granular cells are positive for CD68, but negative CD163, which is easily misinterpreted as macrophage lesion, but that lesion has a distinct histological appearance and is characterized by aggressive clinical behavior [27]. Lipidized cells with foamy cytoplasm are another pattern of GBM. The cells

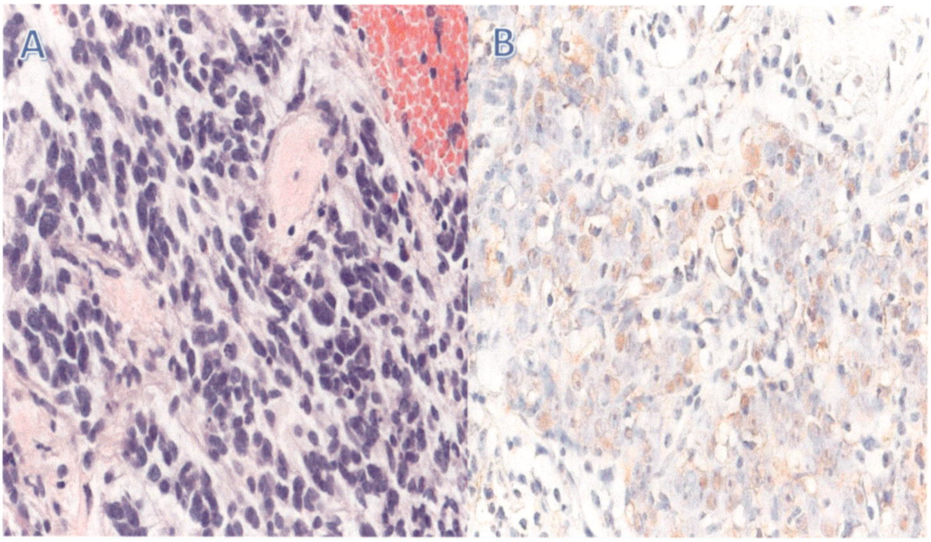

Figure 4.
(H&E 200x) PNET-like pattern in GBM may have a similar cell morphology to those of medulloblastomas and neuroblastoma (A). BRAF is positive in epithelioid tumor cells (B, IHC stain, X200).

may be grossly enlarged; adipose tissue-like tumor cells may be lobules or diffuse patterns [25]. GBMs with a primitive neuroectodermal tumor (PNET) component present a nest of immature cells with markedly increased cellularity, high N/C ratios, and active mitotic figures. The nodular cells differentiated into neuronal, medulloblastoma-like, even showing Homer-Wright rosettes, and the anaplastic cytology of that is similar to CNS embryonal tumors. These tumors were reported that had increased frequency of cerebrospinal fluid dissemination, like Ewing sarcoma (**Figure 5**) [28].

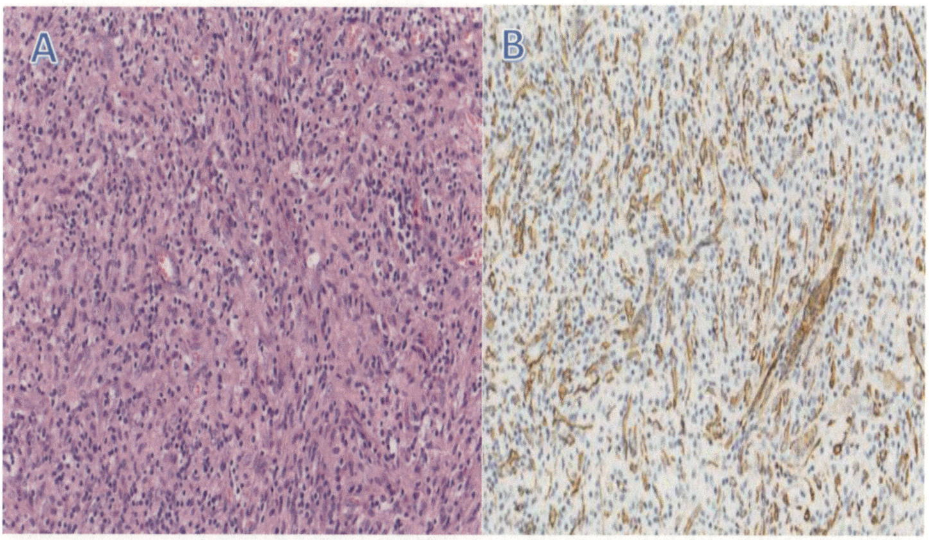

Figure 5.
A mixture of gliomatous and sarcomatous tissues in gliosarcoma. There are many inflammatory cells infiltration in the background (A, H&E x200). (B) the GFAP IHC stain highlights glioma components of gliosarcoma (IHC 200x).

3. Molecular genetic bases of GBMs

At molecular level, GBM has at least two subtypes, primary and secondary. In 1996, Watanabe et al. first reported the evidence that primary and secondary GBMs were with distinct genetic alterations [29]. *TP53* mutations were found to be uncommon in primary GBMs but occurred more commonly in secondary GBMs. *EGFR* overexpression was primarily in primary GBMs but was rare in secondary GBMs. Further studies showed *TP53*, and *IDH1* mutation and *EGFR* overexpression are mutually exclusive events, suggesting two different genetic pathways in the development of GBMs [29]. This hypothesis was further confirmed by additional studies, which provided additional evidence that primary and secondary GBMs develop through distinct molecular pathways [28, 30]. Typical for primary GBMs are *EGFR* amplification or mutation, *PTEN* mutation, and entire loss of chromosome 10 [28, 30]; while genetic alterations more common in secondary GBMs include *TP53* and *IDH1* mutations and 19q loss [28, 30]. Especially, the *IDH1* mutation is currently considered as the most characteristic change for the secondary GBMs, as well as those lower-grade gliomas, including both astrocytomas and oligodendrogliomas (**Figure 6**).

Primary GBM occurs in elderly patients with no history of previous existing lower-grade gliomas, and the tumor is driven by amplification of *EGFR* and/or mutation of *EGFRvIII*, while the secondary GBM, the patients had a history of low-grade gliomas and the tumor is under the mutations of *IDH1*, and *p53*.

3.1 1p/19q co-deletion

The loss of chromosome arms 1p and 19q is an established genetic hallmark of oligodendroglial tumors; it can be detected in up to 80% of oligodendrogliomas (WHO grade II) and up to 80% in anaplastic oligodendrogliomas (WHO grade III) by a few large scale studies [29, 30].

The co-deletion of 1p/19q has been shown its great prognostic value as the tumors with this type of co-deletion respond much better to chemotherapy, which led to a better prognosis and a longer tumor-free survival time. The co-deletion is not only associated with the patient's age, but also the tumor's anatomic locations. For age, the younger the patient, the higher chance of co-deletion. Tumors in frontal lobes carry the highest percentage of co-deletion, followed by the parietal lobe, and occipital lobe, while tumors in the temporal lobe is with the lowest chance of co-deletion. In addition, morphologically the tumor is more typical to the oligodendroglioma, it has more chance to have co-deletion. If the tumor has only one deletion, 1p deletion appears clinically more important than 19q deletion in some early studies. It should be noted that research demonstrated that at least 5% astrocytic neoplasms, including GBMs also have this type of chromosomal deletion, and the astrocytic neoplasms with the co-deletion have shown the same response clinically as the oligodendrogliomas, with better prognosis, better chemotherapy response, and longer tumor-free survival time. Therefore, the test of 1p/19q co-deletion becomes a part of the routine supplementary test in GBM diagnosis, since nowadays, the glial tumor diagnosis requests molecular analysis in our practice, as oncologists request those results for making a treatment plan. Various techniques are available to detect 1p/19q co-deletion; however, fluorescent in situ hybridization (FISH) is often used in many laboratories due to its technical ease, and this type of co-deletion involved the entirely loss of the short arm of chromosome 1 and the long arm of chromosome 19, which makes the FISH test an easy approach (**Figure 7**). FISH is a pathologist's favored method in practice,

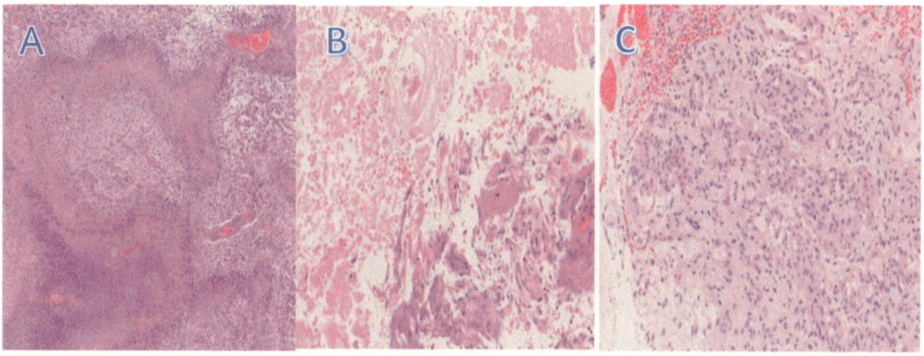

Figure 6.
Picture of glioblastoma is composed of sinuous and hypercellular band of cells, which traces the border of necrotic zones in what is known as pseudopalisading (A, H&E x200). Necrosis in GBM involves both tumor cells and blood vessels. Necrosis in GBMs does not necessarily have pseudopalisading. Either type of necrosis serves WHO 4 tumors as grading criterion (B, H&E x200). Glomeruloid vascular proliferation is a classic histological feature in GBM, multilayered intravascular endothelial cells gathering together (C, H&E x 200).

and can be used directly on formalin-fixed and paraffin-embedded tissue and does not require additional tissue from the patient. Another frequently used method is loss of heterozygosity (LOH), which is a PCR-based test that compares tumor DNA to the patient's "normal" DNA as a control, usually from peripheral blood.

3.2 IDH mutations

First identifiend in 2008, isocitrate dehydrogenases 1 and 2, (IDH1 and IDH2), are homologous, NADP+ – dependent cytoplasmic and mitochondrial enzymes, respectively. The function of these enzymes is the conversion of Isocitrate to α-ketoglutarate with the simultaneous reduction of NADP+ to NADPH. IDH1 has recently been discovered to be mutated in a vast majority of astrocytic and oligodendroglial neoplasms with WHO grade 2–3, as well as in secondary GBM (WHO grade 4). IDH 1 mutation is very rare in primary GBM and has not been detected in pediatric pilocytic astrocytomas (WHO grade 1).

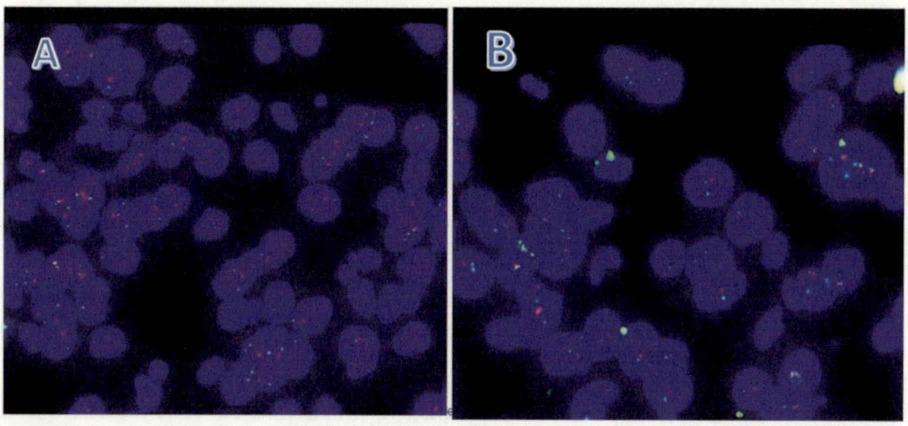

Figure 7.
1p/19q codeletion by FISH (A, 1p deletion red; B, 19q deletion red).

The most common mutation is heterozygous point mutation with substitution of arginine by histidine at codon 132 (R132H), located in the substrate-binding site. This IDH 1-R132H mutation has a reported rate of 50–93% in gliomas. IDH1 mutation is currently considered the initial step of tumorigenesis in glial neoplasms, including both astrocytic and oligodendral gliomas, although the IDH1 mutation-related gliomagenesis is not fully understood, it appears to be multifactorial. The product and byproduct of the reaction, α-ketoglutarate, and NADPH, both defend against cellular oxidative stress. Therefore, with decreased quantities of these compounds, the cell may be more susceptible to oxidative damage. In addition to the tumorogenetic property conferred by the inability to perform the conversion, it appears that the IDH1 mutation confers an enzymatic gain of function. With the IDH1 mutations, the cancer cell has the gained ability to convert α-ketoglutarate into 2-hydroxyglutarate (2HG). This reaction will not only further decrease α-ketoglutarate store, but will also reduce NADPH to NADP+, further increasing the cell's susceptibility to oxidative stress. The overproduction of 2HG in the brain has been oncogenic with an increased risk of brain tumors. Furthermore, there is an association between the IDH1 mutation and increases hypoxia-induced factor-1α. Hypoxia-induced factor-1α is a transcription factor associated with tumorigenesis, such as the upregulation of vascular endothelial growth factor, and stimulating tumor angiogenesis. Interestingly, as a matter of factor, vascular proliferation is one of the histopathological features of GBM.

IDH-wild-type GBMs show a widespread anatomical distribution, while IDH-mutant GBMs favor the frontal lobe, which offers the surgeons more wildly resection of the tumors and provides the potential for a better prognosis. In addition, those IDH-mutant gliomas, no matter lower-grade astrocytomas or oligodendrogliomas with 1p/19q co-deletion all favor this location, supporting the hypothesis that these gliomas develop from a distinct population of common precursor cells [14].

IDH1 mutation has been shown to be a strong, independent prognostic biomarker not only in GBMs, but also in diffuse gliomas of lesser grades (grade 2 or 3) as well. There is no difference yet to be seen in terms of the point mutation, R132H verse others, regarding patients' outcome. While the IDH1 mutation conveys a better patients' outcome, unlike 1p/19q co-deletion, it does not predict a better response of the glioma to chemotherapy. In addition to its prognostic value, the identification of IDH mutations could be used diagnostically to determine tumor verse reactive conditions. Analysis of IDH1/2 mutations could be utilized in the separation of primary and secondary GBMs and for the challenging cases of differentiating pilocytic astrocytoma from cystic GBM.

Recently, IHC staining by using a specific antibody against mutant IDH1-R132H was developed, which can be applied to routine paraffin-embedded tissue. This has been proved to be a tumor-specific marker differentiating reactive from neoplastic cells in grade II and III gliomas. However, selecting a good antibody is important for practice, since some antibodies on the market lack the sensitivity and specificity requested by pathological diagnosis. In addition, detection of IDH1/2 mutations can also be achieved by PCR techniques and direct sequencing.

Key points:

- Associated with a better outcome and younger age.
- Found in secondary glioblastoma, rarely in primary.
- Also found in grades II-III diffuse gliomas.

- Used for prognosis and diagnosis.

By 2016, WHO classification of tumors of the central nervous system [14], GBM was separated into IDH-wild-type and IDH mutant subtypes based on the mutation status of *IDH1/2* genes that encode Isocitrate dehydrogenases 1 and 2 (IDH1 and IDH2).

It was requested as part on the diagnosis of gliomas currently. Adult diffuse gliomas (used to be grade II or III) have at least three molecular subtypes by new WHO classification of tumors of CNS [1]. The first, tumors with IDH mutation and 1p/19q co-deletion, this type tumors are more likely with oligodendroglial differentiation and good prognosis. The second are those tumors with IDH mutation and *p53* mutation, are likely with astrocytic differentiation and slightly better prognosis. The third one are those tumors with IDH wild type and more likely astrocytic differentiation and higher grade with poor prognosis. For example, a brain mass biopsied shows infiltrating astrocytoma with active mitoses but no definitive histological features of necrosis and vascular proliferation. IDH1 status was negative by IHC stain and PCR, the tumor was with EGFR amplification and TERT promoter mutation. Despite the histologic absence of tumor necrosis and microvascular proliferation (traditionally diagnosed as grade 2 or 3 astrocytoma), this molecular profile is now considered to be in keeping with an IDH-wild type GBM (CNS WHO grade 4) by the 2021/5th edition of WHO Classification of CNS Tumors [1].

3.3 P53

P53 was one of the first identified tumor suppress genes and is involved in many neoplasms, from carcinomas of lung and breast, sarcomas, to brain tumors. *TP53* gene is located on the short arm of chromosome 17. The major function of P53 is to control cell cycle progression, promote apoptosis, DNA integrity, and the survival of cells exposed to DNA damaging agents. In an activated status, P53 acts as a transcription regulator leading to the upregulation of *p21*. The protein P21 is the stop protein responsible for binding to the cyclin-dependent kinase and inhibiting cell proliferation. Thus, a mutated *p53* will be unable to prevent cell replication, resulting in uncontrolled tumor growth.

In most human cancers, *PT53* is inactivated by gene alteration, which results in the loss of the protein's tumor suppressor function.

The majority of mutations involving *p53* lead to missense mutations, and there is a resultant prolongation of the protein half-life, which accumulates in the nucleus of the cells. Therefore, by IHC stains for P53 highlight the nuclei of the cells and are used as a surrogate marker for identifying cells affected by a mutation in this pathway.

The significance of the detection of P53 overexpression in gliomas is inconsistent. Some reports indicated that diffused positive of nuclear PT53 stain might correlate IDH1 mutation in secondary GBMs. In terms of diagnosis, p53 would be a less favorable marker than others in distinguishing primary from secondary GBMs given that P53 overexpression has been reported in up to 25% of primary GBMs. As a prognostic marker, p53 has been shown inconsistent results. While some reports indicate a shorter survival time for gliomas overexpressing P53, this finding has not been confirmed by several meta-analyses yet.

3.4 EGFR

EGFR is one of the well-unknown tumor growth factors receptor, and which is involved in many malignancies, from carcinomas of the lung and breast to uncommon sarcomas. The receptor tyrosine kinase (RTK) of EGFR is frequently altered in

IDH-wildtype GBM. Overall, about 60% of tumors show evidence of *EGFR* amplification, mutation, rearrangement, or altered splicing. The most frequent of these alterations is *EGFR* amplification., which occurs in about 40% of IDH-wild type GBMs and in 60% of GBMs in the DNA methylation group. In the majority of cases, EGFR amplification is associated with a second EGFR alteration, such as extracellular domain mutations or in-frame intragenic deletions encoding either EGFRvIII or other alternative transcripts [1]. Like most growth factor receptors, it is composed of three major parts, an extracellular ligand-binding domain, a transmembrane domain, and an intracellular domain with tyrosine kinase activity. Each those tumor carries a different EGFR mutation. In primary GBM, besides EGFR amplification, the *EGFR* mutation is characterized by in-frame deletion of exons 2–7, resulting in a truncated extracellular domain with the inability to bind a ligand but retains ligand-independent tonic and constitutive activities to stimulate the tumor nuclei to promote tumor cell proliferation. This mutation is named as EGFRvIII (EGFR variant III), which plays an important role in tumorigenesis by activating Mitogen Active Protient Kinase (MAPK) and phosphoinositide-3-kinase (PI3K-Akt) pathways, leading to cell proliferation, decreased apoptosis, angiogenesis, and aggressive tumor invasion [31]. In most primary GBMs, EGFR amplification and mutation occur simultaneously, which offers the tumor cells a great proliferation advantage, aggressive clinical behavior as well a bad prognosis. EGFR amplification and mutation can be detected by FISH (**Figure 8**) as well as PCR techniques.

3.5 PTEN alteration and 10q LOHs

Phosphatase and tensin homolog (*PTEN*), located at 10q23, is a tumor suppressor gene with a role in opposing the PI3K-Akt pathway. In gliomas with a mutant *PTEN* gene, there is an associated increase in PI3-Akt pathway signaling, which may contribute to the tumor's malignant behavior of aggressively invasion and infiltration. Mutations at the *PTEN* gene are found in 15–40% of primary GBMs but are absent in IDH1 mutated secondary GBMs and other lower-grade gliomas.

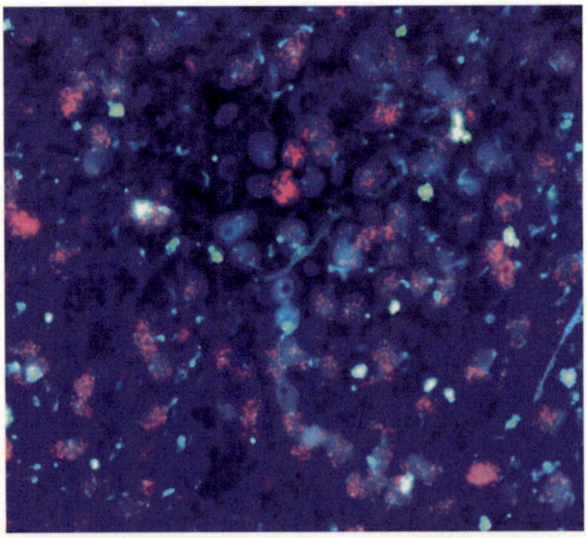

Figure 8.
Amplification of EGFR by FISH (red color) is one of characteristic molecular changes of primary GBM.

PTEN mutation and 10q LOH both carry the same negative prognostication for GBMs. LOH analysis or FISH can be used for this type of mutation evaluation [31].

Loss of heterozygosity (LOH) at chromosome 10q23 occurs commonly in a different type of human tumors. In GBMs, approximately 70% of GBMs are with *PTEN* alterations. PTEN is a negative regulator of the phosphoinositide 3 kinase pathway, a major signaling stimulating cellular proliferation in response to growth factor stimulation. *PTEN* deletions were more common in GBMs, but not in lower-grade, like grade II/III gliomas. *PTEN* deletion was very common across all gene expression subtypes, but absent in IDH1 mutant tumors [32]. *PTEN* loss was associated with AKT pathway activity [33]. Several studies demonstrated that patients with loss of PTEN generally had shorter survival than patients with PTEN retention, However, PTEN loss was not associated with worse survival in newly diagnosed GBMs patients of the TMZ era [34].

3.6 TERT promoter mutation in GBMs

Telomerase reverse transcriptase (TERT) in gliomagenesis has been recently further strengthened by the frequent occurrence of TERT promoter mutations (TERTp-mut) in gliomas and many other malignant neoplasms.

The telomerase reverse transcriptase (*TERT)* gene encodes a highly specialized reverse transcriptase, which adds hexamer repeats to the 3′ end of chromosomes. The increased telomerase activity seen in cancer leads to the preservation of telomeres, allowing tumors to avoid induction of apoptosis.

The promoter region of *TERT* contains two hotspots for point mutation; with most GBM (about 80% in one study) carry these mutations. They are more common in IDH1-wild type GBMs but rare in secondary (IDH1 mutant) GBMs and other astrocytomas. *TERT* mutation are also common in oligodendrogliomas. TERTp-mutation is associated with poor outcomes in patients with GBM [35]. A study found that about 75% GBMs were associated with TERTp-mutation, TERTp-mut was associated with IDH-wt, EGFR amplification, CDKN2A deletion, and chromosome 10q loss, but not with MGMT promoter methylation (Combined analysis). TERTp-mutation was an independent factor for poor prognosis. TERTp mutation can be detected by sequencing and RT-PCR [35].

3.7 MGMT status

Epigenetic gene silencing by DNA methylation is another common mechanism of inactivating genes. The MGMT gene encodes a DNA repair protein and is transcriptional silenced by promoter methylation [1]. The interplay between epigenetic regulation (post-translational modification) and GBM tumorigenesis has several modalities. Epigenetic modifiers can be oncogenic or tumor suppressors affected by genetic alteration of gain and loss-of-function, which results in the disruption of epigenetic regulatory processes by affecting histone modification, DNA methylation, and chromatin remodeling. The MGMT (O^6-methylguanine-DNAethyltransferase) gene at 10q26 encodes for a DNA repair protein. In gliomas of different grades, the MGMT gene is silenced by promoter hypermethylation, impeding transcription, and thus, resulting in a decreased expression of the MGMT protein. This epigenetic modification has been associated with increased sensitivity to alkylating chemotherapy. In alkylating therapies such as temozolomide (TMZ), a methyl group is added to the O^6-position of the nucleotide guanine, resulting in DNA damage and apoptosis [31]. A full-functioning MGMT would remove this methyl group, however with reduced expression of the protein secondary to promoter hypermethylation the cell has a decreased ability to repair alkylated DNA. Therefore,

Cell of origin	
EGFR ampl/mutation	*IDH* mutation
PETN mutation	*p53* mutation
Monosomy10	10q loss
Primary GBM	**Secondary GBM**

Table 1.
A summary of the major genetic pathway for primary and secondary GBMs.

MGMT expression analysis can be used to predict which tumors may have a more favorable response to alkylating chemotherapeutic agents, like TMZ. Testing of MGMT can be applied to pediatric gliomas as well. MGMT promoter methylation has been found in up to 40% of primary GBMs and 40–60% of secondary GBMs. The aberration is also present in other diffuse gliomas, with a preponderance of oligodendrogliomas at 60–93% [1, 31].

While studies have shown that MGMT promoter methylation results in a significantly longer survival time for patients with GBM treated with concomitant treatment of temozolomide and radiotherapy, there have been discordant reports regarding MGMT methylation as a predictor for increased survival in patients receiving radiotherapy alone. However, in gliomas of lesser grades there is a clear prognostic association between MGMT methylation status and sole radiotherapy. The underlying mechanism by which MGMT methylation would offer a favorable prognosis when not in relation to chemotherapy is a bit more difficult to clarify. As mentioned previously, gliomas often contain multiple molecular aberrancies and thus it may be the result of another molecular change, or the summation of several changes, that convey this prognostic significance to radiotherapy.

The most common method utilized to assess the MGMT promoter methylation status is a methylation-specific PCR analysis, which applies primers composed of differing quantities of CpG sites to allow differentiation between methylated and unmethylated DNA. Methylation-specific pyrosequencing has also been employed with strong sensitivity. Other DNA-based methods are available such as combined bisulfite restriction analysis (COBRA) and methylation-specific multiplex ligation-dependent probe amplification (MS-MLPA) [31, 34].

Key points:

- Predictive for a better response of glioblastomas to alkylating chemotherapy.
- Associated with better prognosis in diffuse gliomas treated with radiotherapy, alkylating chemotherapy, or combination therapy.
- Can be found in all glioma types.

In summary, in primary and secondary GBMs, each has its own genetic pathway, which are summarized in the following table for easy reference (**Table 1**).

4. Conclusion

Glioblastoma (GBM) is a malignant tumor of the central nervous system with a very poor prognosis even with current treatment including surgery, chemo, and radiotherapy. Most patients with GBMs have only 15 to 20 months of survival time. In the last two decades, the rapid development of molecular genetic techniques helped us to move our understanding of the GBM into a new level [36, 37]. It is believed that further research will identify new and more important and reliable biomarkers of GBM, which enable us to develop more sensitive target treatment, and eventually, we can overcome this challenging neoplasm.

Abbreviations

GBM	Glioblastoma
FISH	Fluorescent in situ hybridization
IHC	Immunohistochemistry
LOH	Loss of heterozygosity
EGFR	Epidermal growth factor receptor
TMZ	Temozolomide
TERT	Telomerase reverse transcriptase
TERTp-mut	TERT promoter mutation
IDH	Isocitrate dehydrogenase
MGMT	O^6-methylguanine-DNA methyltransferase
PTEN	Phosphatase and tensin homolog
NGS	next-generation sequencing
WHO	World Health Organization
CNS	Central nerve system
PNET	primitive neuroectodermal tumor
GFAP	Glial fibrillary acidic protein

Author details

Frank Y. Shan[1,2*], Dachun Zhao[3], Carlos A. Tirado[1], Ekokobe Fonkem[2], Yi-lu Zhang[2], Dong-xia Feng[2] and Jason H. Huang[2]

1 Department of Anatomic Pathology, Texas A&M University, Baylor Scott and White Health, College of Medicine, Temple, TX, USA

2 Department of Neurosurgery, Texas A&M University, Baylor Scott and White Health, College of Medicine, Temple, TX, USA

3 Department of Pathology, Peking Union Medical College Hospital, Chinese Academy of Medical Sciences and Peking Union Medical College, DongCheng District, Beijing, P.R. China

*Address all correspondence to: yshan918@gmail.com

References

[1] Louis DN et al. The 2021 WHO classification of tumors of the central nervous system: A summary. Neuro-Oncology. 2021;**23**(8):1231-1251

[2] Tamai S, Kinoshita M, Sabit H, et al. Case of metastatic glioblastoma with primitive neuronal component to the lung. Neuropathology. 2019;**39**(3):218-23

[3] Burger PC, Kleihues P. Cytologic composition of the untreated glioblastoma with implications for evaluation of needle biopsies. Cancer. 1989;**63**(10):2014-23

[4] Haddad SF, Moore SA, Schelper RL, et al. Vascular smooth muscle hyperplasia underlies the formation of glomeruloid vascular structures of glioblastoma multiforme. Journal of Neuropathology & Experimental Neurology. 1992;**51**(5):488-92

[5] Nagashima T, Hoshino T, Cho KG. Proliferative potential of vascular components in human glioblastoma multiforme. Acta Neuropathologica. 1987;**73**(3):30-5

[6] Clara CA, Marie SK, de Almeida JR, et al. Angiogenesis and expression of PDGF-C, VEGF, CD105 and HIF-1a in human glioblastoma. Neuropathology. 2014;**34**(4):343-52

[7] Rong Y, Durden DL, Van Meir EG, et al. 'Pseudopalisading' necrosis in glioblastoma: A familiar morphologic feature that links vascular pathology, hypoxia, and angiogenesis. Journal of Neuropathology and Experimental Neurology. 2006;**65**(6):529-39

[8] Spinelli C, Tawil N, Adnani L, Rak J, Choi D. Extracellular vesicle mediated vascular pathology in glioblastoma. Sub-Cellular Biochemistry. 2021;**97**:247-73

[9] Unruh D, Schwarze SR, Khoury L, et al. Mutant IDH1 and thrombosis in gliomas. Acta Neuropathologica. 2016;**132**(6):917-30

[10] Zulch KJ. Histological Typing of Tumours of the Central Nervous System. Vol. 21. Geneva: World Health Organization; 1979

[11] Kleihues P, Burger PC, Scheithauer BW. Histological Typing of Tumours of the Central Nervous System. Berlin: Springer-Verlag; 1993

[12] Kleihues P, Cavenee WK. World Health Organization Classification of Tumours of the Nervous System. Lyon: WHO/IARC; 2000

[13] Louis DN, Ohgaki H, Wiestler OD, Cavenee WK. World Health Organization Histological Classification of Tumours of the Central Nervous System. 4th ed. Lyon: International Agency for Research on Cancer; 2007

[14] Louis DN, Ohgaki H, Wiestler OD, Cavenee WK. World Health Organization Classification of Tumours of the Central Nervous System. 4th ed., updated ed. Lyon: International Agency for Research on Cancer; 2016

[15] Margetts JC, Kalyan-Raman UP. Giant-celled glioblastoma of brain. A clinico-pathological and radiological study of ten cases (including immunohistochemistry and ultrastructure). Cancer. 1989;**63**(3):524-31

[16] Ortega A, Nuho M, Walia S, Mukherjee D, Black KL, Patil CG. Treatment and survival of patients harboring histological variants of glioblastoma. Journal of Clinical Neuroscience. 2014;**21**(10):1709-13

[17] Shinojima N, Kochi M, Hamada J, Nakamura H, Yano S, Makino K, et al. The influence of sex and the presence of giant ceils on postoperative long-term survival in adult patients with supratentorial glioblastoma multiforme. Journal of Neurosurgery. 2004;**101**(2):219-26

[18] Rodriguez FJ, Scheithauer BW, Giannini C, et al. Epithelial and pseudoepithelial differentiation in glioblastoma and gliosarcoma: A comparative morphologic and molecular genetic study. Cancer. 2008;**113**(10):2779-89

[19] Rosenblum MK, Erlandson RA, Budzilovich GN. The lipid-rich epithelioid glioblastoma. The American Journal of Surgical Pathology. 1991;**15**(10):925-34

[20] Korshunov A, Chavez L, Sharma T, et al. Epithelioid glioblastomas stratify into established diagnostic subsets upon integrated molecular analysis. Brain Pathology. 2018;**28**(5):656-62

[21] Tada T, Katsuyama T, Aoki T, Kobayashi S, Shigematsu H. Mixed glioblastoma and sarcoma with osteoid-chondral tissue. Clinical Neuropathology. 1987;**6**(4):460-63

[22] Khanna M, Siraj F, Chopra P, Bhalla S, Roy S. Gliosarcoma with prominent smooth muscle component (gliomyosarcoma): A report of 10 cases. Indian Journal of Pathology & Microbiology. 2011;**54**(1):51-54

[23] Gherardi R, Baudrimont M, Nguyen JP, et al. Monstrocellular heavily lipidized malignant glioma. Acta Neuropathologica. 1986;**69**(1-2):28-32

[24] Oh JE, Ohta T, Nonoguchi N, et al. Genetic alterations in gliosarcoma and giant cell glioblastoma. Brain Pathology. 2016;**26**(4):517-22

[25] Hinrichs BH, Newman S, Appin CL, et al. Farewell to GBM-O: Genomic and transcriptomic profiling of glioblastoma with oligodendroglioma component reveals distinct molecular subgroups. Acta Neuropathologica Communications. 2016;**4**:4

[26] Perry A, Aldape KD, George DH, Burger PC. Small cell astrocytoma: An aggressive variant that is dinicopathologically and genetically distinct from anaplastic oligodendroglioma. Cancer. 2000;**101**(10):2318-26

[27] Brat DJ, Scheithauer BW, Medina-Flores R, Rosenblum MK, Burger PC. Infiltrative astrocytomas with granular cell features (granular cell astrocytomas): A study of histopathologic features, grading, and outcome. The American Journal of Surgical Pathology. 2002;**26**(6):750-7

[28] Ohgaki H, Dessen P, Jourde B, Horstmann S, Nishikawa T, DiPatre PL, et al. Genetic pathwaysto glioblastoma: Apopulation-based study. Cancer Research. 2004;**64**:6892-9

[29] Watanabe K, Tachibana O, Sato K, Yonekawa Y, Kleisues P, Ohgaki H. Overexpression of the EGF receptor and *p53* mutations are mutually exclusive in the evaluation of primary and secondary glioblastomas. Brain Pathology. 1996;**6**:217-224

[30] Ohgaki H, Kleihues P. Genetic pathways to primary and secondary glioblastoma. The American Journal of Pathology. 2007;**170**:1445-53

[31] Kresak J, Shan Y. Molecular diagnostics of gliomas. In: Coppola D, editor. Molecular Diagnostics of Cancers. Dordrecht, Heidelberg, New York, London: Springer; 2013. pp. 1-18. ISBN: 978-94-07-7191-8

[32] Dang L, White DW, Gross S, Bennett BD, Bittinger BD, Drigger EM. Cancer-associated IDH1 mutations produce 2-hydroxyglutarate. Nature. 2009;**462**:739-44

[33] Toedt G, Barbus S, Wolter M, Felsberg J, Tews B, Blond F. Molecular signatures classify astrocytic gliomas by IDH1 mutation status. International Journal of Cancer. 2011;**128**:177-83

[34] Christebsen BC, Smith AA, Zhang S, Koestle DC, Houseman EA, Marsit CJ. DNA methylation, Isocitrate dehydrogenase mutation, and survival in glioma. Journal of the National Cancer Institute. 2011;**103**:143-53

[35] Labussiere M, Di Stefano AL, Gleize V, Boisselier B, Giry M, Mangesius S, et al. TERT promoter mutations in gliomas, genetic associations and clinic-pathological correlations. British Journal of Cancer. 2014;**111**:2024-2032

[36] Ohgaki H, Kleihues P. The definition of primary and secondary glioblastoma. Clinical Cancer Research. 2012;**19**(4):764-772

[37] Li Q-J, Cal J-Q, Liu C-Y. Evolving molecular genetics of glioblastoma. Chinese Medical Journal. 2016;**129**(4):464-471

Chapter 3

Perspective Chapter: Glioblastoma of the Corpus Callosum

Daulat Singh Kunwar, Ved Prakash Maurya, Balachandar Deivasigamani, Rakesh Mishra and Amit Agrawal

Abstract

Glioma is the most common malignant tumour of the brain, in which glioblastoma (GBM) is the most aggressive form which infiltrates through the white fibre tracts. Corpus callosum (CC) is most invaded by GBM, it carries poor prognosis as mostly these tumours are not touched upon due to the belief of post operative cognitive decline, or there is incomplete resection leading to tumour recurrence. However current advancement in technology, operative techniques and better understanding of nature of CC-GBM, maximal safe resection is being carried out with better outcomes in comparison with the GBM without infiltration of CC.

Keywords: butterfly glioma, butterfly glioblastoma, corpus callosum, glioma, glioblastoma, surgical resection, survival

1. Introduction

Glioblastoma multiforme originates in the cerebral white matter, accounts for 12–15% of all intracranial neoplasms and is the most common primary intra-axial malignancies [1]. Corpus callosum is the largest interhemispheric commissure connecting two identical cortical areas, and it acts as a white matter bridge between two hemispheres for tumour cells to migrate [2]. These are often reported arising from frontal and parietal lobes. Butterfly gliomas involving the corpus callosum characteristically appear as "butterfly" on imaging as the tumour has contiguous extension through the corpus callosum into both the cerebral hemispheres [1, 3, 4]. The incidence of butterfly glioma ranges from 3 to 14% of all high-grade gliomas [5, 6], and the isolated corpus callosum GBM is a relatively unusual variant of butterfly glioblastoma and account for 3% of all GBM [7]. The butterfly GBM of the corpus callosum can be anterior involving genu or less commonly can be posterior involving splenium [1]. Involvement of the corpus callosum can be on one side or either side involving both cerebral hemispheres (butterfly GBM) [8, 9]. Involvement of the corpus callosum makes the resection difficult and carries a poorer prognosis [10]. In this chapter, we discuss the pathology, clinical and imaging characteristics of glioblastomas involving the corpus callosum and review the management and outcome of these subgroup of tumours.

2. Clinical features

Glioblastoma of the corpus callosum is characterised by a rapidly progressive deteriorating clinical course [11]. Progressive tumour growth in CC causes mass effect and white matter network connectivity changes (due to oedema or direct infiltration) [12]. Because of its location corpus callosum, glioblastomas involve the highly eloquent area of the brain, leading to impaired higher mental function, severe neurological deterioration and features of raised intracranial pressure (headache, vomiting and altered sensorium) [11, 13]. The myriad of symptoms of corpus callosum involvement includes non-specific headaches, paresis, seizures, depression, mutism, ataxia, behavioural abnormalities and Cotard's syndrome [14–16]. Tumours involving the splenium can lead to memory and cognitive function as several associative pathways pass through this area making the outcome further poorer [17].

3. Imaging

CT scan with contrast administration can be used as screening tool; however, post-contrast MRI is the investigation of choice for detail evaluation and

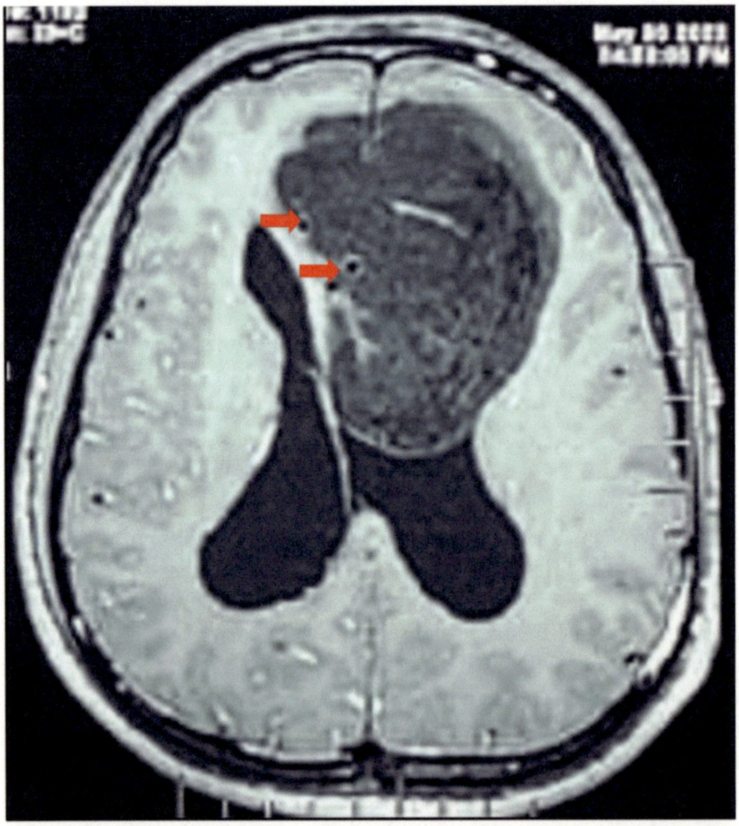

Figure 1.
Axial T1WI with contrast showing lesion involving the corpus callosum (at the genu) with main bulk towards the left side and crossing the midline to invade the right frontal lobe. The red arrows indicate the pushed anterior cerebral arteries towards the right side due to mass effect.

management including surgical planning [7, 18, 19]. Typically, corpus callosal GBM appears as a butterfly-shaped lesion with heterogeneous enhancement with areas of necrosis and haemorrhages with irregular postcontrast peripheral enhancement (**Figure 1**) [7, 18]. Coronal as well as sagittal fluid-attenuated inversion recovery images shall help in delineating the lesion and their relationship with surrounding structures better, [18] and diffusion tensor imaging shall help for the identification of white fibre tracts [20]. Pre-operative planning of tumour removal based on connectomics (machine learning-based algorithm which incorporates DTI and important cerebral network) is also available now [21].

4. Differential diagnosis

A number of pathologies those involve corpus callosum can mimic butterfly glioblastomas including other lesser grade variants of gliomas involving corpus callosum, [22–25] lymphoma, metastasis, [26] toxoplasmosis, [27] demyelinating butterfly pseudo glioma, [28] and neuronal ceroid-lipofuscinosis (Kufs' disease) [29] because of its multiplanar capability, MRI with contrast enhancement and FLAIR sequence [7, 18] can help to differentiate these lesions from each other; however, in doubtful cases the biopsy shall help to make the diagnosis.

5. Management

The aim of management is to improve patient's functionality and quality of life by relieving the symptoms and minimising the complications. Even though there are advances in immunotherapy, targeted therapy and oncolytic viral therapy most patients with CC-GBM suffer from limited survival. Currently, maximal safe resection with adjuvant chemo-radiotherapy remains gold standard [30–32]. Recent advances in the management of brain tumours have made resection of the corpus callosum glioblastomas preferred, possible and safe [33, 34]. Surgery improves overall survival, and it is superior to biopsy [4, 35, 36]. Surgical approaches help in reducing the tumour burden [11, 35, 37, 38] and also provide tissue sample for pathologic and molecular characterisation of the tumour (IDH 1/2 mutation or MGMT promoter methylation or both), thus guiding the further adjuvant management approaches [35]. Surgical resection can also be facilitated by intraoperative magnetic resonance imaging MRI-guided laser interstitial thermal therapy (LITT) techniques as this will increase the efficacy and safety of the procedure [37, 39–41]. Evidence suggests that preoperative KPS score, adjuvant radio chemotherapy and extent of surgical resection (EoR) have impact on survival besides patient's age. In a systematic review done by Palmisciano *et al.* [12], they say that resection of glioma infiltrating the corpus callosum has no significant changes in the post operative complications. Gross total resection of the tumour increases overall survival. Foster *et al.* [42] say that many patients with glioma infiltrating the corpus callosum rarely undergo surgical removal in fear of the post op neuropsychological sequelae. Authors hypothesise that the neuropsychological deficits are mainly due to tumour. Removing tumour reduces the mass effect and improves the microenvironment of the surrounding neurons; this may improve the neurocognitive and neurological function. In a prospective analysis done by them in 21 patients, they found that the neurocognitive decline post operatively was present in 75% of patients who presented with a median KPS of 100%.

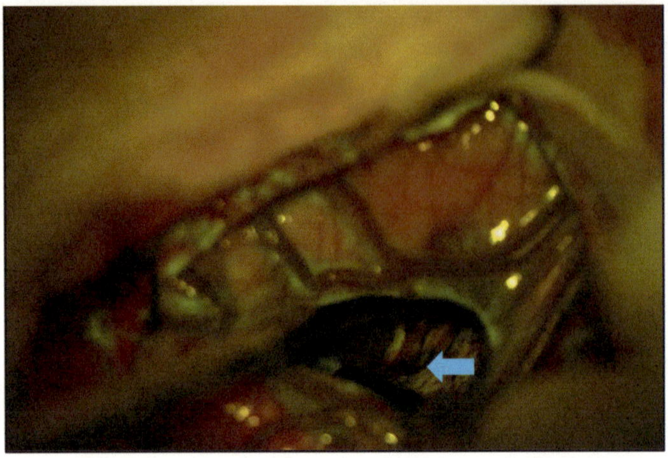

Figure 2.
Intraoperative photograph of tumour resection with the use of sodium fluorescence dye. The blue arrow indicates the plane of tumour-brain interface which was obvious after sodium fluorescence dye administration and facilitated the tumour decompression.

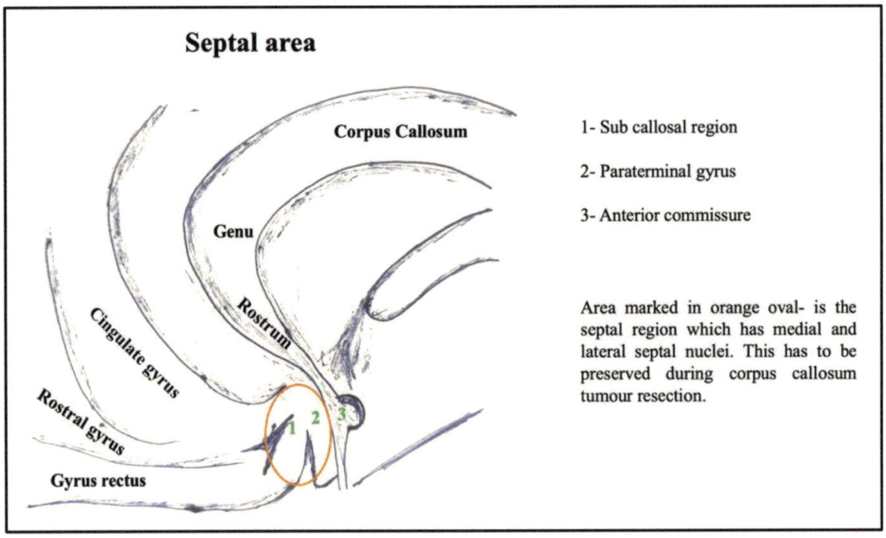

Figure 3.
Representative sketch depicting the corpus callosum and related neuroanatomical structures encountered during surgical resection. The septal nuclei (under orange oval area) need to be preserved during tumour decompression.

But surprisingly after 6 months a very few had impairment in attention, executive functioning, memory and depression. Authors strongly suggest that surgical resection of tumour might outweigh morbidity. Complications like motor deficits, cognitive decline post operatively is due to manipulation of the white fibres of CC and post operative edema (**Figure 2**) [36, 43].

Photo dynamic tumour visualisation technology is very helpful in achieving maximal extent of resection (i.e. supra marginal resection) which is the only modifiable factor linked with overall survival of the patients. Sodium fluorescein (**Figure 2**) and 5-Aminolevulinic acid (5-ALA) are the agents currently being used. In a recent study

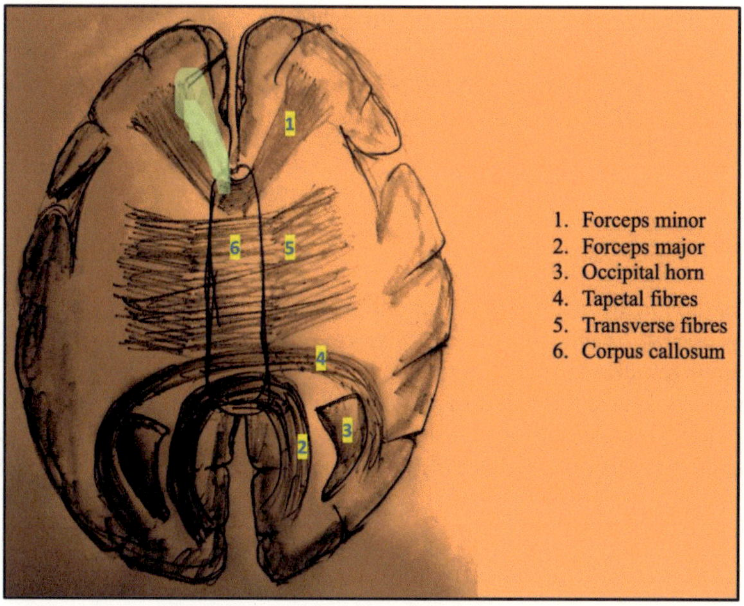

Figure 4.
Figure demonstrating white fibres through which tumour cells from one part of the brain reaching corpus callosum and travels to other side. The light green colour lesion is representing a lesion in the right frontal lobe infiltrating the forceps minor and traversing towards the opposite side.

done on peritumoral region, they found that 5-ALA staining extends beyond the sodium fluorescein-stained areas, even then there are tumour positive cells beyond this region [44]. Combining both fluorescein sodium and 5-ALA gives very good background information of the glioma cells and is more effective in supra marginal resection [33, 45, 46] current understanding is that fluorescein and 5-ALA should be supplemented with supplemented with intra-operative neurophysiological monitoring for better clinical outcome as well as overall survival [44].

In cases of glioma infiltrating the genu and rostrum of the corpus callosum, one should be careful not to enter the subcallosal region (contains septal nucleus) during resection (**Figures 3** and **4**). As this may cause psychiatric disturbances along with cognitive decline, this has been pointed out by Sughrue *et al.* [34].

However, because of its unique location and spread, in comparison with other GBMs, the conservative resection of corpus callosum is possible, thus reducing the chances of overall survival [9–12]. Temozolomide alone or in combination has been shown as a safer alternative in elderly population [26, 28, 42, 43].

6. Outcome

In spite of advances in maximal safe surgical resection techniques, availability of adjuvant radiotherapy and temozolomide chemotherapy, as for other glioblastomas the prognosis in cases of corpus callosal glioblastomas is dismal [3, 4, 19, 25, 35, 39, 47]. In literature, the overall survival in cases of butterfly glioblastomas is in weeks to months, and the median survival of 3 months and a six-month survival is only 38% [3, 19, 22, 24]. Median overall survival of a CC infiltrated glioblastomas is 10.7 months, whereas it is 13.2 months in a non-CC infiltrated glioblastoma [36]. In a series of 215 patients where the corpus callosum was involved, overall survival was less than <6 months [48]. It is also observed that there are higher rates of recurrence in whom the infiltrated part of tumour in corpus callosum was not removed [36, 49]. However, their isolated case of long-term survival, in a report the patient survived the disease for 5 years and 2 months after the initial diagnosis [50].

7. Conclusion

Glioblastoma infiltrating the corpus callosum is rare yet highly invasive. With the improved intra-operative adjuncts, surgical techniques and concepts, there is higher tumour resection rates with minimal complications. While managing corpus callosal tumours, one should always aim for safe maximal resection with multimodal approach if the situation permits. However, in spite of the advances in the diagnosis and management techniques, there is not much improvement in the overall outcome of these patients.

Author details

Daulat Singh Kunwar[1*], Ved Prakash Maurya[2], Balachandar Deivasigamani[3], Rakesh Mishra[4] and Amit Agrawal[5]

1 Department of Radiotherapy and Clinical Oncology, Government Doon Medical College, Dehradun, Uttarakhand, India

2 Department of Neurosurgery, Sanjay Gandhi Post Graduate Institute of Medical Sciences, Lucknow, India

3 Department of Neurosurgery, Apollo Cancer Centre, Chennai, India

4 Department of Neurosurgery, Institute of Medical Sciences, Trauma Centre and Mahamana Centenary Superspeciality Hospital, Banaras Hindu University, Varanasi, India

5 Department of Neurosurgery, All India Institute of Medical Sciences, Bhopal, Madhya Pradesh, India

*Address all correspondence to: daulatsinghk@yahoo.com

References

[1] Kiely F, Twomey F. Butterfly glioma involving splenium of corpus callosum. IJCMI. 2015;**2015**:1000277. DOI: 10.4172/2376-0249.1000277

[2] Mickevicius NJ, Carle AB, Bluemel T, Santarriaga S, Schloemer F, Shumate D, et al. Location of brain tumor intersecting white matter tracts predicts patient prognosis. Journal of Neuro-Oncology. 2015;**125**:393-400

[3] Dayani F, Young JS, Bonte A, Chang EF, Theodosopoulos P, McDermott MW, et al. Safety and outcomes of resection of butterfly glioblastoma. Neurosurgical Focus. 2018;**44**:E4

[4] Chaichana KL, Jusue-Torres I, Lemos AM, Gokaslan A, Cabrera-Aldana EE, Ashary A, et al. The butterfly effect on glioblastoma: Is volumetric extent of resection more effective than biopsy for these tumors? Journal of Neuro-Oncology. 2014;**120**:625-634

[5] Balana C, Capellades J, Teixidor P, Roussos I, Ballester R, Cuello M, et al. Clinical course of high-grade glioma patients with a "biopsy-only" surgical approach: A need for individualised treatment. Clinical and Translational Oncology. 2007;**9**:797-803

[6] Dziurzynski K, Blas-Boria D, Suki D, Cahill DP, Prabhu SS, Puduvalli V, et al. Butterfly glioblastomas: A retrospective review and qualitative assessment of outcomes. Journal of Neuro-Oncology. 2012;**109**:555-563

[7] Sharma R, Tiwari T, Goyal S. Classical imaging finding in callosal glioblastoma multiforme. BMJ Case Reports. 2021;**14**

[8] Nazem-Zadeh M-R, Saksena S, Babajani-Fermi A, Jiang Q, Soltanian-Zadeh H, Rosenblum M, et al. Segmentation of corpus callosum using diffusion tensor imaging: Validation in patients with glioblastoma. BMC Medical Imaging. 2012;**12**:1-16

[9] Kallenberg K, Goldmann T, Menke J, Strik H, Bock HC, Stockhammer F, et al. Glioma infiltration of the corpus callosum: Early signs detected by DTI. Journal of Neuro-Oncology. 2013;**112**:217-222

[10] Talos I-F, Zou KH, Ohno-Machado L, Bhagwat JG, Kikinis R, Black PM, et al. Supratentorial low-grade glioma resectability: Statistical predictive analysis based on anatomic MR features and tumor characteristics. Radiology. 2006;**239**:506

[11] Franco P, Delev D, Cipriani D, et al. Surgery for IDH1/2 wild-type glioma invading the corpus callosum. Acta Neurochirurgica. 2021;**163**:937-945

[12] Palmisciano P, Ferini G, Watanabe G, et al. Gliomas infiltrating the Corpus callosum: A systematic review of the literature. Cancers. 2022;**14**:2507

[13] Witoonpanich P, Bamrungrak K, Jinawath A, Wongwaisayawan S, Phudhichareonrat S, Witoonpanich R. Glioblastoma multiforme at the corpus callosum with spinal leptomeningeal metastasis. Clinical Neurology and Neurosurgery. 2011;**113**:407-410

[14] Zhang J, Xing S, Li J, Chen L, Chen H, Dang C, et al. Isolated astasia manifested by acute infarct of the anterior corpus callosum and cingulate gyrus. Journal of Clinical Neuroscience. 2015;**22**:763-764

[15] Yapıcı-Eser H, Onay A, Öztop-Çakmak Ö, Egemen E,

Vanlı-Yavuz EN, Solaroğlu İ. Rare case of glioblastoma multiforme located in posterior corpus callosum presenting with depressive symptoms and visual memory deficits. Case Reports. 2016;**2016**:bcr2016

[16] Boaro A, Harary M, Chukwueke U, Valdes Quevedo P, Smith TR. The neurocognitive evaluation in the butterfly glioma patient. A systematic review. Interdisciplinary Neurosurgery. 2019;**18**:100512

[17] Sammler D, Kotz SA, Eckstein K, Ott DV, Friederici AD. Prosody meets syntax: The role of the corpus callosum. Brain. 2010;**133**:2643-2655

[18] Uchino A, Takase Y, Nomiyama K, Egashira R, Kudo S. Acquired lesions of the corpus callosum: MR imaging. European Radiology. 2006;**16**:905-914

[19] Agrawal A. Butterfly glioma of the corpus callosum. Journal of Cancer Research Therapy. 2009;**5**:43

[20] Tench C, Morgan P, Wilson M, Blumhardt L. White matter mapping using diffusion tensor MRI. Magnetic Resonance in Medicine: An Official Journal of the International Society for Magnetic Resonance in Medicine. 2002;**47**:967-972

[21] Yeung JT, Taylor HM, Nicholas PJ, Young IM, Jiang I, Doyen S, et al. Using quicktome for intracerebral surgery: Early retrospective study and proof of concept. World Neurosurgery. 2021;**154**:e734-e742

[22] Zakrzewska M, Szybka M, Zakrzewski K, Biernat W, Kordek R, Rieske P, et al. Diverse molecular pattern in a bihemispheric glioblastoma (butterfly glioma) in a 16-year-old boy. Cancer Genetics and Cytogenetics. 2007;**177**:125-130

[23] Kappos L. What is your diagnosis? Butterfly glioma originating from the corpus callosum. Schweizerische Rundschau fur Medizin Praxis= Revue Suisse de Medecine Praxis. 1992;**81**:785-786

[24] Arora M, Praharaj SK. Butterfly glioma of corpus callosum presenting as catatonia. The World Journal of Biological Psychiatry. 2007;**8**:54-55

[25] Bourekas EC, Varakis K, Bruns D, Christoforidis GA, Baujan M, Slone HW, et al. Lesions of the corpus callosum: MR imaging and differential considerations in adults and children. American Journal of Roentgenology. 2002;**179**:251-257

[26] Garber ST, Khoury L, Bell D, Schomer DF, Janku F, McCutcheon IE. Metastatic adenoid cystic carcinoma mimicking butterfly glioblastoma: A rare presentation in the splenium of the Corpus callosum. World Neurosurgery. 2016;**95**(621):e13-e19

[27] Lee H-J, Williams R, Kalnin A. Toxoplasmosis of the corpus callosum: Another butterfly. American Journal of Roentgenology. 1976;**166**:1280-1281

[28] Scozzafava J, Johnson E, Blevins G. Demyelinating butterfly pseudo-glioma. Journal of Neurology, Neurosurgery & Psychiatry. 2008;**79**:12-13

[29] Hammersen S, Brock M, Cervós-Navarro J. Adult neuronal ceroid lipofuscinosis with clinical findings consistent with a butterfly glioma: Case report. Journal of Neurosurgery. 1998;**88**:314-318

[30] Brown TJ, Brennan MC, Li M, Church EW, Brandmeir NJ, Rakszawski KL, et al. Association of the extent of resection with survival in glioblastoma: A systematic review

and meta-analysis. JAMA Oncology. 2016;**2**:1460-1469

[31] Sanai N, Berger MS. Surgical oncology for gliomas: The state of the art. Nature Reviews Clinical Oncology. 2018;**15**:112-125

[32] Bi J, Chowdhry S, Wu S, Zhang W, Masui K, Mischel PS. Altered cellular metabolism in gliomas—An emerging landscape of actionable co-dependency targets. Nature Reviews Cancer. 2020;**20**:57-70

[33] Coburger J, Engelke J, Scheuerle A, Thal DR, Hlavac M, Wirtz CR, et al. Tumor detection with 5-aminolevulinic acid fluorescence and Gd-DTPA–enhanced intraoperative MRI at the border of contrast-enhancing lesions: A prospective study based on histopathological assessment. Neurosurgical Focus. 2014;**36**:E3

[34] Sughrue ME. The Glioma Book. Leipzig, Germany: Georg Thieme Verlag; 2020

[35] Opoku-Darko M, Amuah JE, Kelly JJ. Surgical resection of anterior and posterior butterfly glioblastoma. World Neurosurgery. 2018;**110**:e612-e620

[36] Boaro A, Kavouridis VK, Siddi F, Mezzalira E, Harary M, Iorgulescu JB, et al. Improved outcomes associated with maximal extent of resection for butterfly glioblastoma: Insights from institutional and national data. Acta Neurochirurgica. 2021;**163**:1883-1894

[37] Beaumont TL, Mohammadi AM, Kim AH, Barnett GH, Leuthardt EC. Magnetic resonance imaging-guided laser interstitial thermal therapy for glioblastoma of the corpus callosum. Neurosurgery. 2018;**83**:556-565

[38] Stupp R, Mason WP, Van Den Bent MJ, Weller M, Fisher B, Taphoorn MJ, et al. Radiotherapy plus concomitant and adjuvant temozolomide for glioblastoma. New England Journal of Medicine. 2005;**352**:987-996

[39] Cui M, Chen H, Sun G, Liu J, Zhang M, Lin H, et al. Combined use of multimodal techniques for the resection of glioblastoma involving corpus callosum. Acta Neurochirurgica. 2022;**164**:689-702

[40] Mohammadi AM, Hawasli AH, Rodriguez A, Schroeder JL, Laxton AW, Elson P, et al. The role of laser interstitial thermal therapy in enhancing progression-free survival of difficult-to-access high-grade gliomas: A multicenter study. Cancer Medicine. 2014;**3**:971-979

[41] Hawasli AH, Bagade S, Shimony JS, Miller-Thomas M, Leuthardt EC. Magnetic resonance imaging-guided focused laser interstitial thermal therapy for intracranial lesions: Single-institution series. Neurosurgery. 2013;**73**:1007-1017

[42] Forster M-T, Behrens M, Lortz I, Conradi N, Senft C, Voss M, et al. Benefits of glioma resection in the corpus callosum. Scientific Reports. 2020;**10**:16630

[43] Dadario NB, Zaman A, Pandya M, Dlouhy BJ, Gunawardena MP, Sughrue ME, et al. Endoscopic-assisted surgical approach for butterfly glioma surgery. Journal of Neuro-Oncology. 2022;**156**:635-644

[44] Yano H, Nakayama N, Ohe N, Miwa K, Shinoda J, Iwama T. Pathological analysis of the surgical margins of resected glioblastomas excised using photodynamic visualization with both 5-aminolevulinic acid and fluorescein sodium. Journal of Neuro-Oncology. 2017;**133**:389-397

[45] Molina ES, Wölfer J, Ewelt C, Ehrhardt A, Brokinkel B, Stummer W. Dual-labeling with 5–aminolevulinic acid and fluorescein for fluorescence-guided resection of high-grade gliomas: Technical note. Journal of Neurosurgery. 2017;**128**:399-405

[46] Della Puppa A, Munari M, Gardiman MP, Volpin F. Combined fluorescence using 5-aminolevulinic acid and fluorescein sodium at glioblastoma border: Intraoperative findings and histopathologic data about 3 newly diagnosed consecutive cases. World Neurosurgery. 2019;**122**:e856-e863

[47] Chen K-T, Wu T-WE, Chuang C-C, Hsu Y-H, Hsu P-W, Huang Y-C, et al. Corpus callosum involvement and postoperative outcomes of patients with gliomas. Journal of Neuro-Oncology. 2015;**124**:207-214

[48] Fyllingen EH, Bø LE, Reinertsen I, Jakola AS, Sagberg LM, Berntsen EM, et al. Survival of glioblastoma in relation to tumor location: A statistical tumor atlas of a population-based cohort. Acta Neurochirurgica. 2021;**163**:1895-1905

[49] Duffau H, Khalil I, Gatignol P, Denvil D, Capelle L. Surgical removal of corpus callosum infiltrated by low-grade glioma: Functional outcome and oncological considerations. Journal of Neurosurgery. 2004;**100**:431-437

[50] Finneran M, Marotta DA, Altenburger D, Nardone E. Long-term survival in a patient with butterfly glioblastoma: A case report. Cureus. 2020;**2020**:e6914. DOI: 10.7759/cureus.6914

Chapter 4

Canine Glioma as a Model for Human Glioblastoma

Nicole M. Yost and James M. Angelastro

Abstract

Glioblastoma, a high-grade diffuse glioma, carries a poor clinical prognosis despite decades of extensive research on the genetic and molecular features of disease and investigation of experimental therapeutics. Because spontaneous canine glioma and human glioblastoma share many clinicopathologic characteristics, recent efforts have focused on utilizing companion dogs as a preclinical model for both research and therapeutic development. A detailed investigation of the canine disease, with particular attention to the genetic and molecular profile, is important in order to allow translation of specific clinical findings from canines to humans and vice versa. In this chapter, we investigate the most common genetic, molecular, and epigenetic alterations associated with canine and human glioma. Appropriate implementation of the canine glioma model may provide valuable information to improve both human and veterinary patient care.

Keywords: glioma, glioblastoma, canine, spontaneous model, translational neuro-oncology, comparative biology, genetics, molecular pathology

1. Introduction

Gliomas are the most common type of malignant primary central nervous system (CNS) neoplasm in humans within the United States [1]. Glioblastoma (GBM), a World Health Organization (WHO) grade IV glioma, is a particularly aggressive tumor, and it accounts for nearly half of the malignant CNS tumors in humans, with an average incidence of over 12,000 cases each year [1, 2]. Even with intensive therapy involving surgery, radiation therapy, chemotherapy, and the most recent FDA-approved therapy utilizing antimitotic alternating electrical fields, the median survival time for patients with GBM is less than 2 years [3].

Companion dogs also spontaneously develop gliomas, including high grade variants that are similar to human glioma and glioblastoma [4]. These canine gliomas share many clinicopathologic features with human disease, such as comparable imaging characteristics, genetic and molecular aberrations, tumor microenvironments, and histopathologic characteristics [5–9]. Correspondingly, the Comparative Oncology Program within the National Cancer Institute developed a Comparative Brain Tumor Consortium (CBTC) to further investigate and utilize spontaneously arising brain tumors in dogs as a model of the human disease with specific emphasis on comparative glioma [10]. As such, the spontaneous canine glioma model has gained attraction as a preclinical tool to improve the success of human clinical trials by bridging the gap between laboratory models of glioma and human patients.

Subsequent large-scale studies have greatly improved our diagnostic classification and molecular understanding of canine gliomas and have allowed more direct comparisons to human glioma and glioblastoma [11, 12]. While many similarities continue to exist between canine and human glioma, it is also important to characterize the differences between the canine and human disease to ensure that the model is utilized effectively and appropriately. Further investigation into canine glioma, with a focus on comparative molecular and genetic characteristics, can help establish which novel therapeutics can best harness the canine spontaneous glioma model and allow maximal possible benefit to both human and animal patients with gliomas.

2. Overview of canine glioma

Gliomas are the second most common primary intracranial tumor among dogs [4, 13] and have an overall prevalence of 0.9% in the canine population [4]. Gliomas tend to occur in adult dogs, with a median age of diagnosis of approximately 8 years and an increasing prevalence with increasing age [4, 14]. No significant difference in the frequency of intracranial tumors in male versus female dogs have been shown [13], although several recent studies have documented a slightly higher rate of diagnosis in males [14, 15]. Brachycephalic dog breeds, including Boston Terriers, French Bulldogs, English Bulldogs, Boxers, and English Toy Spaniels, are at significantly higher risk of developing gliomas [4] and are overrepresented, collectively comprising 78% of all cases of canine glioma [14]. A recent genome-wide association study identified a genetic locus and 3 candidate genes that are linked to glioma susceptibility in dogs and may have been under selection among brachycephalic breeds [16].

Common clinical signs among dogs with gliomas include: seizure, gait abnormalities, and mentation and behavior changes [14]. Seizures are particularly common among dogs with a specific type of glioma called oligodendroglioma, and these patients are 3 times more likely to experience seizures than dogs with any other type of primary CNS tumor [13]. Cerebrospinal fluid analysis results are variable among dogs with primary brain tumors, as both inflammatory profiles and normal protein and cell counts have been documented in canine gliomas [13, 14]. Although extracranial metastasis of primary gliomas has not been reported in thoracic and abdominal imaging nor post-mortem analysis at necropsy [13, 14], other unrelated concurrent neoplastic processes have been identified both antemortem and at necropsy in canine glioma patients [13].

Computed tomography (CT) and magnetic resonance imaging (MRI) are the two most widely used imaging modalities to aid in the diagnosis and assessment of canine gliomas. MRI is generally considered the preferred modality for identification of intracranial disease, although CT has been shown to detect mass lesions within the brain in 90% of primary brain tumor cases [13] and has similar ability to measure tumor margins as MRI [17]. On MRI, canine gliomas are generally hypointense on T1-weighted images (T1WI) and hyperintense on T2-weighted images (T2WI) [7]; however some reports note that canine gliomas on T1WI and T2WI are also commonly isointense and of mixed intensity [18]. Generally, low grade canine gliomas have lower levels of contrast enhancement, are less commonly associated with cystic structures, and are located more superficially than high grade gliomas [19]. Overall, MRI is relatively sensitive (approximately 90%) at identifying canine intracranial tumors [18]; however, both MRI and CT are inaccurate predictors of canine glioma type and grade, and ultimately biopsy with histopathology is required for diagnosis [17].

The histopathologic classification scheme of gliomas in both humans and dogs has undergone significant changes in the past several years [2, 11], but generally, gliomas are defined as tumors that resemble glial cells histologically [20]. The two most common types of gliomas are oligodendrogliomas and astrocytomas, and in humans, these gliomas are graded from a scale of grade I to IV based on increasing characteristics of malignancy, as defined by WHO [20, 21]. Molecular and genetic characteristics have been incorporated into the human glioma grading scheme and are expected to be added to the recently revised canine histopathologic glioma classification system [2, 11]. Currently, the three types of gliomas in dogs are oligodendroglioma, astrocytoma, and undefined glioma. These subtypes are then classified as either low- or high-grade based on factors such as necrosis, microvascular proliferation, amount of mitotic activity, and cellular features of malignancy [11].

One important difference between the human and canine disease is the relative frequency of glioma subtypes among patients. The vast majority of human gliomas (approximately 78%) are astrocytic tumors, with 58% of those being the highly malignant GBM [1]. A recent necropsy report utilizing the updated canine glioma classification system reports that astrocytomas may make up as low as 19% of all canine gliomas, with the majority of astrocytomas and oligodendrogliomas being high grade (94% and 84%, respectively) [14]. However, the percentage of canine glioma samples diagnosed as astrocytoma is variable within the literature, with some necropsy reports noting that 35% and 60% of all canine gliomas are astrocytic tumors [4, 13].

Similar treatments options exist for canine glioma, including surgery, radiation therapy, and chemotherapy [15, 22, 23]. In a systematic review of treatment modalities in canine brain tumors, the median survival time of dogs with suspected intracranial gliomas is reported as 226 days [24]. However, euthanasia is also commonly elected for companion dogs diagnosed with gliomas, and one study found that nearly half of all dogs with glioma were euthanized on the day of diagnosis [14]. As such, canine spontaneous glioma is a disease that is associated with significant morbidity and mortality, and novel treatments to improve survival times are clearly still needed.

3. Comparative genetic and molecular signature

Our understanding of the molecular aberrations associated with gliomas has dramatically expanded over the last several decades. In humans, it was found that specific genetic and molecular characteristics are closely linked to glioma biologic behavior and prognosis [20]. Thus, the WHO CNS tumor classification criteria began to incorporate molecular parameters in addition to classic histopathological characteristics into the glioma grading scheme in the 2016 update [2]. In alignment with the goal to utilize canine glioma patients as a model of the human disease, the CBTC assembled a Glioma Pathology Board to revise the canine glioma classification system in a way such that genomic data can be incorporated, mirroring the human classification system [11].

In order to assess the extent to which the spontaneous canine glioma model can be utilized as a model of the human disease, a detailed investigation of what is known about the genetic landscape of canine gliomas is warranted. Genetic alterations that are commonly encountered in human glioblastoma and canine glioma will be discussed, including dysregulation of the receptor tyrosine kinase (RTK)/Ras/

phosphoinositide 3-kinase (PI3K) pathway, the p53 pathway, and the retinoblastoma (Rb) pathway, as well as other specific genes, proteins, and epigenetic factors involved in canine and human glioma. See **Table 1** for a list of abbreviations used for oncogenes and tumor suppressor genes discussed. See **Table 2** for a summary of the comparative somatic mutation rates among common glioma drivers in humans and dogs.

3.1 RTK/Ras/PI3K pathway

Tyrosine kinase receptors are commonly altered in human glioblastoma. Brennan et al. found that at least one RTK is either amplified or mutated in 67% of

EGFR	Epidermal growth factor receptor
PDGFRA	Platelet-derived growth factor receptor A
VEGF	Vascular endothelial growth factor receptor
FGFR	Fibroblast growth factor receptor
NF1	Neurofibromin 1
PTEN	Phosphatase and tensin homolog
PIK3CA	Phosphatidylinositol 3-kinase catalytic subunit alpha
PIK3R1	Phosphatidylinositol 3-kinase regulatory subunit 1
TP53	Tumor protein 53
CDKN2A	Cyclin-dependent kinase inhibitor 2A
MDM2	Mouse double minute 2 homolog
RB1	Retinoblastoma 1
CDK4	Cyclin-dependent kinase 4
IDH1	Isocitrate dehydrogenase 1
ATF5	Activating transcription factor 5

Table 1.
Abbreviations of oncogenes and tumor suppressor genes discussed.

	Canine Glioma (Amin et al.) [12]	**Adult Glioblastoma (Brennan et al.) [25]**
EGFR	4%	26%
PDGFRA	21%	4%
NF1	7%	11%
PTEN	<1%	31%
PIK3CA	14%	11%
PIK3R1	1%	11%
TP53	5%	29%
RB1	1%	9%

Table 2.
Somatic mutation rates of selected genes commonly altered in canine glioma and human glioblastoma.

human GBM cases [25]. The most frequently mutated RTK in human GBM is *EGFR* (epidermal growth factor receptor) with a somatic mutation rate of 26%, followed by *PDGFRA* (platelet-derived growth factor receptor A) with a somatic rate of 4% [25]. Both genetic alterations have also been documented in canine glioma; however, the relative frequency is reversed, with a somatic mutation rate of 4% and 21% for *EGFR* and *PDGFRA*, respectively [12]. Utilizing estimates of clonal driver mutations within gliomas, Amin et al. found that clonal *PDGFRA* and *EGFR* mutations occur early on during gliomagenesis within both human and canine gliomas, suggesting molecular similarity among canine and human glioma [12].

EGFR gene amplification is rarely identified in canine glioma, with one report documenting *EGFR* amplification in 3% of cases [8], but overexpression of EGFR protein among dogs with glioma is common. Approximately half of all dogs with gliomas have been reported to have overexpression of EGFR, with significantly greater expression levels among high grade compared to low grade gliomas [26]. Although EGFR mRNA overexpression is seen consistently across both canine astrocytomas and oligodendrogliomas [27], EGFR protein overexpression tends to be more common among astrocytomas and more rarely identified in canine oligodendrogliomas [28].

The *PDGFRA* K385I/M mutation found in a subset of canine gliomas is one of the drivers of glioma in dogs [12]. *PDGFRA* gene amplification is present in nearly half of all canine glioma cases and is particularly common in oligodendrogliomas due to a large gain on canine chromosome 13 [8]. One study found overexpression of PDGFRA mRNA among all canine oligodendrogliomas and nearly half of canine astrocytomas [27]. PDGFRA protein expression patterns are similar, with the highest frequency of PDGFRA overexpression among high grade oligodendrogliomas and fewer numbers of samples overexpressing PDGFRA among canine astrocytomas. Canine astrocytoma PDGFRA overexpression frequency decreases in parallel with decreasing tumor grade [28].

Although genetic alterations in other tyrosine kinase receptors are less common than in EGFR and PDGFRA, many of these receptors have also been investigated as potential targets for glioma therapeutics [29], and will thus be briefly discussed. VEGFR (vascular endothelial growth factor receptor)-1 and VEGFR-2 mRNA overexpression is present in nearly all canine gliomas, with significantly increasing expression correlating with increasing astrocytoma grade [27]. Amplification or mutations involving *FGFR* (fibroblast growth factor receptor) is uncommon in human glioblastoma, with an alteration rate of 3.2% [25], and while the somatic mutation rate for canine gliomas is similarly low, around 1–2% [12], the frequency of *FGFR-1* amplification in canine glioma is notably higher, around 30% [8].

Downstream signaling molecules in the RTK/Ras/PI3K pathway also play important roles in both human and canine glioma and will be investigated further in this section. Somatic mutations involving the tumor suppressor gene *NF1* (neurofibromin 1) occur with similar frequency in human and canine glioma, at a rate of about 11% and 7%, respectively [12, 25]. *NF1* frameshift mutations tend to be late events in the development of gliomas in both humans and dogs [12]. Homozygous losses of *NF1* are uncommon in canine gliomas, being present in about 3% of cases [8]. In a study investigating oligodendrogliomas in brachycephalic breeds, NF1 was not differentially expressed in tumor cells and had similar to expression levels in normal tissue [30].

The tumor suppressor gene *PTEN* (phosphatase and tensin homolog) is the most frequently altered gene in human glioblastoma, with a somatic mutation rate of 31% [25]. Although somatic mutations have not been documented involving *PTEN* in canine gliomas, copy number losses are present in approximately 15% of canine gliomas [8]. With regards to PTEN protein expression, variable expression among canine gliomas and normal CNS tissue has been observed, with a lack of differential expression in tumor tissue [5, 30].

The second most commonly encountered somatic mutation in canine glioma involves the gene *PIK3CA* (phosphatidylinositol 3-kinase catalytic subunit alpha), which is altered in 14% of cases [12]. *PIK3CA* is also mutated with similar frequency in human glioblastoma, with a somatic mutation rate of 11% [25]. The *PIK3CA* H1047R/L mutation found in a subset of canine gliomas is one of the drivers of glioma in dogs [12]. Mutations involving *PIK3CA* are characterized as early mutations driving tumor formation in canine and pediatric but not adult glioma [12]. However, a closely related gene, *PIK3R1* (phosphatidylinositol 3-kinase regulatory subunit 1), is more frequently altered in human glioblastoma than in canine glioma with somatic mutation rates of 11% and 1% [12, 25].

3.2 p53 and Rb pathways

TP53 (tumor protein 53), a tumor suppressor gene, is one of the most frequently altered genes in human glioblastoma, with a somatic mutation rate of 29% [25]; however *TP53* is infrequently mutated in canine glioma, with a somatic mutation rate of only 5% [12]. Although *TP53* somatic mutations among dogs with glioma are rare, focal somatic copy number alterations are slightly more common, at a rate of 12% [12]. TP53 protein expression is most common in canine astrocytic tumors, with more variable and decreased expression among dogs with oligodendrogliomas [5]. TP53 mRNA expression is upregulated relative to normal tissue in brachycephalic breeds with oligodendrogliomas [30]. *CDKN2A* (cyclin-dependent kinase inhibitor 2A) deletions are commonly seen in human GBM, at a rate of 58% [25]. While *CDKN2A* deletions are also present in canine glioma, these mutations are only in astrocytomas and occur at a lower rate of approximately 12% [12]. Although *MDM2* (mouse double minute 2 homolog) amplifications in canine gliomas have not been documented, *MDM4* is amplified in 42% of canine gliomas [8]. Overall p53 pathway copy number alterations are present in 76% of canine gliomas [8], which is similar to the frequency of p53 pathway alterations in 85% of human glioblastomas [25].

RB1 (retinoblastoma 1) somatic mutations are present in human GBM at a rate of 9% [25], while canine glioma *RB1* somatic mutations are much less common, with only 1% of samples affected [12]. Although *RB1* somatic mutations among dogs with glioma are rare, focal somatic copy number alterations are more common, at an overall rate of 21% [12]. *RB1* deletions are most common among canine oligoastrocytomas, followed by oligodendrogliomas and astrocytomas, with gene losses occurring in 80%, 60%, and 27% of samples, respectively [8]. RB1 protein levels in canine glioma are overexpressed, and most of the RB1 protein is dephosphorylated [5]. *CDK4* (cyclin-dependent kinase 4) is not amplified in canine glioma, and *CDK6* is only amplified in 3% of canine glioma samples [8]. Overall Rb pathway copy number alterations are present in 79% of canine gliomas [8], which exactly mirrors the rate (79%) at which human glioblastomas contain Rb pathway alterations [25].

3.3 Other genetic and epigenetic alterations involved in canine and human Glioma

The classic *IDH1* (isocitrate dehydrogenase 1) R132H mutation commonly seen in human low grade gliomas and secondary recurring human GBM [31] has not been observed in canine glioma [32, 33]. However, mutations involving *IDH1* are found infrequently in canine gliomas, with a mutation rate of 4%, and the *IDH1*

R132C mutation found in a small subset of canine gliomas is one of the drivers of glioma in dogs [12].

The transcription factor ATF5 (activating transcription factor 5), has been shown to be overexpressed in several types of cancers in humans [34, 35], and ATF5 mRNA and protein are overexpressed in human low grade astrocytoma and GBM, with the highest expression in GBMs [36]. ATF5 protein expression is also elevated in canine gliomas, with the highest levels of expression in canine GBM [37].

Canine glioma is reportedly more similar to human pediatric glioma than adult glioma with respect to several different factors. Both canine and human pediatric glioma cases contain at least 1 significantly mutated gene in approximately half of the cases; this is contrasted with adult human gliomas, which carry at least 1 significantly mutated gene over 90% of the time [12]. Although canine glioma has a relatively low mutational burden, aneuploidy (characterized by arm-level copy gains) is common in canine gliomas. The median percent of the canine genome affected by copy number alterations in canine glioma is 25%, which is similar to human pediatric glioma (19–26% of the genome); both of which were higher than adult glioma (8–18% of the genome) [12]. The DNA methylation pattern of canine gliomas was found to be characterized as pediatric glioma in 78% of samples analyzed, with the other remaining 13% and 9% of cases being classified as IDH wild-type adult and IDH-mutant adult glioma, respectively [12].

4. Conclusion

Both human glioblastoma and canine glioma are diseases that carry a grim prognosis for patients. Because dogs develop gliomas spontaneously and with similar frequencies and clinicopathologic features of disease, canine glioma has recently been proposed as a preclinical model for both research efforts and novel therapeutic development prior to clinical trials in humans. In order to best utilize this model, a thorough investigation into what is currently known about canine glioma is of paramount importance.

While many similarities exist between human and canine glioma, several key differences are essential to document so that this model can be used appropriately. The key differences between human and canine glioma that are highlighted in this review include: the relative frequency of glioma histologic subtypes, the frequency of specific genetic variants among drivers of glioma formation, the overall genomic mutational burden, the relative frequency of aneuploidy, and the pattern of DNA methylation. With regards to aneuploidy and epigenetic changes, canine glioma appears to be more similar to pediatric than adult glioma.

These differences are particularly important to consider with respect to investigational therapeutics. New drugs and other therapies that specifically target or otherwise harness these features of glioma to treat the disease may yield different results among canines and humans with gliomas. Additionally, canine glioma may serve as a more reliable model for human pediatric glioma in certain genetic and epigenetic studies.

Acknowledgements

Funding was provided by the Students Training in Advanced Research (STAR) Program through a National Institutes of Health T35 grant (OD010956).

Conflict of interest

J.M. Angelastro was on the scientific advisory board member of Sapience Therapeutics (2016–2020), which has licensed the ATF5 technology to treat one of the cancers, glioblastoma, from Columbia University, and is co-inventor on patents owned by Columbia University (New York, NY) and patents owned by Columbia University and the University of California, Davis (Davis, CA).

Author details

Nicole M. Yost[1,2] and James M. Angelastro[3]*

1 School of Veterinary Medicine, University of California, Davis, CA, USA

2 Center for Comparative Medicine, Baylor College of Medicine, Houston, TX, USA

3 Department of Molecular Biosciences, School of Veterinary Medicine, University of California, Davis, CA, USA

*Address all correspondence to: jmangelastro@ucdavis.edu

References

[1] Ostrom QT, Cioffi G, Waite K, Kruchko C, Barnholtz-Sloan JS. CBTRUS statistical report: Primary brain and other central nervous system tumors diagnosed in the United States in 2014-2018. Neuro-Oncology. 2021;**23**:III1-I105

[2] Louis DN, Perry A, Reifenberger G, von Deimling A, Figarella-Branger D, Cavenee WK, et al. The 2016 World Health Organization classification of tumors of the central nervous system: A summary. Acta Neuropathologica. 2016;**131**(6):803-820

[3] Stupp R, Taillibert S, Kanner A, Read W, Steinberg DM, Lhermitte B, et al. Effect of tumor-treating fields plus maintenance temozolomide vs maintenance temozolomide alone on survival in patients with glioblastoma a randomized clinical trial. JAMA. 2017;**318**(23):2306-2316

[4] Song RB, Vite CH, Bradley CW, Cross JR. Postmortem evaluation of 435 cases of intracranial neoplasia in dogs and relationship of neoplasm with breed, age, and body weight. Journal of Veterinary Internal Medicine. 2013;**27**(5):1143-1152

[5] Boudreau CE, York D, Higgins RJ, LeCouteur RA, Dickinson PJ. Molecular signalling pathways in canine gliomas. Veterinary and Comparative Oncology. 2017;**15**(1):133-150

[6] Candolfi M, Curtin JF, Nichols WS, Muhammad AKMG, King GD, Pluhar GE, et al. Intracranial glioblastoma models in preclinical neuro-oncology: Neuropathological characterization and tumor progression. Journal of Neuro-Oncology. 2007;**85**(2):133-148

[7] Young BD, Levine JM, Porter BF, Chen-Allen AV, Rossmeisl JH, Platt SR, et al. Magnetic resonance imaging features of intracranial astrocytomas and oligodendrogliomas in dogs. Veterinary Radiology & Ultrasound. 2011;**52**(2):132-141

[8] Dickinson PJ, York D, Higgins RJ, Le Couteur RA, Joshi N, Bannasch D. Chromosomal aberrations in canine gliomas define candidate genes and common pathways in dogs and humans. Journal of Neuropathology and Experimental Neurology. 2016;**75**(7):700-710

[9] Lipsitz D, Higgins RJ, Kortz GD, Dickinson PJ, Bollen AW, Naydan DK, et al. Glioblastoma multiforme: Clinical findings. Magnetic Resonance Imaging, and Pathology in Five Dogs. 2003;**40**(6):659-669

[10] Leblanc AK, Mazcko C, Brown DE, Koehler JW, Miller AD, Miller CR, et al. Creation of an NCI comparative brain tumor consortium: informing the translation of new knowledge from canine to human brain tumor patients. Neuro-Oncology. 2016;**18**(9):1209-1218

[11] Koehler JW, Miller AD, Miller CR, Porter B, Aldape K, Beck J, et al. A revised diagnostic classification of canine glioma: Towards validation of the canine glioma patient as a naturally occurring preclinical model for human glioma. Journal of Neuropathology and Experimental Neurology. 2018;**77**(11):1039-1054

[12] Amin SB, Anderson KJ, Boudreau CE, Martinez-Ledesma E, Kocakavuk E, Johnson KC, et al. Comparative molecular life history of spontaneous canine and human gliomas. Cancer Cell. 2020;**37**(2):243-257.e7

[13] Snyder JM, Shofer FS, Van Winkle TJ, Massicotte C. Canine intracranial primary neoplasia: 173 cases (1986-2003). Journal of Veterinary Internal Medicine. 2006;**20**(3):669-675

[14] José-López R, Gutierrez-Quintana R, de la Fuente C, Manzanilla EG, Suñol A, Pi Castro D, et al. Clinical features, diagnosis, and survival analysis of dogs with glioma. Journal of Veterinary Internal Medicine. 2021;**35**(4):1902-1917

[15] Hubbard ME, Arnold S, Bin Zahid A, McPheeters M, Gerard O'Sullivan M, Tabaran AF, et al. Naturally occurring canine glioma as a model for novel therapeutics. Cancer Investigation. 2018;**36**(8):415-423. DOI: 10.1080/07357907.2018.1514622

[16] Truvé K, Dickinson P, Xiong A, York D, Jayashankar K, Pielberg G, et al. Utilizing the dog genome in the search for novel candidate genes involved in glioma development—genome wide association mapping followed by targeted massive parallel sequencing identifies a strongly associated locus. PLoS Genetics. 2016;**12**(5):1-22

[17] Stadler KL, Ruth JD, Pancotto TE, Werre SR, Rossmeisl JH. Computed tomography and magnetic resonance imaging are equivalent in mensuration and similarly inaccurate in grade and type predictability of canine intracranial gliomas. Frontiers in Veterinary Science. 2017;**4**(SEP):1-7

[18] Ródenas S, Pumarola M, Gaitero L, Zamora À, Añor S. Magnetic resonance imaging findings in 40 dogs with histologically confirmed intracranial tumours. Veterinary Journal. 2011;**187**(1):85-91

[19] Bentley RT, Ober CP, Anderson KL, Feeney DA, Naughton JF, Ohlfest JR, et al. Canine intracranial gliomas: Relationship between magnetic resonance imaging criteria and tumor type and grade. Veterinary Journal. 2013;**198**(2):463-471. DOI: 10.1016/j.tvjl.2013.08.015

[20] Chen R, Smith-Cohn M, Cohen AL, Colman H. Glioma subclassifications and their clinical significance. Neurotherapeutics. 2017;**14**(2):284-297

[21] Louis DN, Ohgaki H, Wiestler OD, Cavenee WK, Burger PC, Jouvet A, et al. The 2007 WHO classification of tumours of the central nervous system. Acta Neuropathologica. 2007;**114**(2):97-109

[22] Magalhães TR, Benoît J, Néčová S, North S, Queiroga FL. Outcome after radiation therapy in canine intracranial meningiomas or gliomas. In Vivo (Brooklyn). 2021;**35**(2):1117-1123

[23] Moirano SJ, Dewey CW, Wright KZ, Cohen PW. Survival times in dogs with presumptive intracranial gliomas treated with oral lomustine: A comparative retrospective study (2008-2017). Veterinary and Comparative Oncology. 2018;**16**(4):459-466

[24] Hu H, Barker A, Harcourt-Brown T, Jeffery N. Systematic review of brain tumor treatment in dogs. Journal of Veterinary Internal Medicine. 2015;**29**(6):1456-1463

[25] Brennan CW, Verhaak RGW, McKenna A, Campos B, Noushmehr H, Salama SR, et al. The somatic genomic landscape of glioblastoma. Cell. 2013;**155**(2):462

[26] Fraser AR, Bacci B, le Chevoir MA, Long SN. Epidermal growth factor receptor and Ki-67 expression in canine gliomas. Veterinary Pathology. 2016;**53**(6):1131-1137

[27] Dickinson PJ, Roberts BN, Higgins RJ, Leutenegger CM, Bollen AW,

Kass PH, et al. Expression of receptor tyrosine kinases VEGFR-1 (FLT-1), VEGFR-2 (KDR), EGFR-1, PDGFRa and c-Met in canine primary brain tumours. Veterinary and Comparative Oncology. 2006;**4**(3):132-140

[28] Higgins RJ, Dickinson PJ, Lecouteur RA, Bollen AW, Wang H, Wang H, et al. Spontaneous canine gliomas: Overexpression of EGFR, PDGFRα and IGFBP2 demonstrated by tissue microarray immunophenotyping. Journal of Neuro-Oncology. 2010;**98**(1):49-55

[29] Pearson JRD, Regad T. Targeting cellular pathways in glioblastoma multiforme. Signal Transduction and Targeted Therapy. 2017;**2**(June):1-11. DOI: 10.1038/sigtrans.2017.40

[30] Filley A, Henriquez M, Bhowmik T, Tewari BN, Rao X, Wan J, et al. Immunologic and gene expression profiles of spontaneous canine oligodendrogliomas. Journal of Neuro-Oncology. 2018;**137**(3):469-479. DOI: 10.1007/s11060-018-2753-4

[31] Cohen AL, Holmen SL, Colman H. IDH1 and IDH2 mutations in gliomas. Current Neurology and Neuroscience Reports. 2013;**13**(5):1-7

[32] Fraser AR, Bacci B, le Chevoir MA, Long SN. Isocitrate dehydrogenase 1 expression in canine gliomas. Journal of Comparative Pathology. 2018;**165**:33-39. DOI: 10.1016/j.jcpa.2018.09.005

[33] Reitman ZJ, Olby NJ, Mariani CL, Thomas R, Breen M, Bigner DD, et al. IDH1 and IDH2 hotspot mutations are not found in canine glioma. International Journal of Cancer. 2010;**127**(1):245-246

[34] Ishihara S, Yasuda M, Ishizu A, Ishikawa M, Shirato H, Haga H. Activating transcription factor 5 enhances radioresistance and malignancy in cancer cells. Oncotarget. 2015;**6**(7):4602-4614

[35] Kong X, Meng W, Zhou Z, Li Y, Zhou B, Wang R, et al. Overexpression of activating transcription factor 5 in human rectal cancer. Experimental and Therapeutic Medicine. 2011;**2**(5):827-831

[36] Feldheim J, Kessler AF, Schmitt D, Wilczek L, Linsenmann T, Dahlmann M, et al. Expression of activating transcription factor 5 (ATF5) is increased in astrocytomas of different WHO grades and correlates with survival of glioblastoma patients. Oncotargets and Therapy. 2018;**11**:8673-8684

[37] York D, Sproul CD, Chikere N, Dickinson PJ, Angelastro JM. Expression and targeting of transcription factor ATF5 in dog gliomas. Veterinary and Comparative Oncology. 2018;**16**(1):102-107

Chapter 5

Systemic Treatment in Glioblastoma

María Ángeles Vaz, Sonia Del Barco Berrón, Raquel Luque, María Villamayor, Juan Manuel Sepúlveda Sánchez and María Vieito

Abstract

Glioblastoma is the most common primary brain tumor and the initial treatment with maximal safe resection is not curative. In order to improve the prognosis, surgery is completed with radiotherapy and temozolomide, an oral chemotherapy, but overall survival remains poor. Therefore, new efforts are needed to improve these results. In fact, different systemic treatments have been tested but, nevertheless, few advances have been reached despite the development of large clinical trials. This chapter will review the most important findings, achievements, and main studies in this pathology. Standard of care in newly diagnosed and recurrent glioblastoma will be reassessed with the results of clinical trials with targeted agents and immunotherapy. Ongoing studies are evaluating advanced treatments, with chimeric antigen receptor T-cells, biospecific T-cell antibodies, tumor vaccines, and oncolytic viruses, although results are pending, a wide review of these new-generation agents is important to better understand the advances in glioblastoma in the coming years.

Keywords: glioblastoma, chemotherapy, immunotherapy, clinical trials

1. Introduction

Glioblastoma is the most frequent primary brain tumor in adults.

The median age of diagnosis is 64 years and the average age-adjusted incidence rate is 3.2 per 100.000 population [1].

Initial treatment includes maximal safe resection, radiotherapy, and chemotherapy with temozolomide based on a phase III pivotal study published in 2005.

Despite all of this, the prognosis remains poor with a median overall survival of 14 months [2].

Therefore, new efforts are needed to improve these results.

Systemic treatments have been tested in different clinical trials. Nevertheless, few advances have been reached.

This chapter will review the most important achievements and main studies in this pathology.

To understand the difficulties to advance in glioblastomas, here we expose some characteristics of this tumor.

Glioblastoma is characterized by the presence of several mechanisms of resistance to different treatments.

One of them is the presence of the blood-brain barrier (BBB). The BBB is composed of a neurovascular structure, with specialized capillary endothelial cells adhered with tight junctions, a basal lamina, and a complex of astrocytic endfeet, pericytes, and intermittent end of neurons. Only small molecules can passively diffuse across this barrier. Other molecules need mechanisms such as pinocytosis or receptor or carried-mediated transcytosis.

Moreover, several drug-resistance proteins (such as P-glycoprotein and multidrug resistance-1) are expressed in the vessel wall to reinforce this barrier.

In glioblastoma, the BBB is heterogeneously disrupted with reduced tight junctions, altered pericytes, and astrocytic end-feet, leading to tumoral areas with different blood permeability to the different drugs [3].

Another mechanism of resistance is tumor heterogeneity, which is perhaps the most challenging obstacle to finding successful treatments for glioblastoma. At a cellular level, glioblastoma tumors are composed of various groups of cells and glioma stem cells (GSCs), each with a specific transcriptional signature.

Moreover, glioblastoma is also characterized by spatial heterogeneity due to the presence of diverse hypoxia gradients and heterogeneity of the tumoral microenvironment.

On the other hand, primary and recurrent glioblastoma can have subclonal genetic alterations, with the presence of regions with different drug sensitivity [3].

Other studied factors that have contributed to systemic treatment failure are related to mechanisms of chemoresistance such as the presence of unmethylated DNA repair enzyme O6Meg DNA methyltransferase (MGMT) [4].

Although the increased knowledge of molecular alteration in this disease, a lack of success has been reported in different approaches to targeted therapy probably related to the tumoral heterogeneity and signaling-pathway redundancy [5, 6] as well as the absence of a biomarker selection.

All of these considerations should be taken into account in the design of the clinical trials, given that several trials fail to demonstrate a clinical benefit for this disease.

As a result of these difficulties, today the standard of care is a maximal initial resection followed by concurrent radiation and temozolomide.

About 70% of GM will experience recurrence within one year of diagnosis with less than 5% of patients surviving after diagnosis.

In recurrent glioblastoma, there is no standard of treatment. The USA Food and Drug Administration (FDA) has approved bevacizumab (but not by EMA) and TTF.

2. Systemic treatment in newly diagnosed glioblastoma: positive trials

The EORTC/NCIC clinical trial demonstrated the clinical benefit of adding chemotherapy to the treatment of surgery and radiotherapy in patients with glioblastoma.

In this study, 573 patients were randomized to receive involved-field radiation therapy alone or radiation plus concurrent temozolomide followed up to six cycles of adjuvant temozolomide.

A statistically significant benefit was observed with the addition of temozolomide, with a median overall survival (OS) of 14.6 months vs. 12.1 months [2]. Since the publication of this study, the standard of care (SOC) in newly diagnosed glioblastoma is temozolomide 75 mg/m2 daily during RT followed by 6 adjuvant cycles of 150–200 mg/m2 on days 1-5/28.

A retrospective analysis of 206 patients has been done to determine the MGMT methylation status. In 45% of the cases, MGMT was methylated and the benefit of the treatment with temozolomide was greater (median overall survival 21.7 months vs. 15.3 months).

In non-methylated patients, there was a survival benefit that was not statistically significant [4].

3. Systemic treatment in newly diagnosed glioblastoma: negative results

Since the publication of the previously mentioned study, by Roger Stupp [2], of what is now the standard of care (SOC), there have been few advances. Furthermore, despite a better understanding of the biology of the tumor, this has not translated into progress in first-line therapy or newly diagnosed GBM. However, this does not mean that efforts to search for new targets and/or therapeutic strategies for improving the prognosis of these patients have been null or void. It must be said that there has been a titanic effort and that the negative results of trials have helped us to steer the research path. Therefore, we are going to review the negative studies with the greatest impact.

3.1 Antiangiogenics

The rationale for the use of drugs that inhibit vascular endothelial growth factors, such as bevacizumab, was based on the concept that the tumor vasculature could be normalized. This would lead to a decrease in tumor interstitial pressure and, therefore, better access to cytotoxic drugs. Moreover, with increased oxygen supply, the efficacy of radiotherapy would also be improved [7]. On the other hand, it is known that GBM overexpresses vascular endothelial growth factor A (VEGF-A), a key regulator of tumor-associated angiogenesis, and these tumors are highly vascularized [8].

Given that bevacizumab has demonstrated activity in patients with recurrent GBM and there was evidence that indicates the combination of bevacizumab with SOC therapy was active for patients with newly diagnosed GBM, two studies were initiated for first-line patients.

In the **AVAglio trial** [9], 921 patients were randomized to receive bevacizumab (10 mg per kilogram of body weight every 2 weeks) or placebo, plus SOC: radiotherapy (2 Gy 5 days a week; maximum, 60 Gy) and temozolomide (75 mg per square meter of body-surface area per day) for 6 weeks. After a 28-day treatment break, maintenance bevacizumab (10 mg per kilogram intravenously every 2 weeks) or placebo, plus temozolomide (150 to 200 mg per square meter per day for 5 days), was continued for six 4-week cycles, followed by bevacizumab monotherapy (15 mg per kilogram intravenously every 3 weeks) or placebo until progression or unacceptable toxicity. Even though PFS was longer in the bevacizumab group (10.6 months vs. 6.2 months; stratified hazard ratio for progression or death, 0.64; 95% confidence interval [CI], 0.55 to 0.74; $P < 0.001$), the OS did not differ between groups (stratified hazard ratio for death, 0.88; 95% CI, 0.76 to 1.02; $P = 0.10$). Maintenance of quality of life and performance status were observed with bevacizumab even though the bevacizumab group had more adverse events (arterial thromboembolic events, hypertension, and complications of wound healing). No predictive influence of MGMT status or any other subgroup variable was observed concerning progression-free survival or overall survival.

The addition of bevacizumab to SOC was also investigated in the Radiation Therapy Oncology Group **(RTOG)-0825 study** [10]. It showed a similar trend toward improvement in PFS (HR 0.79; 95% CI, 0.66 to 0.94; P = 0.007), with a 3.4-month extension of PFS; the difference was not significant according to the prespecified alpha level (P < 0.004) and there was also no statistically significant difference in OS (HR, 1.13; 95% CI, 0.93 to 1.37; P = 0.21).

Finally, the exhaustive review by Cochrane concluded that there is insufficient evidence to support the use of antiangiogenic therapy for people with newly diagnosed glioblastoma [11].

3.2 Integrin inhibition

Integrins are adhesion molecules involved in several tumorigenic processes such as survival, proliferation, migration, invasion, and angiogenesis [12]. Cilengitide is a selective inhibitor of αvβ3 and αvβ5 integrins that are expressed both in GBM tumor cells and in the vasculature. Moreover, several studies demonstrated a potentiation or synergy when cilengitide is combined with radiation therapy and chemotherapy. That was the rationale for exploring cilengitide in newly diagnosed GBM.

The first trial, **CENTRIC EORTC 26071-22072**, was carried out in methylated MGMT promoter tumors. Cilengitide, 200 mg intravenously twice weekly, was added to SOC, maintenance temozolomide was given for up to six cycles, and cilengitide was given for up to 18 months or until disease progression or unacceptable toxic effects. The primary endpoint was overall survival [13]. Unfortunately, the addition of this drug did not improve the outcome: OS was 26·3 months in both arms (HR,1·02;95%CI,0·81–1·29;p = 0·86) and PFS 10·6 months in the cilengitide arm and 7·9 months in the control arm (HR, 0·92; 95% CI, 0·75–1·12;p = 0·41).

Later, data were published on unmethylated tumors [13]. It offered the opportunity to use dose intensification as a means of overcoming resistance. Patients were randomized to standard cilengitide (2000 mg twice weekly until progression) or intensive cilengitide (2000 mg daily for 5 days during radiotherapy followed by twice weekly until progression) with radiotherapy and temozolomide or a control arm with SOC. Median PFS was 5.6 months and 5.9 months in the standard and intensive cilengitide arms, respectively, versus 4.1 months in the control arm. The median OS was 13.4 months (range, 0–30 mo) in the control arm, 16.3 months (range, 0–29) in the standard cilengitide arm, and 14.5 months (range, 0–29) in the intensive cilengitide arm, which is statistically nonsignificant. No benefit was observed despite dose escalation and most striking was the improvement in OS in patients who were expected to have a worse prognosis as they were unmethylated. The study was underpowered to consider the 3-month improvement in OS was enough. In addition, we do not have a biomarker to select responders.

Integrins are an important target in GBM, but a better understanding of the interaction between the tumor and the extracellular matrix is needed [14].

3.3 PARP inhibitors

Half of the patients with GBM have methylated MGMT and there is a rationale for combining PARP inhibitors with temozolomide, based on the importance of PARP in mediating basic tissue repair as well as homologous recombination.

The combination of veliparib and SOC did not provide benefits [15]. In ASCO 2022, the **Alliance A071102 trial** was presented [16]. Total of 447 patients with MGMT promoter hypermethylated GBM after radiotherapy and temozolomide were randomized to receive adjuvant temozolomide, given on days 1 to 5 every 28 days, combined with either placebo (n = 224) or veliparib (n = 223), given on days 1 to 7 every 28 days. Treatment was continued for up to six cycles. For phase II, PFS was the primary endpoint. The results were disappointing as the PFS was similar in both groups: 13.2 months with veliparib versus 12.1 months with placebo (HR 1.05, 95% confidence interval 0.86–1.29, p = .31). Median OS was 28.1 months with veliparib and 24.8 months with placebo (hazard ratio 0.89, 95% confidence interval 0.71–1.11, P = .15). The study is negative despite the different hypotheses put forward by the authors about improved survival at intermediate time points.

Effective biomarkers are needed to identify patients who are most likely to benefit from the addition of veliparib.

3.4 ANTI EGFR therapies

Epidermal growth factor receptor (EGFR) gene amplification on chromosome 7 (EGFR-amp) is expressed in 50% of GBMs. The EGFR variant 3 mutation (EGFRvIII), a tumor-specific deletion of exons (2–7), is active and is observed in approximately 50% of GBMs with EGFR (~25% overall) [17]. Nevertheless, EGFR-targeted treatments in GBM have been disappointing.

3.5 Antibody-drug conjugate

Depatuxizumab mafodotin (depatux-m) is an antibody-drug conjugate composed of a monoclonal antibody that binds to activated EGFR and is bound to a microtubule inhibitor toxin. It was tested in a phase III trial, adults with centrally confirmed, EGFR-amp newly diagnosed GBM [18]. Patients were randomized to receive SOC plus depatux-m at 2.0 mg/kg during RT, then 1.25 mg/kg on days 1 and 15/28, and continue until disease progression versus SOC. The trial was a phase III with OS as the primary endpoint. There was no improvement with the addition of the antibody; OS for depatux-m over placebo (median 18.9 vs. 18.7 months, HR 1.02,95% CI 0.82–1.26, 1-sided p = 0.63). PFS was longer for depatux-m than placebo (median 8.0 vs. 6.3 months; HR 0.84, 95% confidence interval [CI] 0.70–1.01, p = 0.029), particularly among those with EGFRvIII-mutant (median 8.3 vs. 5.9 months, HR 0.72, 95% CI 0.56–0.93, 1-sided p = 0.002) or MGMT unmethylated (HR 0.77, 95% CI 0.61–0.97; 1-side p = 0.012) tumors but without an OS improvement. One of the most peculiar toxicities of this drug is the corneal epitheliopathy that occurred in 94% of depatux-m-treated patients (61% grade 3–4), causing 12% to discontinue.

4. Pharmacologic treatment of recurrent glioblastoma

In the recurrence set, the prognosis of these patients is poor, with an estimated survival of about 6 months [19].

Compared to newly diagnosed glioblastoma, the management of the recurrent disease is not curative and less standardized without randomized trials. Different approaches should be considered including systemic agents (chemotherapy and target therapy) or locoregional treatments (radiation therapy and surgery) [20].

There is limited evidence for the systemic therapy of recurrent GB (rGB).

Several prognostic factors should be taken into account to select the patients that can benefit from systemic treatment after recurrence. Some of these factors are tumor size, location, performance status, and administration of steroids.

It is recommended to enroll these patients in a clinical trial whenever possible.

Outside a clinical trial, a second-line treatment could be considered.

The most commonly used agents are nitrosoureas, bevacizumab, and temozolomide, but none is approved by EMA because most of the time the evidence was derived from small to no randomized studies [21]. Bevacizumab has been approved by the FDA for recurrent high-grade glioma.

Treatments as promising as immunotherapy and drugs against EGFR are not superior to the treatments cited. Several novel treatments are undergoing evaluation in clinical trials.

4.1 Nitrosoureas

Nitrosoureas (lomustine, carmustine, fotemustine) have shown activity in phase II trials in rGB.

Lomustine (CCNU) is an oral nitrosourea. It has shown a modest improvement in overall survival (median OS 7.1–9.8 months).

Lomustine has never been shown to be superior to other drugs in randomized studies but represents the control treatment arm in randomized clinical trials. Lots of new drugs, especially multitarget tyrosine kinase inhibitors, have been tried alone or in association with lomustine or against lomustine without any benefit in overall survival [22].

Fotemustine is a new intravenous nitrosourea with a better toxicity profile. It has proven activity in glioblastoma in several phase II studies and is mainly used in Europe [23].

4.2 Antiangiogenic agents

Bevacizumab (BV) is a VEGF-A (vascular endothelial growth factor A) targeting monoclonal antibody. It was a very promising agent in rGB. In phase II, studies showed a PFS-6 rate ranging from 18–42% and median OS from 6.5 to 9.2 months. However, in randomized clinical trials, it has not been proven to have better results than lomustine.

In the phase II randomized trial BELOP (5) the combination of BV and lomustine showed an OS benefit over lomustine. Nevertheless, the phase III EORTC 26102 study randomized more than 400 patients with rGB to BV plus lomustine versus lomustine. The results showed a significant difference in PFS, but without any impact on OS, which was the main endpoint [24]. It is not yet known, which subgroup of patients could benefit from BV and its real impact on OS. Combinations of BV with other agents do not appear to be superior to monotherapy.

Regorafenib, an oral multi-kinase inhibitor, has been investigated versus lomustine in the randomized phase II trial REGOMA. The primary endpoint was overall survival in the intention-to-treat population, which was higher in the experimental arm. However,the planned statistical design did not have enough power to estimate survival advantage. Therefore, the authors concluded that phase III is needed to confirm this benefit [20].

4.3 Temozolomide

Temozolomide rechallenge can be considered an option in patients who have tumor recurrence beyond four to six months from the end of the first-line treatment with temozolomide and have a methylated MGMT promotor.

Another strategy consists of the administration of temozolomide in an extended regimen. Extended schedules had been developed to overcome TMZ resistance in phase II studies [25].

There are small studies that yield modest results in rGB (PFS-6 rates 17–50%) [21].

4.4 AntiEGFR therapy

About 50% of all GB patients present an amplification of the epidermal growth factor receptor (EGFR) gene. Agents targeting this receptor failed to show a significant survival impact on patients with rGB.

The most promising agent has been depatuxizumab mafodotin, an antibody-drug conjugate, that consists of an antibody directed against EGFR and EGFRvIII, conjugated to a toxin (monomethyl auristatin F). The INTELLANCE-2 /EORTC 1410 phase II randomized study [26] investigated depatux-M in combination with temozolomide or as a single agent in recurrent EGFR amplified GB. Patients who received depatux-M and temozolomide had a trend toward improved survival but did not reach statistical significance.

4.5 Future promising agents

It is necessary to improve the design of clinical trials in GB.

Personalized treatments based on the tumor's molecular characteristics have had promising results.

There are small studies with inhibitors of NTRK (neurotrophic tropomyosin receptor kinase), BRAF (B-Raf proto-oncogene), FGFR (fibroblast growth factor receptor), PDGFR (platelet-delivered growth factor receptor), IDH (isocitrate dehydrogenase), and histones, mainly, that are showing interesting preliminary results.

Other types of immunotherapy, such as chimeric antigen receptor T-cells (CAR-Ts), chimeric antigen receptor macrophages (CAR-Ms), oncolytic viruses, and vaccines, are under evaluation [27].

5. Recurrence glioblastoma: radiotherapy and surgery

Despite systemic treatment, other options could be considered for recurrence.

As previously referred, in this context, treatment decisions must be individualized.

One of the most important prognostic factors for benefit from local treatment is the previous performance status. Other useful factors include young age, the extent of the disease, the histologic grade, the relapse-free interval, the recurrence pattern (i.e., local versus diffuse), and the extent of the second surgical resection [28].

A negative factor is ependymal involvement, which is independent of performance status, tumor size, and extent of resection [29].

Patients with a localized recurrence are better candidates for reoperation or reirradiation interventions than those with primary refractory disease or diffuse or multifocal relapse.

It is important to point out that these patients should be referred to a multidisciplinary brain tumor center with a multidisciplinary team to revise images, evolution, and options of treatment [28, 30, 31].

In conclusion, the best candidates for reoperation are patients with large but well-circumscribed, symptomatic tumors that are amenable to complete or near-complete resection, particularly if the tumor has recurred after an extended interval.

The benefit of reirradiation of glioblastoma is uncertain and can be considered in selected patients. Occasionally used in patients with a localized or out-of-field glioblastoma recurrence. Instead, patients with a poor performance status have poor prognostic, and the risks of receiving subsequent treatment outweigh the benefits [32, 33].

5.1 Reoperation

Approximately, only 20 to 30 percent of patients with recurrent glioblastoma are candidates for a re-operation [19, 34, 35].

The technics used are the same as for primary resection and included 5-aminolevulinic acid (5-ALA) guided resection that showed benefit in recurrent glioblastoma [36–38].

There is no evidence to suggest that these results are better than and can be expected with radiation and/or chemotherapy alone.

Two meta-analyses have analyzed surgery as a treatment approach in recurrent glioblastoma.

The first study assessed eight observational studies for a total of 1906 patients with glioblastoma who underwent primary surgery and 709 patients with secondary surgery. The pooled hazard ratio (HR) showed a longer OS for patients receiving surgery at the time of recurrence (HR: 0.722; p: 0.001).

The second meta-analysis selected nine studies for a total of 1507 patients with glioblastoma and 1335 patients treated with re-intervention.

Among these studies, OS after repeat surgery ranged from 8 to 13 months. Maximal safe resection appears to confer a significant OS benefit (HR 0.59, p: 0.1). Radiographic confirmed gross total resection was the most prognostic variable related to the extent of surgery and was associated with longer OS (HR 0.52, p: 0.01) [39].

Another interesting option is carmustine polymer wafers. A review revealed three trials in which patients with glioblastoma who received carmustine wafers had statistically significant longer overall survival. Overall results of these trials seem to suggest that carmustine wafer implantation demonstrates promise as an effective and tolerable treatment strategy for GBM [40]. Daily practice is not commonly used due to potential surgical complications.

In conclusion, surgery should be included in the treatment algorithm for recurrent glioblastoma. It should be proposed when it is technically safe and associated with a feasible total resection, especially in patients with good performance status. Optimal management after surgery is still unknown, and prospective studies are ongoing to study different strategies, such as RESURGE trial [41].

5.2 Reirradiation

Salvage reirradiation has been utilized in the treatment of recurrent diseases for years. The role of reirradiation in patients with recurrent glioblastoma is uncertain, and there is little prospective data. For this reason, participation in clinical trials is encouraged.

As most recurrences occur within the high-dose radiation field (90–95%), reirradiation is generally poorly considered as a treatment option due to the high risk of toxicity.

The adequate selection of patients suitable for reirradiation is a key issue. Age, performance status, target volume, time to progression, type of progression, and site of recurrence are essential elements to consider. Different techniques can be used: conventionally fractionated radiotherapy (RT), hypofractionated stereotactic radiosurgery (HFSRT), and stereotactic radiosurgery (SRS) [42].

Based on mostly retrospective series, selected patients with small recurrent tumors and a good performance status may benefit from repeat radiation using modern high-precision techniques to deliver total doses of 30 to 35 Gy in 5 to 15 fractions [43].

Reirradiation with conventional involved field radiation at therapeutic doses (54 to 60 Gy) is not recommended in patients with relapsed disease due to treatment-related toxicity. The most common form used is fractionated radiosurgery or hypofractionated radiotherapy (e.g., 30 to 35 Gy in 5 to 15 fractions). Selection is based on the preference of the treating radiation oncologist and local availability since there are no clear differences in efficacy [44].

Reirradiation can be given with both concurrent or sequential administration of systemic therapy (TMZ, bevacizumab, and immunotherapy). The available data in patients with recurrent glioblastoma generally suggest that reirradiation modestly improves progression-free survival compared with systemic therapy alone, but overall survival is similar [45].

A few prospective data are available in a phase II trial 182 patients with recurrent glioblastoma were randomized to receive bevacizumab alone or in combination with radiation treatment (35 Gy in 10 fractions). The combination of radiation therapy and bevacizumab prolonged the PFS of these patients without significant improvement in OS [45].

The risk of radionecrosis should also be considered [46].

The benefit of the addition of bevacizumab to radiotherapy treatment was published in a recent systematic review. Data from a total of 1399 patients, were analyzed (954 patients receiving RT alone and 445 patients receiving RT and bevacizumab). Multivariate analysis showed that bevacizumab was associated with significantly improved. Patients receiving BVZ also had significantly lower rates of radionecrosis (2.2% vs. 6.5%) [47].

Other initial trials (phase I) studied the combination of RT, bevacizumab, and immunotherapy with promising results, but further controlled studies are needed to confirm these effects [48, 49].

Interstitial brachytherapy has been used in patients with recurrent high-grade gliomas, with several observational studies suggesting a survival benefit. However, brachytherapy is associated with a high incidence of radiation necrosis [50, 51].

An alternate form of brachytherapy uses an inflatable balloon catheter containing a liquid I-125 radioisotope (GliaSite) inserted at the time of surgical resection, which allows delivery of a quantifiable high dose of radiation to the tissue. No randomized clinical trials have been reported comparing this form of brachytherapy with other approaches. The role of brachytherapy is diminishing as experience with SRS and fractionated localized limited field radiation evolves [52, 53].

6. Immnunotherapy

Historically, the central nervous system (CNS) was considered to be immunologically isolated. However, today we know that the immunity system of the CNS is different but not incapable. There are functional lymphatic vessels and there are antigen-presenting cells: microglia, macrophages, astrocytes, and classical APCs such as dendritic cells [54].

Glioblastoma is a cold tumor, with a low mutational burden; furthermore, as detailed below, it has demonstrated a poor response to immune stimulation therapies, such as immune checkpoint blockade. Even when T-cell responses are induced in CNS tumors by means such as vaccination, as discussed above, the number of antigen-specific TILs can remain relatively low, and the cells that are present often show a depleted phenotype. The reduced number and limited activity of T-cells in CNS tumors are largely due to the unique immunosuppressive immune environment of the brain [55].

The final step of the immune response in glioblastoma is the destruction by the active T-lymphocyte of the GBM cells after binding to their tumor antigen on MHC-I *via* the T-cell receptor (TCR). These T-cells are activated after recognizing the GBM cells, secreting inflammatory cytokines, and inducing GBM cell death.

Glioblastomas are characterized as tumor with a low median TMB and a lack of infiltrating lymphocytes [56]. Current approaches focus on: (1) Increasing glioma immunogenicity and activating the adaptative immune response by using tumor vaccines and oncolytic viruses, (2) Revert T-cell energy and promote a more inflamed tumor microenvironment by using immune cytokines, chemokines, and cytokine modulators, and (3) Overcome the lack of resident tumor infiltrating lymphocytes by directly engaging T-cells through direct activators such as CAR T-cells, TCBs, and bispecific T-cell engager antibodies.

6.1 Checkpoint inhibitor

GBM overexpresses PDL1, leading to PD-L1 binding to PD-1 and thus inhibiting the immune response [55].

Treatment with immune checkpoint blockade has shown improved survival in murine glioma models. However, data from phase III studies with the anti-PD-L1 nivolumab did not meet their primary endpoint of OS in the final analysis.

For newly diagnosed patients with MGMT-methylated or indeterminate GBM, the SOC therapy was compared with the same scheme plus nivolumab [57]. The trial included 716 patients who were required to have a centrally assessed methylated MGMT promoter, a Karnofsky performance status (KPS) of ≥70, and ≤ 3 mg dexamethasone at baseline. This study had two primary endpoints: PFS and OS. Regrettably, there were no significant differences observed for the 2 primary endpoints of the study. The median PFS for patients on the nivolumab arm was 10.6 months, compared with 10.3 months for the control arm. For patients not on corticosteroids, the median OS was 31.3 months for the nivolumab arm and 33.3 months for the control arm.

Nivolumab was also investigated for MGMT unmethylated GBM [58]. The trial compared nivolumab concurrent with RT followed by nivolumab until disease progression or unacceptable toxicity versus SOC. The addition of nivolumab did not improve efficacy. A total of 560 patients were randomized; median OS was 13.4 months (95% CI, 12.6–14.3) with NIVO+RT and 14.9 months (95% CI, 13.3–16.1) with TMZ + RT (HR, 1.31; 95% CI, 1.09–1.58; P = 0.0037). Median PFS was 6.0 months (95% CI, 5.7–6.2) with NIVO+RT and 6.2 months (95% CI, 5.9–6.7) with TMZ + RT (HR, 1.38; 95% CI, 1.15–1.65). A subgroup analysis based on established prognostic factors, including age, KPS, and degree of surgery, showed no significant benefit for the addition of nivolumab in any patient subgroup. One interesting feature was the baseline PD-L1 expression in tumor tissue: <1% in >55% of RT-TMZ and > 62% of RT-nivolumab patients. Although debate still rages regarding the role and predictive value of this biomarker as well as optimal threshold, such a high level of lack-of expression of a key mechanistic molecule is worrisome.

Limitations of immune-based therapy may be related to tumor-associated factors, such as poor immunogenicity and tumor-induced immune tolerance, but it is important that treatment (SOC) induced immune regulatory effects may also play major roles, both adversely and beneficially [54]. In recurrent glioblastoma:

The CheckMate 143 trial included Cohort 1 in which patients with refractory glioblastoma were randomized to nivolumab monotherapy at 3 mg/kg every 2 weeks (10 pts), or nivolumab 1 mg/kg + ipilimumab 3 mg/kg every 3 weeks (10pts) and a non-randomized cohort 1b of 20 pts. that received nivolumab 3 mg/kg + ipilimumab 1 mg/kg Q3W for 4 doses, followed by nivolumab 3 mg/kg Q2W. A total of 3 pts. achieved a partial response (1 pt. with monotherapy and 2 with the combination). Based on the similar OS, RR and the lower degree of G3/4 toxicity, monotherapy with nivolumab was chosen as the treatment strategy for further development.

In the phase III trial, 369 patients were randomized to receive either nivolumab 3 mg/kg Q2W or bevacizumab 10 mg/kg Q2W. This study was negative for its principal objective of overall survival (OS of 9.8 months vs. 10 months and hazard ratio 1.04). OR and PFS favored bevacizumab, but ORR in the nivolumab was 7.8% and the duration of response was better than the one achieved with bevacizumab (11.1 versus 5.3 months) [59].

Other similar trials with checkpoint inhibitor monotherapy worth mentioning are the KEYNOTE-028 trial and the NCT01375842 trial of Atezolizumab. The KEYNOTE-028 [60] included 26 pts with bevacizumab-naïve recurrent glioblastoma have received pembrolizumab 10 mg/kg Q2W for a maximum of 24 months. 2 patients achieved partial responses (ORR of 7.6%) that lasted 8.3 and 22.8 months respectively and the 6 months PFS was 37.7%. On the NCT01375842 [61], 1 of 16 patients with recurrent glioblastoma showed a partial response (ORR of 6.25%).

The fact that in the Checkmate 143 trial nivolumab achieved similar outcomes to Bevacizumab (which is considered an active treatment in the recurrent setting), and the preclinical found that VEGF can mediate immunosuppression on the tumor stroma, the combination of immunotherapy with antiangiogenics could be worth investigating in the recurrent GBM setting. Three different clinical trials that have combined pembrolizumab with bevacizumab [62], avelumab with axitinib [63] or durvalumab with bevacizumab [64], have failed to show better results to those reported with antiangiogenic monotherapy.

Only a selected number of patients with recurrent glioblastoma will be considered candidates for a secondary resection, and as a consequence, the studies in the neoadjuvant setting have included a small number of patients. One small study with nivolumab [65] showed an increase in infiltrating T cells and an increase in the IFN response, while a similar one with pembrolizumab [66] failed to show any changes in the number of CD8 positive cells.

Intriguingly, the duration of response in some patients was high, but the expression of PD1 or the presence of hypermutation has not been associated with response to immunotherapy in gliomas.

6.2 Oncolytic viruses and tumor vaccines

Apart from the direct tumor cell killing that occurs after tumor cells are infected, oncolytic viruses have the potential of increasing immunogenicity in glioblastoma by delivering PAMPs (pathogenic associated molecular patterns) and facilitating the release of tumor-antigens by dying virus-infect cells.

HSV is the most studied virus in immunotherapy [67]. It can function as both an oncolytic agent and a transgene vector, which can be armed with immunomodulatory or angiogenic modulatory genes (i.e., GM-CSF in TVEC and IL2 in G47delta).

Results with G47delta injected intratumorally in patients with recurrent glioblastoma have shown issues with immediate enlargement of the contrast-enhanced area of the target lesion on MRI caused by the treatment, that is produced tumor destruction and lymphocyte infiltration, but the results in terms of OS (1-year OS of 38.5%) and especially the presence of a subset of patients with longer OS seem promising [68].

To create the DNX-2401 adenovirus, a 24-base pair deletion in the E1A gene that renders the virus unable to infect non-tumoral cells was introduced alongside an RGD-motif that enables the virus to infect integrin-rich cells, that are enriched in the tumor cells. Preliminary results of a phase I study show that 20% of patients with recurrent glioblastoma treated with intratumoral injection achieve OS 3y [69].

Another pilot study in patients with pediatric DIPG (a terrible disease where the historic series show a median OS of around 12 months) showed a reduction in tumor size in 9/12 patients, a 25% OR, and a median OS of 17.8 months [70].

Poliovirus PSRIVO is introduced in the tumor area through convention-enhanced delivery and recognizes the poliovirus receptor CD155, which is widely expressed in neoplastic cells in comparison with normal tissues. In a dose-finding study that included 61 patients with glioblastoma, also benefited a subset of patients (21%) that achieved long-term control at 24 and 36 months [71].

Compared with other tumors, the low TMB burden leads to a lower potential of Tumor-specific antigens (TSAs), mutant proteins expressed exclusively in tumor cells. Most studies using peptidic vaccines have focused either on personalized vaccines, with only two small pilot projects being published [72, 73], or vaccination against Tumor-associated antigens(TAAs), proteins present in normal tissues but overexpressed in tumors. A vaccine, called rindopepimut, designed to target the EGFRvIII, which is present in 30% of GBM cases was recently tested in a randomized phase III, after showing immunogenicity, safety, and activity in earlier clinical trials [74]. A phase III study, that randomized 745 patients that had completed their initial chemoradiation without progression showed negative results for OS (20.0 vs 20.1 m) in both patients with and without residual disease [75].

In comparison with peptidic vaccines, DC vaccines have the potential of being generated directly from coculture with tumor lysates, allowing the co-targeting of both TSAs and TAAs. Preclinical studies on glioblastoma have demonstrated that DC vaccines can reduce tumor growth, prolong survival and induce tumor-specific IFN-γ, and cytotoxic T-lymphocytes responses associated with T-cell infiltration of tumors.

Several small clinical trials have shown that this approach is safe and feasible [76–78], and the preliminary results of the largest clinical trial to date, testing DC-Vax, vs placebo with crossover at progression in 331 patients seem promising. But the final unblinded results have yet to be published [79]. Another potential source of dendritic vaccines is the ones generated by exposing cells to pp65, which is a major structural protein of CMV a virus that is frequently present in glioblastoma cells. Although studies using pp65 vaccines are small the median PFS of 25.3 m and OS of 41.1 m are intriguing [80].

6.3 Immunocytokines, chemokines, and other cytokine modulators

Immunocytokines are molecules that target immunostimulating cytokines such as TNF or IL-2 to the tumor microenvironment using signals that direct them to the tumor cells, immune infiltrating cells, or components of the tumor stroma. One potential therapeutic agent in this class is L19TNF, a multimer of TNF fused to the antibody L19 that binds a tumor-specific epitope of the extracellular matrix protein fibronectin. Preliminary studies have shown the safety, feasibility, and intriguing preliminary clinical results in both combinations with lomustine in refractory GBM, and combination with chemoradiation in front-line patients.

TGF-B upregulation in glioblastoma has been linked to increases in the migratory potential, promoting EMT, inducing a CSC-like drug-resistant phenotype, and an immunosuppressive microenvironment [81]. Despite some patients treated with TGFB inhibitors in clinical trials showing prolonged responses [82, 83], the overall results with oral TGFBR have been disappointing [84] most likely due to insufficient target inhibition due to concerns over cardiotoxicity.

CSF-1R inhibitors are cytokine modulators that try to repress tumor-associated myeloid cells that form a substantial proportion of the immunosuppressive glioblastoma microenvironment, by downregulating CSF1R, an important receptor for macrophage differentiation and survival. However clinical trials both in first-line patients combined with chemoradiation and in patients with recurrent disease in both monotherapy and combination with checkpoint inhibitors show limited clinical efficacy.

6.4 CAR T-cells, TCBs, and bispecific T-cell engager antibodies

CAR-T cell treatment share with vaccines the necessity of identifying targets that are primarily present in tumor cells with low expression in normal tissues (TAAs/TSAs).

Accordingly, EGFRvIII has also been chosen as a target for CAR T-cell treatment. One potential issue is that although most patients treated with CAR T-cells developed noticeable peripheral levels of EGFRvIII-directed CAR T-cells when their tumors were resected half of the patients had lost their baseline expression of EGFRvIII [85].

Subsequent small trials with second and third-generation trials including expression of costimulatory proteins show only minimal signs of activity in a few patients [86].

IL13Rα2 CAR-T has also been tested in small clinical trials, with some patients achieving clinical benefit, including 1 patient presenting a complete response. Finally.

HER2 CAR-T cells were deemed to be safe in the phase I clinical trial that included 17 patients, including 1 patient with partial response and 3 with disease stabilization for more than 4 months [87].

Another potential way to overcome the lack of antigen presentation and infiltrating T-Cell is by the use of bispecific antibodies that target at the same time a target present in immune cells, that many times is CD3 and a TSA or TAA. Several modifications to the bispecific antibody structure can be made to modify its protein and characteristics. For example, AMG 596 is composed of two single-chain variable fragments one binding to CD3, and the other to EGFRvIII, while RO7428731 contains both variable regions against EGFRvIII and CD3 and an IgG structure [88].

Author details

María Ángeles Vaz[1*], Sonia Del Barco Berrón[2], Raquel Luque[3], María Villamayor[1], Juan Manuel Sepúlveda Sánchez[4] and María Vieito[5]

1 Ramón y Cajal University Hospital, Madrid, Spain

2 Josep Trueta University Hospital, Gerona, Spain

3 Virgen de Las Nieves University Hospital, Granada, Spain

4 12 Octubre University Hospital, Madrid, Spain

5 Vall D'Hebron University Hospital, Barcelona, Spain

*Address all correspondence to: mavaz4@gmail.com

References

[1] Ostrom QT, Cioffi G, Waite K, Kruchko C, Barnholtz-Sloan JS. CBTRUS statistical report: Primary brain and other central nervous system tumors diagnosed in the United States in 2014-2018. Neuro-Oncology. 2021;**23**(12 Suppl 2):iii1-iii105. DOI: 10.1093/neuonc/noab200

[2] Stupp R et al. Radiotherapy plus concomitant and adjuvant temozolomide for glioblastoma. The New England Journal of Medicine. 2005;**352**(10):987-996. DOI: 10.1056/NEJMoa043330

[3] Ou A, Yung WKA, Majd N. Molecular mechanisms of treatment resistance in glioblastoma. International Journal of Molecular Sciences. 2020;**22**(1):E351. DOI: 10.3390/ijms22010351

[4] Hegi ME et al. MGMT gene silencing and benefit from temozolomide in glioblastoma. The New England Journal of Medicine. 2005;**352**(10):997-1003. DOI: 10.1056/NEJMoa043331

[5] Klingler S et al. Development of resistance to EGFR-targeted therapy in malignant glioma can occur through EGFR-dependent and -independent mechanisms. Cancer Research. 2015;**75**(10):2109-2119. DOI: 10.1158/0008-5472.CAN-14-3122

[6] Ma DJ et al. A phase II trial of everolimus, temozolomide, and radiotherapy in patients with newly diagnosed glioblastoma: NCCTG N057K. Neuro-Oncology. 2015;**17**(9):1261-1269. DOI: 10.1093/neuonc/nou328

[7] Thompson EM, Frenkel EP, Neuwelt EA. The paradoxical effect of bevacizumab in the therapy of malignant gliomas. Neurology. 2011;**76**(1):87-93. DOI: 10.1212/WNL.0b013e318204a3af

[8] Hicklin DJ, Ellis LM. Role of the vascular endothelial growth factor pathway in tumor growth and angiogenesis. Journal of Clinical Oncology. 2005;**23**(5):1011-1027. DOI: 10.1200/JCO.2005.06.081

[9] Chinot OL et al. Bevacizumab plus radiotherapy-temozolomide for newly diagnosed glioblastoma. The New England Journal of Medicine. 2014;**370**(8):709-722. DOI: 10.1056/NEJMoa1308345

[10] Gilbert MR et al. A randomized trial of bevacizumab for newly diagnosed glioblastoma. The New England Journal of Medicine. 2014;**370**(8):699-708. DOI: 10.1056/NEJMoa1308573

[11] Ameratunga M, Pavlakis N, Wheeler H, Grant R, Simes J, Khasraw M. Anti-angiogenic therapy for high-grade glioma. Cochrane Database of Systematic Reviews. 2018;**11**:CD008218. DOI: 10.1002/14651858.CD008218.pub4

[12] Desgrosellier JS, Cheresh DA. Integrins in cancer: Biological implications and therapeutic opportunities. Nature Reviews. Cancer. 2010;**10**(1):9-22. DOI: 10.1038/nrc2748

[13] Stupp R et al. Cilengitide combined with standard treatment for patients with newly diagnosed glioblastoma with methylated MGMT promoter (CENTRIC EORTC 26071-22072 study): A multicentre, randomised, open-label, phase 3 trial. The Lancet Oncology. 2014;**15**(10):1100-1108. DOI: 10.1016/S1470-2045(14)70379-1

[14] Mason WP. End of the road: Confounding results of the CORE trial terminate the arduous journey of cilengitide for glioblastoma. Neuro-Oncology. 2015;**17**(5):634-635. DOI: 10.1093/neuonc/nov018

[15] Sim H-W et al. A randomized phase II trial of veliparib, radiotherapy, and temozolomide in patients with unmethylated MGMT glioblastoma: The VERTU study. Neuro-Oncology. 2021;**23**(10):1736-1749. DOI: 10.1093/neuonc/noab111

[16] Sarkiria JN, Ballman KV, Kizilbash SH, et al. Randomized phase II/III trial of veliparib or placebo in combination with adjuvant temozolomide in newly diagnosed glioblastoma (GBM) patients with MGMT promoter hymertmethylation (Alliance A071102). Journal of Clinical Oncology. 2022;**40**(16_suppl):2001-2001

[17] Lassman AB et al. Comparison of biomarker assays for EGFR: Implications for precision medicine in patients with glioblastoma. Clinical Cancer Research. 2019;**25**(11):3259-3265. DOI: 10.1158/1078-0432.CCR-18-3034

[18] Lassman AB et al. Depatuxizumab-mafodotin in EGFR-amplified newly diagnosed glioblastoma: A phase III randomized clinical trial. Neuro-Oncology. 2022:noac173. DOI: 10.1093/neuonc/noac173

[19] Wong ET et al. Outcomes and prognostic factors in recurrent glioma patients enrolled onto phase II clinical trials. Journal of Clinical Oncology. 1999;**17**(8):2572-2578. DOI: 10.1200/JCO.1999.17.8.2572

[20] Di Nunno V et al. Treatment of recurrent glioblastoma: State-of-the-art and future perspectives. Expert Review of Anticancer Therapy. 2020;**20**(9):785-795. DOI: 10.1080/14737140.2020.1807949

[21] Martínez-Garcia M et al. SEOM clinical guidelines for diagnosis and treatment of glioblastoma (2017). Clinical & Translational Oncology. 2018;**20**(1):22-28. DOI: 10.1007/s12094-017-1763-6

[22] Seystahl K, Wick W, Weller M. Therapeutic options in recurrent glioblastoma—An update. Critical Reviews in Oncology/Hematology. 2016;**99**:389-408. DOI: 10.1016/j.critrevonc.2016.01.018

[23] Tosoni A, Franceschi E, Poggi R, Brandes AA. Relapsed glioblastoma: Treatment strategies for initial and subsequent recurrences. Current Treatment Options in Oncology. 2016;**17**(9):49. DOI: 10.1007/s11864-016-0422-4

[24] Taal W et al. Single-agent bevacizumab or lomustine versus a combination of bevacizumab plus lomustine in patients with recurrent glioblastoma (BELOB trial): A randomised controlled phase 2 trial. The Lancet Oncology. 2014;**15**(9):943-953. DOI: 10.1016/S1470-2045(14)70314-6

[25] Perry JR, Rizek P, Cashman R, Morrison M, Morrison T. Temozolomide rechallenge in recurrent malignant glioma by using a continuous temozolomide schedule: The "rescue" approach. Cancer. 2008;**113**(8):2152-2157. DOI: 10.1002/cncr.23813

[26] Van Den Bent M et al. INTELLANCE 2/EORTC 1410 randomized phase II study of Depatux-M alone and with temozolomide vs temozolomide or lomustine in recurrent EGFR amplified glioblastoma. Neuro-Oncology. 2020;**22**(5):684-693. DOI: 10.1093/neuonc/noz222

[27] Rong L, Li N, Zhang Z. Emerging therapies for glioblastoma: Current state and future directions. Journal of Experimental & Clinical Cancer Research. 2022;**41**(1):142. DOI: 10.1186/s13046-022-02349-7

[28] Lu VM, Jue TR, McDonald KL, Rovin RA. The survival effect of repeat

surgery at glioblastoma recurrence and its trend: A systematic review and meta-analysis. World Neurosurgery. 2018;**115**:453-459.e3. DOI: 10.1016/j.wneu.2018.04.016

[29] Chang SM et al. Perioperative complications and neurological outcomes of first and second craniotomies among patients enrolled in the glioma outcome project. Journal of Neurosurgery. 2003;**98**(6):1175-1181. DOI: 10.3171/jns.2003.98.6.1175

[30] Park C-K et al. A practical scoring system to determine whether to proceed with surgical resection in recurrent glioblastoma. Neuro-Oncology. 2013;**15**(8):1096-1101. DOI: 10.1093/neuonc/not069

[31] Park JK et al. Scale to predict survival after surgery for recurrent glioblastoma multiforme. Journal of Clinical Oncology. 2010;**28**(24):3838-3843. DOI: 10.1200/JCO.2010.30.0582

[32] Azoulay M et al. Benefit of re-operation and salvage therapies for recurrent glioblastoma multiforme: Results from a single institution. Journal of Neuro-Oncology. 2017;**132**(3):419-426. DOI: 10.1007/s11060-017-2383-2

[33] Delgado-Fernandez J et al. Usefulness of Reintervention in recurrent glioblastoma: An indispensable weapon for increasing survival. World Neurosurgery. 2017;**108**:610-617. DOI: 10.1016/j.wneu.2017.09.062

[34] Suchorska B et al. Complete resection of contrast-enhancing tumor volume is associated with improved survival in recurrent glioblastoma-results from the DIRECTOR trial. Neuro-Oncology. 2016;**18**(4):549-556. DOI: 10.1093/neuonc/nov326

[35] Zanello M et al. Recurrent glioblastomas in the elderly after maximal first-line treatment: Does preserved overall condition warrant a maximal second-line treatment? Journal of Neuro-Oncology. 2017;**135**(2):285-297. DOI: 10.1007/s11060-017-2573-y

[36] Franceschi E et al. The effect of re-operation on survival in patients with recurrent glioblastoma. Anticancer Research. 2015;**35**(3):1743-1748

[37] Brandes AA, Vastola F, Monfardini S. Reoperation in recurrent high-grade gliomas: Literature review of prognostic factors and outcome. American Journal of Clinical Oncology. 1999;**22**(4):387-390. DOI: 10.1097/00000421-199908000-00013

[38] Brandes AA et al. Patient outcomes following second surgery for recurrent glioblastoma. Future Oncology. 2016;**12**(8):1039-1044. DOI: 10.2217/fon.16.9

[39] Montemurro N, Perrini P, Blanco MO, Vannozzi R. Second surgery for recurrent glioblastoma: A concise overview of the current literature. Clinical Neurology and Neurosurgery. 2016;**142**:60-64. DOI: 10.1016/j.clineuro.2016.01.010

[40] Zhang Y-D, Dai R-Y, Chen Z, Zhang Y-H, He X-Z, Zhou J. Efficacy and safety of carmustine wafers in the treatment of glioblastoma multiforme: A systematic review. Turkish Neurosurgery. 2014;**24**(5):639-645. DOI: 10.5137/1019-5149.JTN.8878-13.1

[41] Brennan PM et al. Second surgery for progressive glioblastoma: A multi-Centre questionnaire and cohort-based review of clinical decision-making and patient outcomes in current practice. Journal of Neuro-Oncology. 2021;**153**(1):99-107. DOI: 10.1007/s11060-021-03748-0

[42] Bunevicius A, Sheehan JP. Radiosurgery for glioblastoma.

Neurosurgery Clinics of North America. 2021;**32**(1):117-128. DOI: 10.1016/j.nec.2020.08.007

[43] Minniti G, Niyazi M, Alongi F, Navarria P, Belka C. Current status and recent advances in reirradiation of glioblastoma. Radiation Oncology. 2021;**16**(1):36. DOI: 10.1186/s13014-021-01767-9

[44] Barney C, Shukla G, Bhamidipati D, Palmer JD. Re-irradiation for recurrent glioblastoma multiforme. Journal of Clinical Oncology. 2017;**6**(4):36. DOI: 10.21037/cco.2017.06.18

[45] Tsien CI et al. NRG oncology/RTOG1205: A randomized phase II trial of concurrent bevacizumab and Reirradiation versus bevacizumab alone as treatment for recurrent glioblastoma. Journal of Clinical Oncology. 2022:JCO2200164. DOI: 10.1200/JCO.22.00164

[46] Bergman D et al. Randomized prospective trial of fractionated stereotactic radiosurgery with chemotherapy versus chemotherapy alone for bevacizumab-resistant high-grade glioma. Journal of Neuro-Oncology. 2020;**148**(2):353-361. DOI: 10.1007/s11060-020-03526-4

[47] Kulinich DP et al. Radiotherapy versus combination radiotherapy-bevacizumab for the treatment of recurrent high-grade glioma: A systematic review. Acta Neurochirurgica. 2021;**163**(7):1921-1934. DOI: 10.1007/s00701-021-04794-3

[48] Hasan S et al. Salvage fractionated stereotactic radiotherapy with or without chemotherapy and immunotherapy for recurrent glioblastoma Multiforme: A single institution experience. Frontiers in Oncology. 2015;5:106. DOI: 10.3389/fonc.2015.00106

[49] Sahebjam S et al. Hypofractionated stereotactic re-irradiation with pembrolizumab and bevacizumab in patients with recurrent high-grade gliomas: Results from a phase I study. Neuro-Oncology. 2021;**23**(4):677-686. DOI: 10.1093/neuonc/noaa260

[50] Gutin PH et al. Brachytherapy of recurrent malignant brain tumors with removable high-activity iodine-125 sources. Journal of Neurosurgery. 1984;**60**(1):61-68. DOI: 10.3171/jns.1984.60.1.0061

[51] Simon JM et al. Brachytherapy of glioblastoma recurring in previously irradiated territory: Predictive value of tumor volume. International Journal of Radiation Oncology, Biology, Physics. 2002;**53**(1):67-74. DOI: 10.1016/s0360-3016(01)02804-8

[52] Chan TA et al. Treatment of recurrent glioblastoma multiforme with GliaSite brachytherapy. International Journal of Radiation Oncology, Biology, Physics. 2005;**62**(4):1133-1139. DOI: 10.1016/j.ijrobp.2004.12.032

[53] Welsh J et al. GliaSite brachytherapy boost as part of initial treatment of glioblastoma multiforme: A retrospective multi-institutional pilot study. International Journal of Radiation Oncology, Biology, Physics. 2007;**68**(1):159-165. DOI: 10.1016/j.ijrobp.2006.11.053

[54] Sampson JH, Gunn MD, Fecci PE, Ashley DM. Brain immunology and immunotherapy in brain tumours. Nature Reviews. Cancer. 2020;**20**(1):12-25. DOI: 10.1038/s41568-019-0224-7

[55] Bausart M, Préat V, Malfanti A. Immunotherapy for glioblastoma: The promise of combination strategies. Journal of Experimental & Clinical Cancer Research. 2022;**41**(1):35. DOI: 10.1186/s13046-022-02251-2

[56] Cristescu R et al. Pan-tumor genomic biomarkers for PD-1 checkpoint blockade-based immunotherapy. Science. 2018;**362**(6411):eaar3593. DOI: 10.1126/science.aar3593

[57] Lim M et al. Phase III trial of chemoradiotherapy with temozolomide plus nivolumab or placebo for newly diagnosed glioblastoma with methylated MGMT promoter. Neuro-Oncology. 2022;**24**(11):1935-1949. DOI: 10.1093/neuonc/noac116

[58] Omuro A et al. Radiotherapy combined with Nivolumab or Temozolomide for newly diagnosed glioblastoma with Unmethylated MGMT promoter: An international randomized phase 3 trial. Neuro-Oncology. 2022:noac099. DOI: 10.1093/neuonc/noac099

[59] Reardon DA et al. Effect of Nivolumab vs bevacizumab in patients with recurrent glioblastoma: The CheckMate 143 phase 3 randomized clinical trial. JAMA Oncology. 2020;**6**(7):1003-1010. DOI: 10.1001/jamaoncol.2020.1024

[60] Reardon DA et al. Treatment with pembrolizumab in programmed death ligand 1-positive recurrent glioblastoma: Results from the multicohort phase 1 KEYNOTE-028 trial. Cancer. 2021;**127**(10):1620-1629. DOI: 10.1002/cncr.33378

[61] Lukas RV et al. Clinical activity and safety of atezolizumab in patients with recurrent glioblastoma. Journal of Neuro-Oncology. 2018;**140**(2):317-328. DOI: 10.1007/s11060-018-2955-9

[62] Nayak L et al. Randomized phase II and biomarker study of Pembrolizumab plus bevacizumab versus Pembrolizumab alone for patients with recurrent glioblastoma. Clinical Cancer Research. 2021;**27**(4):1048-1057. DOI: 10.1158/1078-0432.CCR-20-2500

[63] Awada G et al. Axitinib plus avelumab in the treatment of recurrent glioblastoma: A stratified, open-label, single-center phase 2 clinical trial (GliAvAx). Journal for Immunotherapy of Cancer. 2020;**8**(2):e001146. DOI: 10.1136/jitc-2020-001146

[64] Nayak L et al. Circulating immune cell and outcome analysis from the phase II study of PD-L1 blockade with Durvalumab for newly diagnosed and recurrent glioblastoma. Clinical Cancer Research. 2022;**28**(12):2567-2578. DOI: 10.1158/1078-0432.CCR-21-4064

[65] Schalper KA et al. Neoadjuvant nivolumab modifies the tumor immune microenvironment in resectable glioblastoma. Nature Medicine. 2019;**25**(3):470-476. DOI: 10.1038/s41591-018-0339-5

[66] de Groot J et al. Window-of-opportunity clinical trial of pembrolizumab in patients with recurrent glioblastoma reveals predominance of immune-suppressive macrophages. Neuro-Oncology. 2020;**22**(4):539-549. DOI: 10.1093/neuonc/noz185

[67] Peters C, Rabkin SD. Designing herpes viruses as oncolytics. Molecular Therapy-Oncolytics. 2015;**2**:15010. DOI: 10.1038/mto.2015.10

[68] Todo T, Ino Y, Ohtsu H, Shibahara J, Tanaka M. A phase I/II study of triple-mutated oncolytic herpes virus G47Δ in patients with progressive glioblastoma. Nature Communications. 2022;**13**(1):4119. DOI: 10.1038/s41467-022-31262-y

[69] Lang FF et al. Phase I study of DNX-2401 (Delta-24-RGD) oncolytic adenovirus: Replication and immunotherapeutic effects in recurrent malignant glioma. Journal of Clinical Oncology. 2018;**36**(14):1419-1427. DOI: 10.1200/JCO.2017.75.8219

[70] Tejada S et al. DNX-2401, an oncolytic virus, for the treatment of newly diagnosed diffuse intrinsic pontine gliomas: A case report. Frontiers in Oncology. 2018;**8**:61. DOI: 10.3389/fonc.2018.00061

[71] Desjardins A et al. Recurrent glioblastoma treated with recombinant poliovirus. The New England Journal of Medicine. 2018;**379**(2):150-161. DOI: 10.1056/NEJMoa1716435

[72] Hilf N et al. Actively personalized vaccination trial for newly diagnosed glioblastoma. Nature. 2019;**565**(7738):240-245. DOI: 10.1038/s41586-018-0810-y

[73] Keskin DB et al. Neoantigen vaccine generates intratumoral T cell responses in phase Ib glioblastoma trial. Nature. 2019;**565**(7738):234-239. DOI: 10.1038/s41586-018-0792-9

[74] Schuster J et al. A phase II, multicenter trial of rindopepimut (CDX-110) in newly diagnosed glioblastoma: The ACT III study. Neuro-Oncology. 2015;**17**(6):854-861. DOI: 10.1093/neuonc/nou348

[75] Weller M et al. Rindopepimut with temozolomide for patients with newly diagnosed, EGFRvIII-expressing glioblastoma (ACT IV): A randomised, double-blind, international phase 3 trial. The Lancet Oncology. 2017;**18**(10):1373-1385. DOI: 10.1016/S1470-2045(17)30517-X

[76] Cho D-Y et al. Adjuvant immunotherapy with whole-cell lysate dendritic cells vaccine for glioblastoma multiforme: A phase II clinical trial. World Neurosurgery. 2012;**77**(5-6):736-744. DOI: 10.1016/j.wneu.2011.08.020

[77] Jie X, Hua L, Jiang W, Feng F, Feng G, Hua Z. Clinical application of a dendritic cell vaccine raised against heat-shocked glioblastoma. Cell Biochemistry and Biophysics. 2012;**62**(1):91-99. DOI: 10.1007/s12013-011-9265-6

[78] Yao Y et al. Molecular subgroups and B7-H4 expression levels predict responses to dendritic cell vaccines in glioblastoma: An exploratory randomized phase II clinical trial. Cancer Immunology, Immunotherapy. 2018;**67**(11):1777-1788. DOI: 10.1007/s00262-018-2232-y

[79] Liau LM et al. First results on survival from a large phase 3 clinical trial of an autologous dendritic cell vaccine in newly diagnosed glioblastoma. Journal of Translational Medicine. 2018;**16**(1):142. DOI: 10.1186/s12967-018-1507-6

[80] Batich KA et al. Long-term survival in glioblastoma with cytomegalovirus pp65-targeted vaccination. Clinical Cancer Research. 2017;**23**(8):1898-1909. DOI: 10.1158/1078-0432.CCR-16-2057

[81] Mangani D et al. Limited role for transforming growth factor-β pathway activation-mediated escape from VEGF inhibition in murine glioma models. Neuro-Oncology. 2016;**18**(12):1610-1621. DOI: 10.1093/neuonc/now112

[82] Rodon J et al. First-in-human dose study of the novel transforming growth factor-β receptor I kinase inhibitor LY2157299 monohydrate in patients with advanced cancer and glioma. Clinical Cancer Research. 2015;**21**(3):553-560. DOI: 10.1158/1078-0432.CCR-14-1380

[83] Yap TA et al. First-In-human phase I study of a next-generation, Oral, TGFβ receptor 1 inhibitor, LY3200882, in patients with advanced cancer. Clinical Cancer Research. 2021;**27**(24):6666-6676. DOI: 10.1158/1078-0432.CCR-21-1504

[84] Capper D et al. Biomarker and histopathology evaluation of patients

with recurrent glioblastoma treated with Galunisertib, Lomustine, or the combination of Galunisertib and Lomustine. International Journal of Molecular Sciences. 2017;**18**(5):E995. DOI: 10.3390/ijms18050995

[85] O'Rourke DM et al. A single dose of peripherally infused EGFRvIII-directed CAR T cells mediates antigen loss and induces adaptive resistance in patients with recurrent glioblastoma. Science Translational Medicine. 2017;**9**(399):eaaa0984. DOI: 10.1126/scitranslmed.aaa0984

[86] Goff SL et al. Pilot trial of adoptive transfer of chimeric antigen receptor-transduced T cells targeting EGFRvIII in patients with glioblastoma. Journal of Immunotherapy. 2019;**42**(4):126-135. DOI: 10.1097/CJI.0000000000000260

[87] Ahmed N et al. «HER2-specific chimeric antigen receptor-modified virus-specific T cells for progressive glioblastoma: A phase 1 dose-escalation trial», *JAMA*. Oncologia. 2017;**3**(8):1094-1101. DOI: 10.1001/jamaoncol.2017.0184

[88] Iurlaro R et al. A novel EGFRvIII T-cell bispecific antibody for the treatment of glioblastoma. Molecular Cancer Therapeutics. 2022;**21**(10):1499-1509. DOI: 10.1158/1535-7163.MCT-22-0201

Chapter 6

Noncanonical (Non-R132H) IDH-Mutated Gliomas

Tariq D. Al-Saadi and Roberto J. Diaz

Abstract

Mutations in *IDH1* or *IDH2* confer a significant survival advantage compared to their isocitrate dehydrogenase (IDH) wild-type counterparts and, as such, are the most significant prognostic factors in this group. The mutations in the IDH1 gene are heterozygous and almost always involve only a single residue (arginine 132), which is replaced by histidine in roughly 90% of tumors. Regardless, the non-p.R132H (noncanonical) mutations in the IDH1 gene were also documented in around 20% of mutated glioma. The noncanonical IDH mutations have distinguishing radiological and histological features. The existence of such tumors seems to be associated with a genetic predisposition to cancer development.

Keywords: noncanonical, IDH-mutant, glioma, astrocytoma

1. Introduction

1.1 The 2020 WHO classification of adult gliomas

According to the latest World Health Organization (WHO) classification of CNS tumors, all isocitrate dehydrogenase (IDH)-mutant tumors were classified as either IDH-mutant oligodendrogliomas or astrocytomas and graded as WHO grade 2, 3, or 4 [1]. This classification recognized a grade 4 IDH-mutant astrocytoma and tumors harboring CDKN2A/B homozygous deletion. We favor using the term cancerous glioma to the previous term "Low-Grade Glioma (LGG)," since the current 2020 WHO classification presented major changes that advance the role of molecular diagnostics in CNS tumor classification. With the new classification, there are three groups of adult-type gliomas (**Figure 1**).

Group 1 is the astrocytoma with IDH mutation, group 2 is astrocytoma with no IDH mutation (IDH wild-type), and group 3 is oligodendroglioma, which carries the IDH mutation and 1p/19q co-deletion. Other significant molecular profile findings include IDH1, IDH2, ATRX, TP53, and CDKN2A/B. Group 1 is further classified based on the histopathological grade into 2, 3, and 4. The second group is the astrocytoma with IDH wild-type status, where only one histological grade is given (grade 4) due to the nature of the disease and it is prognosis. A third group is oligodendrogliomas which are characterized by the 1p/19q co-deletion which is unique for this group and considered to be a positive prognostic marker for this particular group [2, 3].

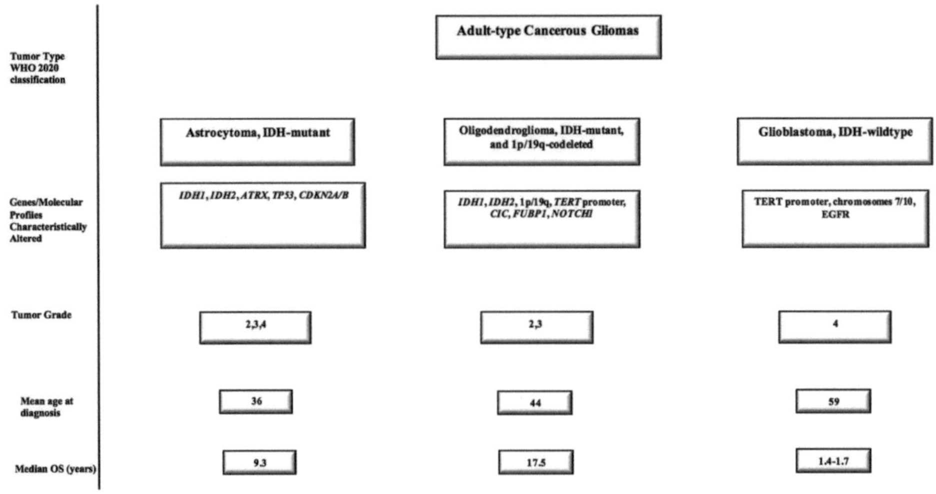

Figure 1.
The 2020 WHO classification of adult gliomas.

2. IDH mutation in glioma

IDH1 mutations are very recurring in World Health Organization (WHO) grade II astrocytomas, anaplastic astrocytomas WHO grade III, low-grade/anaplastic oligodendrogliomas, and secondary glioblastomas (representing 80%, 64%, 66–80%, and 83%, respectively) [4–7]. Several studies have consistently reported a positive association between the IDH1 mutations and the better prognosis for patients with malignant gliomas [7–11]. Yet, for the adult cancerous glioma or (LGGs) vague results have been published so far. Metellus et al. studied a small series of 47 LGGs (85% oligodendroglial and 15% astrocytic tumors) and deduced that IDH1 mutations were positive prognostic values and associated with more prolonged overall survival (OS) and progression-free survival (PFS) [12]. Dubbink et al. analyzed a retrospective series of 49 low-grade astrocytomas for IDH1/2 mutations and found a highly significant correlation between OS and IDH1 status [13]. A more considerable series by Sanson and his colleagues with 100 LGGs (88% oligodendroglial tumors and 12% astrocytomas WHO-II) concluded that IDH1 is a prognostic marker and associated with longer OS only but not with PFS [9]. An association between IDH1 mutation status and OS was also noted in a cohort of 139 LGGs consisting of 61 oligodendroglial and 78 astrocytic tumors [5]. Contrariwise, additional investigations on patients with LGGs did not report any correlation between IDH1 mutation and OS [14–16]. These studies were associated with low hazard ratio (HR); however, a meta-analysis reported later (included the later studies) showed a positive HR between the IDH mutation status and death (with less mortality rate in IDH-mutated glioma compared to the wild-type) [17].

2.1 Biological impact of IDH mutation

In adults, mutations in *IDH1* or *IDH2* confer a significant survival benefit compared to their IDH wild-type counterparts and as such are the most important prognostic factor in this group [9]. Glioma-specific mutations in IDH1 always affect the amino acid arginine in position 132 of the amino acid sequence which belongs to

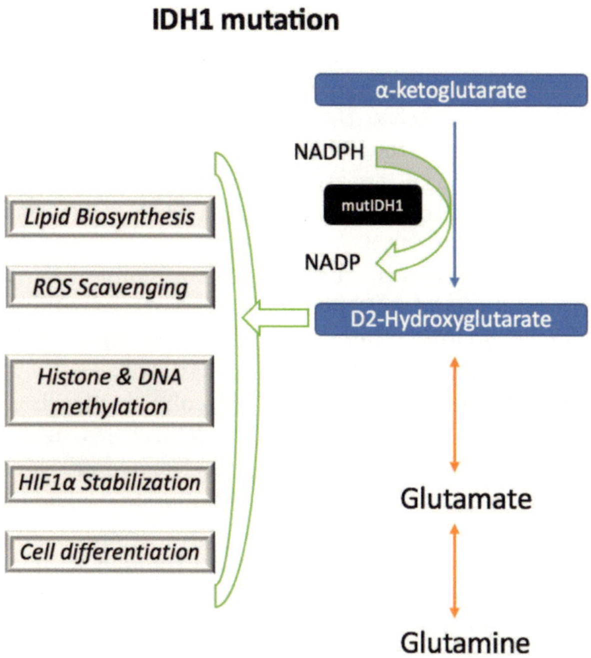

Figure 2.
Biological role of IDH1 mutation [22].

an evolutionary highly conserved region located at the binding site for isocitrate [8]. The role of IDH1 mutations in tumor biology currently is intensely studied. Mutations inactivate enzyme activity and confer the novel function of catalyzing the conversion of alpha-ketoglutarate (αKG) to D-2-hydroxyglutarate (2HG) [5]. The downstream effects of mutant IDH include decreased cellular NADPH and αKG levels, HIF1a stabilization, increased production of 2HG, which competitively inhibits αKG-dependent enzymes such as histone methyltransferases and 5-methylcytosine hydroxylases [18–22], as shown in (**Figure 2**).

3. Noncanonical IDH-mutant gliomas

3.1 Overview and prevalence

Mutations in the IDH1 gene are heterozygous and almost always affect only a single residue (arginine 132), which is replaced by histidine in roughly 90% of tumors [4, 9, 23–25]. Nonetheless, non-p.R132H mutations in the IDH1 gene (e.g. p.R132C) have been documented to accumulate at higher frequencies in histological subtypes of glioma [5] in astrocytomas of Li-Fraumeni patients [26] and in patients with AML [27]. Visani and his co-authors found that around 19% of grade II or III tumors harbored a noncanonical IDH mutation, while in GBM they recognized only the IDH1-R132H mutation [28].

Blass et al. [24] sequenced 685 primary brain tumors to analyze the genomic region spanning wild-type R132 of IDH1. They recognized 221 somatic IDH1 mutations with higher frequency in secondary glioblastomas followed by oligoastrocytomas, oligodendrogliomas, and diffuse astrocytomas (88%, 78%, 69%, and 68% respectively). Exclusively one wild-type allele was detected, and all the mutations were heterozygous. Mutation in codon 132 of IDH1 was detected only and 205 mutations were of the R132H type. Nevertheless, they also encountered leading to R132C, R132S, R132G, R132L, and R132V (eight, four, two, one, and one mutation, respectively), as shown in **Figure 3**. There was no apparent association of the rare mutation types with a distinct tumor entity, although six of the eight R132C mutations were seen in astrocytomas.

Hartmann and his colleagues analyzed 1010 human gliomas for mutations in codons 132 and 172 in the genes for IDH1 and IDH2, respectively [5]. Their series consisted of 1010 diffuse gliomas including diffuse astrocytomas WHO grade II (227), anaplastic astrocytomas WHO grade III (228), anaplastic oligoastrocytomas (177), anaplastic oligodendrogliomas WHO grade III (174), oligodendrogliomas WHO grade II (128), and oligoastrocytomas WHO grade II (76). R132H was the dominant amino acid sequence alteration accounting for 92.7% of the detected mutations followed by R132C, R132S, R132G, and R132L. The type and distribution of the mutations are given in **Figure 4**.

The disparities in the literature regarding the low frequencies of R132S, R132G, and R132L may be due to dissimilarities in sample size and different types of tumors examined. Franceschi and his colleagues lately reviewed 390 patients with an R132H-IDH1 mutation and 34 patients with a non-R132H mutation [29]. Likened to patients with the R132H-IDH1 mutation, patients with non-R132H mutations were discovered to have less frequent 1p19q co-deletion. In addition, they were also younger than those with noncanonical IDH1 mutation ($p < 0.001$). Improved overall survival was correlated to the extent of surgical resection, 1p19 co-deletion existence, and the presence of non-R132H mutation [29].

The prognostic impact of non-R132 mutation is still under study and not fully defined.

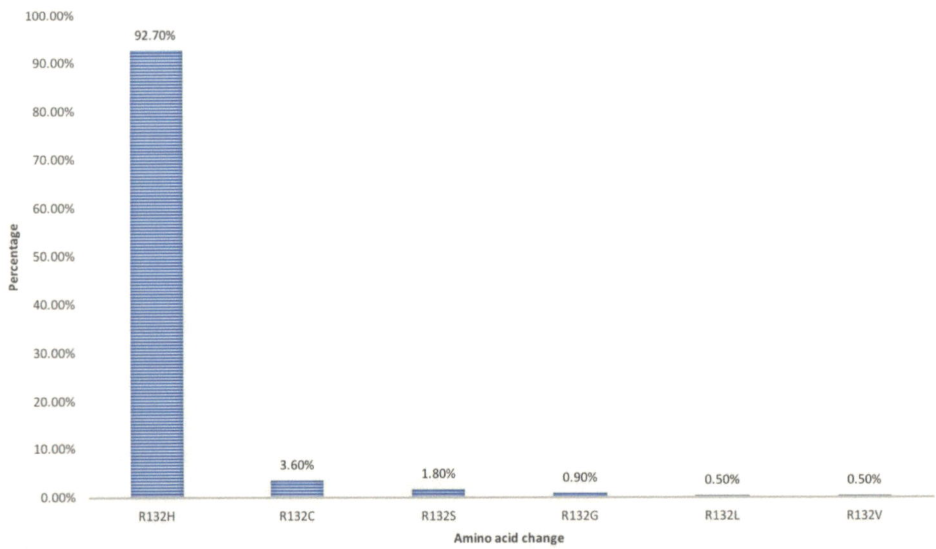

Figure 3.
Type of 221 IDH1 mutations in brain tumors in Blass et al.'s study [24].

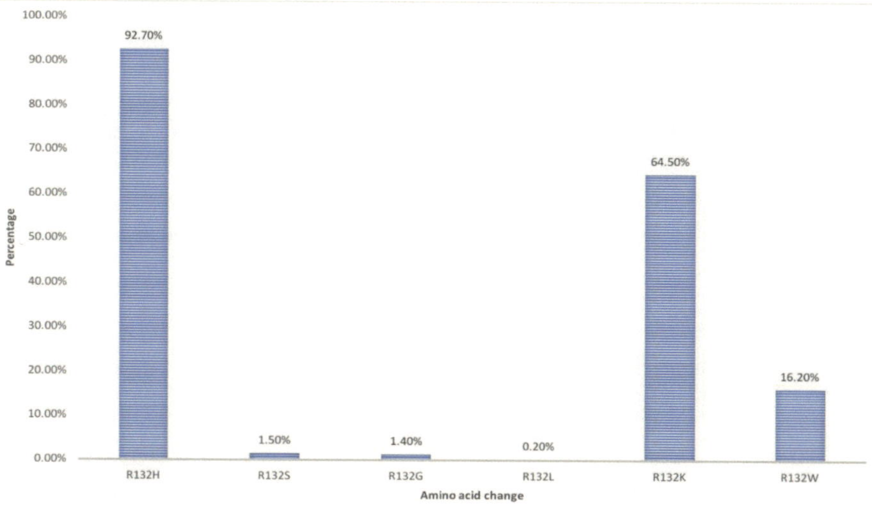

Figure 4.
Type of 716 IDH1 and 31 IDH2 mutations and frequency among mutations in 1010 WHO grades II and III astrocytomas, oligodendrogliomas, and oligoastrocytomas analyzed by Hartmann et al. [5].

Since most mutations affect the same hot spot region of IDH1-R132H, it was naturally presumed that the associated clinical outcomes are similar to that of IDH1-R132H mutated tumors, as implied by the difficulty in culling clinical data for specific noncanonical mutations from documented series. Restricted data are available in the literature concerning the prognosis, overall survival, and role of adjuvant therapies (radiotherapy and/or chemotherapy) in patients with noncanonical IDH mutations. Moreover, the literature also lacks studies that distinguish the IDH-mutant astrocytomas and oligodendrogliomas. The issue with combining the two different groups is that the oligodendrogliomas are characterized by the 1p19q co-deletion with the positive prognostic marker for this group. This might have an influence on the overall conclusion of these studies.

Figure 5a-d displaying a Scopus review of documents that cited the "noncanonical IDH" OR "non-R132" mutated glioma in the title or abstract. There were 10 total articles. The figure shows the overlay visualization of the authors and the connections between the authors. The colors demonstrate the year of publication, and the size of the circle displays the weight of the author in terms of the number of published documents in this domain. The lines indicate the connectivity between the authors. For instance, Franceschi [29] was involved in 3 documents and had a total of 17 connections (**Figure 5b**). The same applies to Brandes (**Figure 5c**) [30]. Nevertheless, Angelini [31] for instance was involved in one document only (smaller circle) and had only a total link of eight (**Figure 5d**).

3.2 Age distribution in noncanonical IDH-mutated glioma

There were only three articles that reported the significance of the age distribution in the IDH-mutated gliomas [5, 29, 32]. Posetsch and Franceschi and their colleagues reported a younger age for patients harboring all types of IDH1 noncanonical mutations as compared to IDH1 canonical mutation (median age 35 vs. 43 years and

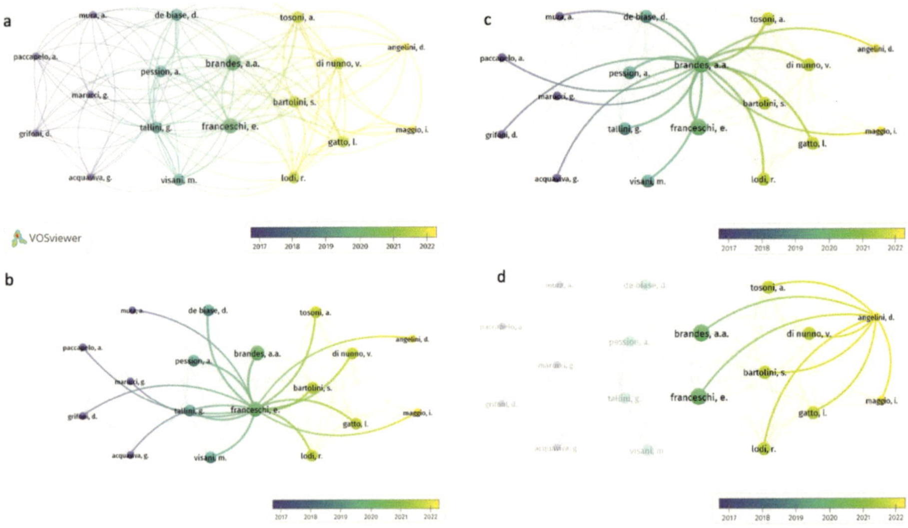

Figure 5.
The overlay visualization of noncanonical IDH-mutated article's authors (Scopus indexed).

29 vs. 39 years) [29, 32]. Yet, Hartmann et al. reported a significantly younger age only for patients with IDH1 R132C noncanonical mutations with a median age of 34.9 vs. 42.9 years [5].

3.3 Patient outcome

A recently published systematic review and meta-analysis aimed to evaluate the clinical role of IDH noncanonical mutations documented a possible favorable prognostic role for IDH noncanonical mutations [33]. Another study reported a prolonged survival for patients with IDH1 noncanonical mutations as compared to IDH canonical mutation [29]. However, two other studies reported no association between the noncanonical mutations and the survival rate [23, 32]. Nevertheless, the later studies were lacking the reporting of the survival hazard ratio (HR) with the confidence interval.

3.4 Current therapy and future direction

One of the most remarkable phenomena noticed in IDH-mutated glioma is the production of 2HG. This oncometabolite was found to be involved in the activation of different cancer-associated signaling pathways in addition to tumorigenesis and tumor progression.

Targeting the mutant enzymes of the IDH1/2 has long been sought as a novel therapeutic strategy to prevent the progression of cancers harboring the IDH1/2 mutation [34]. The benefit of this targeted therapy in glioma using small-molecule inhibitors have been established by several continuing investigations [35, 36]. An example of IDH-R132H enzyme inhibitor is the compound AGI-5198, which is an allosteric, selective inhibitor inhibiting the synthesis of 2HG in mouse and human glioma cells [36, 37]. Researchers also found that mutant IDH1 promotes selective vulnerability by altering NAD+ supply [38]. The expression of Naprt1 (a rate-limiting enzyme within the NAD+ salvage system) can be reduced by the introduction of mutant IDH1 and results in more depressed basal NAD+ levels. Exposure to NAMPT inhibitors thus effectively hinders both NAD+ salvage pathways in IDH1-mutant cells, resulting in a metabolic crisis that activates the energy sensor AMPK and initiation of autophagy. They also highlighted that reduced NAD+ salvage plays a major role in the mechanism of NAMPT inhibitor hypersensitivity [38].

Ongoing phase I/II clinical trials are currently in progress to assess the safety of different IDH-mutant inhibitors in glioma patients. Early clinical results suggest that the IDH1-mutant inhibitor AG-120 (ivosidenib) is an example of an IDH1-mutant inhibitor that is satisfactorily accepted in patients with previously treated non-contrast-enhancing gliomas [39].

4. Conclusion

Noncanonical IDH mutations are observed in only a limited number of all gliomas and are exceedingly rare among glioblastomas. It is unclear if tumors with these mutations are associated with more favorable outcome compared to canonical IDH mutants. Further study of the natural history of noncanonical IDH-mutant cancerous gliomas and analysis of the treatment effect of IDH mutation-specific targeted therapy is needed in the future.

5. Recommended articles

The recommended articles are [1, 4, 5, 15, 24, 29, 31, 32, 34, 39].

Abbreviations

LGG	low-grade glioma
IDH	isocitrate dehydrogenase
WHO	World Health Organization
NADPH	nicotinamide adenine dinucleotide phosphate
aKG	alpha-ketoglutarate

Author details

Tariq D. Al-Saadi[1,2] and Roberto J. Diaz[1,2]*

1 Faculty of Medicine, McGill University, Montreal, Canada

2 Department of Neurology and Neurosurgery, Montreal Neurological Institute, McGill University, Montreal, Canada

*Address all correspondence to: roberto.diaz@mcgill.ca

References

[1] Louis DN, Perry A, Wesseling P, et al. The 2021 WHO classification of tumors of the central nervous system: A summary. Neuro-Oncology. 2021;**23**(8):1231-1251. DOI: 10.1093/neuonc/noab106

[2] Schmidt MC, Antweiler S. Urban N et al impact of genotype and morphology on the prognosis of glioblastoma. Journal of Neuropathology and Experimental Neurology. 2002;**61**:321-328

[3] Boots-Sprenger SHE et al. Significance of complete 1p/19q co-deletion, IDH1 mutation and MGMT promoter methylation in gliomas: Use with caution. Modern Pathology. 2013;**26**(7):922-929

[4] Yan H, Parsons DW, Jin G, et al. IDH1 and IDH2 mutations in gliomas. The New England Journal of Medicine. 2009;**360**:765-773

[5] Hartmann C, Meyer J, Balss J, et al. Type and frequency of IDH1 and IDH2 mutations are related to astrocytic and oligodendroglial differentiation and age: A study of 1,010 diffuse gliomas. Acta Neuropathologica. 2009;**118**(4):469-474. DOI: 10.1007/s00401-009-0561-9

[6] Nobusawa S, Watanabe T, Kleihues P, Ohgaki H. IDH1 mutations as molecular signature and predictive factor of secondary glioblastomas. Clinical Cancer Research. 2009;**15**:6002-6007

[7] van den Bent MJ, Dubbink HJ, Marie Y, et al. IDH1 and IDH2 mutations are prognostic but not predictive for outcome in anaplastic oligodendroglial tumors: A report of the European Organization for Research and Treatment of cancer brain tumor group. Clinical Cancer Research. 2010;**16**:1597-1604

[8] Parsons DW, Jones S, Zhang X, et al. An integrated genomic analysis of human glioblastoma multiforme. Science. 2008;**321**(5897):1807-1812. DOI: 10.1126/science.1164382

[9] Sanson M, Marie Y, Paris S, Idbaih A, Laffaire J, Ducray F, et al. Isocitrate dehydrogenase 1 codon 132 mutation is an important prognostic biomarker in gliomas. Journal of Clinical Oncology. 2009;**27**:4150-4154

[10] Weller M, Felsberg J, Hartmann C, Berger H, Steinbach JP, Schramm J, et al. Molecular predictors of progression-free and overall survival in patients with newly diagnosed glioblastoma: A prospective translational study of the german glioma network. Journal of Clinical Oncology. 2009;**27**(34):5743-5750. DOI: 10.1200/JCO.2009.23.0805

[11] Wick W, Hartmann C, Engel C, Stoffels M, Felsberg J, Stockhammer F, et al. NOA-04 randomized phase III trial of sequential radiochemotherapy of anaplastic glioma with procarbazine, lomustine, and vincristine or temozolomide. Journal of Clinical Oncology. 2009;**27**(35):5874-5880. DOI: 10.1200/JCO.2009.23.6497

[12] Metellus P, Coulibaly B, Colin C, et al. Absence of IDH mutation identifies a novel radiologic and molecular subtype of WHO grade II gliomas with dismal prognosis. Acta Neuropathologica. 2011;**120**:719-729

[13] Dubbink HJ, Taal W, van Marion R, Kros JM, van Heuvel I, Bromberg JE, et al. IDH1 mutations in low-grade astrocytomas predict survival but not response to temozolomide. Neurology. 2009;**73**(21):1792-1795. DOI: 10.1212/WNL.0b013e3181c34ace

[14] Kim YH, Nobusawa S, Mittelbronn M, Paulus W, Brokinkel B, Keyvani K, et al. Molecular classification of low-grade diffuse gliomas. The American Journal of Pathology. 2010;**177**(6):2708-2714. DOI: 10.2353/ajpath.2010.100680

[15] Thon N, Eigenbrod S, Kreth S, Lutz J, Tonn JC, Kretzschmar H, et al. IDH1 mutations in grade II astrocytomas are associated with unfavorable progression-free survival and prolonged postrecurrence survival. Cancer. 2011;**118**(2):452-460. DOI: 10.1002/cncr.26298

[16] Ahmadi R, Stockhammer F, Becker N, Hohlen K, Misch M, Christians A, et al. No prognostic value of IDH1 mutations in a series of 100 WHO grade II astrocytomas. Journal of Neuro-Oncology. 2012;**109**(1):15-22. DOI: 10.1007/s11060-012-0863-y

[17] Di Carlo DT et al. Idh wild-type who grade ii diffuse low-grade gliomas. A heterogeneous family with different outcomes. Systematic review and meta-analysis. Neurosurgical Review. 2020;**43**(2):383-395. DOI: 10.1007/s10143-018-0996-3

[18] Bleeker FE, Lamba S, Leenstra S, et al. IDH1 mutations at residue p.R132 (IDH1(R132)) occur frequently in high-grade gliomas but not in other solid tumors. Human Mutation. 2009;**30**:7-11

[19] Zhao S, Lin Y, Xu W, et al. Glioma-derived mutations in IDH1 dominantly inhibit IDH1 catalytic activity and induce HIF-1alpha. Science. 2009;**324**:261-265

[20] Dang L, White DW, Gross S, et al. Cancer-associated IDH1 mutations produce 2-hydroxyglutarate. Nature. 2009;**462**:739-744

[21] Xu W, Yang H, Liu Y, et al. Oncometabolite 2-hydroxyglutarate is a competitive inhibitor of alpha-ketoglutarate-dependent dioxygenases. Cancer Cell. 2011;**19**:17-30

[22] Alzial G, Renoult O, Paris F, Gratas C, Clavreul A, Pecqueur C. Wild-type isocitrate dehydrogenase under the spotlight in glioblastoma. Oncogene. 2022;**41**(5):613-621. DOI: 10.1038/s41388-021-02056-1

[23] Gravendeel LA, Kloosterhof NK, Bralten LB, van Marion R, Dubbink HJ, Dinjens W, et al. Segregation of non-p.R132H mutations in IDH1 in distinct molecular subtypes of glioma. Human Mutation. 2010;**31**:E1186-E1199

[24] Balss J, Meyer J, Mueller W, et al. Analysis of the IDH1 codon 132 mutation in brain tumors. Acta Neuropathologica. 2008;**116**:597-602

[25] Ichimura K, Pearson DM, Kocialkowski S, Backlund LM, Chan R, Jones DT, et al. IDH1 mutations are present in the majority of common adult gliomas but rare in primary glioblastomas. Neuro-Oncology. 2009;**11**:341-347

[26] Watanabe T, Nobusawa S, Kleihues P, Ohgaki H. IDH1 mutations are early events in the development of astrocytomas and oligodendrogliomas. The American Journal of Pathology. 2009;**174**:1149-1153

[27] Paschka P, Schlenk RF, Gaidzik VI, Habdank M, Kronke J, Bullinger L, et al. IDH1 and IDH2 mutations are frequent genetic alterations in acute myeloid leukemia and confer adverse prognosis in cytogenetically normal acute myeloid leukemia with NPM1 mutation without FLT3 internal tandem duplication. Journal of Clinical Oncology. 2010;**28**:3636-3643

[28] Visani M, Acquaviva G, Marucci G, et al. Non-canonical IDH1 and IDH2

mutations: A clonal and relevant event in an Italian cohort of gliomas classified according to the 2016 World Health Organization (WHO) criteria. Journal of Neuro-Oncology. 2017;**135**:245-254. DOI: 10.1007/s11060-017-2571-0

[29] Franceschi, Enrico, Dario De Biase, Vincenzo Di Nunno, Annalisa Pession, Alicia Tosoni, Lidia Gatto, Giovanni Tallini, et al. 2021. "Idh1 Non-Canonical Mutations and Survival in Patients with Glioma." *Diagnostics (Basel, Switzerland)* 11 (2). doi:10.3390/diagnostics11020342

[30] Brandes AA, Tosoni A, Cavallo G, Reni M, Franceschi E, Bonaldi L, et al. Correlations between O6-methylguanine DNA methyltransferase promoter methylation status, 1p and 19q deletions, and response to temozolomide in anaplastic and recurrent Oligodendroglioma: A prospective GICNO study. Journal of Clinical Oncology. 2006;**24**:4746-4753. DOI: 10.1200/JCO.2006.06.3891

[31] Nunno Vincenzo V et al. Clinical and molecular features of patients with gliomas Harboring Idh1 non-canonical mutations: A systematic review and meta-analysis. Advances in Therapy. 2021;**39**(1):165-177. DOI: 10.1007/s12325-021-01977-3.

[32] Poetsch L, Network P, Bronnimann C, Loiseau H, Frénel JS, Siegfried A, et al. Characteristics of IDH-mutant gliomas with non-canonical IDH mutation. Journal of Neuro-Oncology. 2021;**151**:279-286

[33] Mondesir J, Willekens C, Touat M, de Botton S. IDH1 and IDH2 mutations as novel therapeutic targets: Current perspectives. Journal of Blood Medicine. 2016;**7**:171

[34] Kadiyala P et al. Inhibition of 2-hydroxyglutarate elicits metabolic reprogramming and mutant IDH1 glioma immunity in mice. The Journal of Clinical Investigation. 2021;**131**(4):139542

[35] Urban DJ et al. Assessing inhibitors of mutant isocitrate dehydrogenase using a suite of pre-clinical discovery assays. Scientific Reports. 2017;**7**(1):12758

[36] Turcan S et al. IDH1 mutation is sufficient to establish the glioma hypermethylator phenotype. Nature. 2012;**483**(7390):479-483

[37] Tateishi K et al. Extreme vulnerability of Idh1 mutant cancers to Nad depletion. Cancer Cell. 2015;**28**(6):773-784. DOI: 10.1016/j.ccell.2015.11.006

[38] Mellinghoff IK et al. ACTR-46. AG-120, a first-in-class mutant IDH1 inhibitor in patients with recurrent or progressive IDH1 mutant glioma: Updated results from the phase 1 non-enhancing glioma population. Neuro-Oncology. 2017;**19**(suppl_6):vi10-vi11

[39] Waitkus, Matthew S, et al. "Biological role and therapeutic potential of Idh mutations in cancer." Cancer Cell, vol. 34, no. 2, 2018, pp. 186-195., doi:10.1016/j.ccell.2018.04.011.

Chapter 7

New Approaches in the Treatment of Glioblastoma Multiforme

Lee Roy Morgan, Branko S. Jursic, Marcus Ware and Roy S. Weiner

Abstract

Central nervous system (CNS) malignancies are rare, but commonly fatal and glioblastoma (GBM) is the most common of the primary brain tumors. In contrast to metastatic malignancies involving the CNS, which have external blood supplies that develop when the malignant cells penetrate the blood-brain-barrier (BBB), GBM generates its own intracerebral neovascular support system. Thus, the therapeutic issues as discussed herein review the development of drugs and therapeutics that will penetrate the BBB and are cytotoxic *to* GBM and other brain tumors. Since GBM is a CNS malignancy with minimal effective therapeutic options available, designing drugs and therapeutics as treatment for this malignancy that penetrate, but do not disrupt the BBB is the goal of this chapter. 4-Demethylcholesteryl-4-penclomedine (DM-CHOC-PEN) was designed and developed because of its lipophilic properties that *would* potentiate crossing the BBB and penetrate brain tumors. The drug has now completed Phase I/II clinical trial in humans with primary brain malignancies *demonstrating* objective responses in GBM. In addition, preliminary experiences with naturally occurring polyphenols—curcumin, quercetin, catechins and phloretin and derivatives—are reviewed as potential naturally occurring anti-glioblastoma agents.

Keywords: temozolamide (TMZ), glioblastoma multiforme (GBM), recurrence, radiosurgery, chemotherapy, 4 demethyl-4-cholesteryloxycarbonylpenclomedine, DM-CHOC-PEN, and multimodality treatment

1. Introduction

Approximately 48% of all primary malignant brain tumors are glioblastoma multiforme (GBM), and more than 10,000 people will succumb to the disease in the US each year alone (1). The 5-year relative survival rate for these patients with GBM increased only from 23%, as reported in the mid-1970s, to 36% in the early 2000s [1, 2]. Adding to the complexity of the disease is the cancer's ability to rapidly mutate, so even in different locations in the brain of the same patient, GBMs encompass a mosaic of cancer cell types, posing a major challenge for tumor-targeted therapy [3]. Thus, despite the advancements in the management and treatments for malignancies which we review here, the prognosis for long term survival for glioblastoma (GBM) continue to be dismal [4].

2. History of the disease

For metastatic cancers involving the brain there are cancer-associated-breaks and related neovascular channels in the BBB that allow drug penetration [4]. However, GBMs commonly lack facilitating neovascular changes in the BBB and must rely on drug lipophilicity and/or target transport mechanisms for anti-cancer agents to penetrate the BBB. GBM responses to the present therapies available are dismal and new therapies that penetrate the BBB are needed. Classically GBMs induce their own intracerebral neovascular blood supply within the brain that supplies the tumor mass with blood and nutrients—no extra-BBB blood supplies are involved; thus, the principle issue is penetrating the BBB [2, 5].

The major goal of this article is to initiate new ideas in the management of GBM, as well as other types of CNS malignancy. The core therapeutic challenge is to obtain long term objective responses through mechanisms involving drug penetration of the brain *via* the BBB and utilizing the changes in the chemistry of GBM malignancies.

In the treatment of GBMs, for drug and therapy modalities to be effective, there must be small/diffuse vascular accesses/openings or breaks (surgery sites), or lipophilic target pathways through the BBB secondary to interactions with a receptor or transport mechanism for penetration of the brain and CNS tumor masses [6].

Needless to mention, many treatment approaches that should be useful therapies for GBM also possess toxicities secondary to particle size and/or interaction with inappropriate sites—locally or distant—and unable to reach the tumor masses, and are not employed.

GBM has not been associated with smoking or any other lethal factors. The tumor remains the most common and lethal form of CNS brain cancers and one of the most difficult to manage.

In summary, since GBMs do not induce neoplastic blood support systems, drug and immune tumor targets, immune therapies do not easily penetrate the BBB and GBMs have not responded well to systemic therapies and new therapies should be aggressively evaluated [1, 2, 7, 8].

3. Current drug therapies

The O^6-methylguanine-DNA-methyltransferase (MGMT) gene encodes for an important DNA repair protein which acts by removing alkyl products from the O^6 position on guanine. A so-called “suicide enzyme,” following removal of the alkyl groups, the newly alkylated MGMT protein, is then marked for degradation by ubiquitination [8]. Proper functioning of the gene is important for maintaining cell integrity. Epigenetic silencing of the MGMT gene by methylation of the CpG islands of the promoter region has been shown to correlate with loss of gene transcription and protein expression [9, 10]. Loss of expression of the MGMT protein results in decreased DNA repair and retention of alkyl groups, thereby allowing alkylating agents such as carmustine (BCNU), lomustine (CCNU), and temozolomide to have greater efficacy in patients whose tumors exhibit hypermethylation of the MGMT promoter, reducing the MGMT protein concentration [10–13].

3.1 Temozolamide

Temozolamide (Temadar, TMZ) (**Figure 1**) continues to be the standard therapy +/− radiation for GBMs. However, the benefit of the therapy has been less than

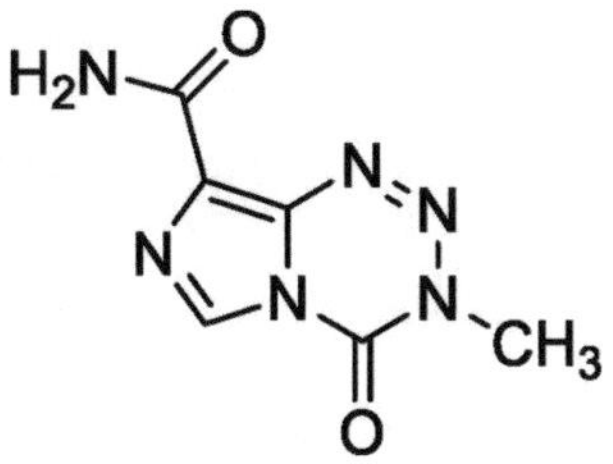

Figure 1.
Temozolamide (Temadar, TMZ).

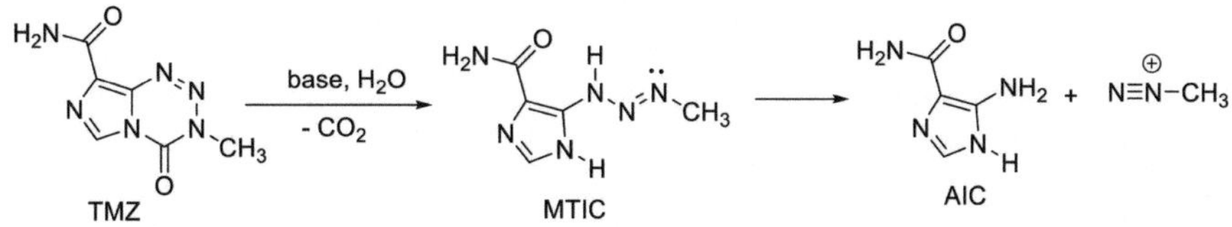

Figure 2.
Mechanism of action for TMZ.

desirable since methylated *MGMT*- GBMs are most sensitive, as well uncommon [11–13]. Once TMZ passes through the BBB its mechanism of action is as follows:

TMZ is quickly and almost completely absorbed from the gut, and readily penetrates the blood– brain barrier and brain. The concentration of drug in the cerebrospinal fluid is approximately 30% of the concentration in the blood plasma. Intake with food decreases maximal plasma concentrations by 33%. TMZ is a prodrug; it is hydrolyzed at physiological pH to 3-methyl-(triazen-1) imidazole-4-carboxamide (MTIC), which further splits into monomethyl hydrazine—likely the active methylating agent—and 5-aminoimidazole-4-carboxamide (AIC) [13].

TMZ also induces breaks in the BBB and transforms several tumor marker receptors [13]. The therapeutic benefit of temozolomide depends on its ability to alkylate/methylate DNA, which most often occurs at the N^7 or O^6 positions of guanine residues *via* the methyl hydrazine metabolite (**Figure 2**).

The time of day that the drug is administered may be of importance. Drug administered early in the AM appears to be more active than when administered in the evening. Since the drug is lipophilic and morning meals are commonly high in lipids may be a possible explanation.

4. Core therapeutic challenges to obtaining long term objective tumor responses

There are numerous challenges to be considered when designing new drugs as therapy for primary CNS malignancies.

- Transport of drugs through the BBB. Although the use of drugs and protocols that are designed to include tumor target markers is becoming popular, the penetration of the BBB is still an issue.

- For focal lesions, surgical resection followed by TMZ plus radiation is acceptable practice.

- The presence of the PD-1 surface antigen in some GBM tumors has proven that the presence of tumor target check point markers may have a role in combination therapy when present. The latter approach is of major interest for future trials.

- Developing new drugs that are small or have unique transport mechanisms

- Identifying surface receptors on the BBB that will assist with drug transport into the brain and GBMs.

- Taking advantage of the BBB's lipophilicity is still a viable option that must be considered in drug/therapeutic design.

Due to the Warburg-associated inductive effects present, cancer cells utilize glucosamine in contrast to glucose in the Krebs cycle for energy [3, 4, 14]. Although breaks in the BBB similar to those seen in metastatic cancers involving the CNS are not observed in the brains with GBM present, microneovascular support is present in the GBM associated para-cerebral environment.

There are new reports regarding tumor-target marker agents that are demonstrating activity against target-negative GBMs, however, more new agents that do not require a tumor-target marker for activity are needed [1]. Drug design needs to take advantage of natural target mechanisms *via* the BBB [3].

In this chapter we discuss several interesting non-tumor target designed agents [2].

4.1 Designing agents to diffuse through the BBB

4-Demethylcholesteryl penclomedine (DM-CHOC-PEN) (**Figure 3.**) was designed and developed because of its lipophilic properties that was anticipated to potentiate crossing the BBB and penetrating brain tumors [3]. The basic nucleus penclomedine was developed at the NCI- Southern Research Institute as treatment for brain tumors, but was withdrawn from clinical trials because of CNS toxicities (seizures) [14, 15]. The cholesteryl ester was added to the penclomedine nucleus at DEKK-TEC (see below) to increase lipophilicity [1].

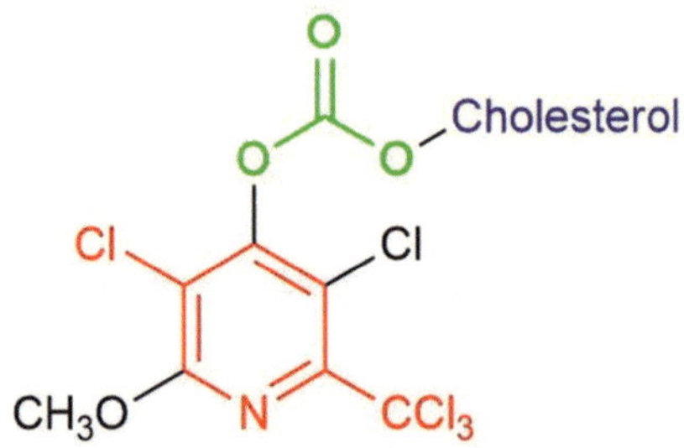

- Pyridine ring w/ bi-functional alkylating groups - a *bis*-alkylator – red
- Lipophilic cholesterol moiety - blue
- Carbonate - high energy linker – green
- Binds to DNA's cytosine/guanine nucleotides in DNA *via* replacements of chlorine groups at positions - 2 and 5.

Figure 3.
DM-CHOC-PEN and functional moieties. [3, 14–16].

4.2 DM-CHOC-PEN—Mechanism of action

During Phase I clinical pharmacodynamics studies when DM-CHOC-PEN was administrated IV, the drug was identified associated with erythrocytes (~50%), which is considered to be the mechanism by which it enters the cerebral circulation (**Figure 3**) and, therefore, available for transport into the tumor bed and the cancer cells resident therein [1, 4, 6]. The drug has been identified in intracranial metastatic NSCLC tissue [1,].

Glucosamine is a component of the mucopolysaccharides that involved in the chemistry of red blood cell (RBCs) surface membranes and DM-CHOC-PEN has an affinity for glucosamine (**Figure 4**) [4]. Association of DM-CHOC-PEN with

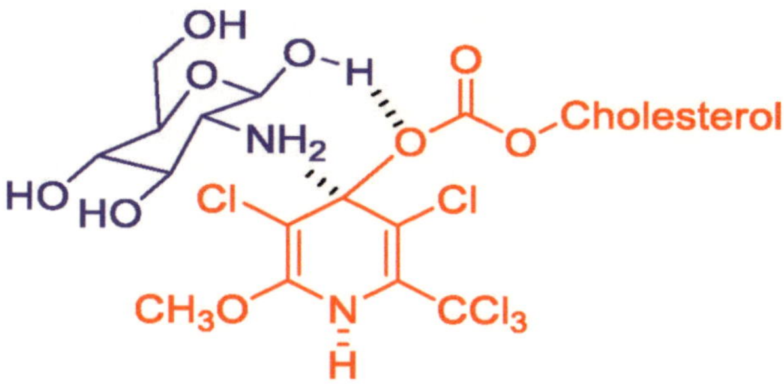

Figure 4.
DM-CHOC-PEN transport into CNS with glucosamine on RBC surfaces.

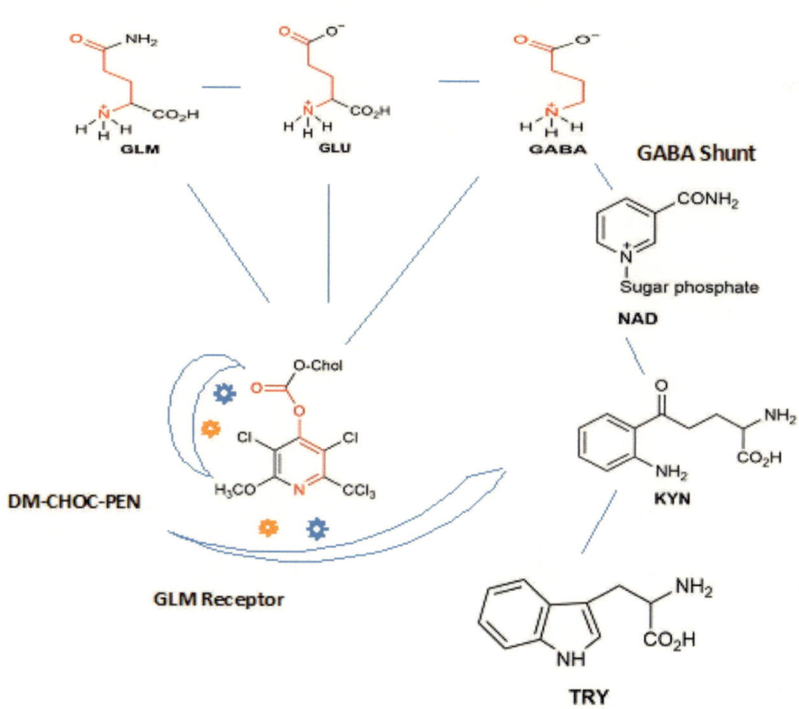

Figure 5.
DM-CHOC-PEN's transport into cells—Similarity with glutamine—Similarity with glutamine. NAD = pyridine nucleotides, KYN = kynurenine, and TRY = tryptophan.

glucosamine allows the drug to form complexes with the surface of RBCs and be transported into the brain (**Figure 4**).

After transportation through the BBB and into the brain, DM-CHOC-PEN is transported into cancer cells with glutamine because of similarities with that structure (**Figure 5**).

Figure 6 represents a possible complex between DM-CHOC-PEN and glutamine that can occur after the former penetrates through the BBB into the brain and transported into GBM cells. Cancer cells, especially GBM, utilize glutamine as a source of C & H for ATP synthesis [4]. The Warburg effect is present in the GBM cells, thus glucose is not utilized for ATP synthesis [4].

Figure 7 continues to be the best explanation of how DM-CHOC-PEN penetrates the BBB and intracerebral GBMs [2–6]. This mechanism was proposed by our group several years ago and continues to be a working model [2–6].

Table 1 reviews the results reported during Phase I/II clinical trial with DM-CHOC-PEN in primary brain tumors in adults [5, 17]. Unfortunately, as noted in **Table 1**, DM-CHOC-PEN is not active in all GBMs treated to date [5, 17].

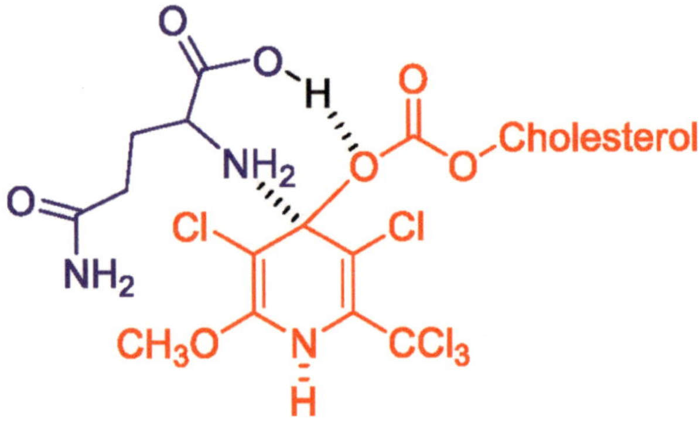

Figure 6.
Complex of DM-CHOC-PEN with glutamine.

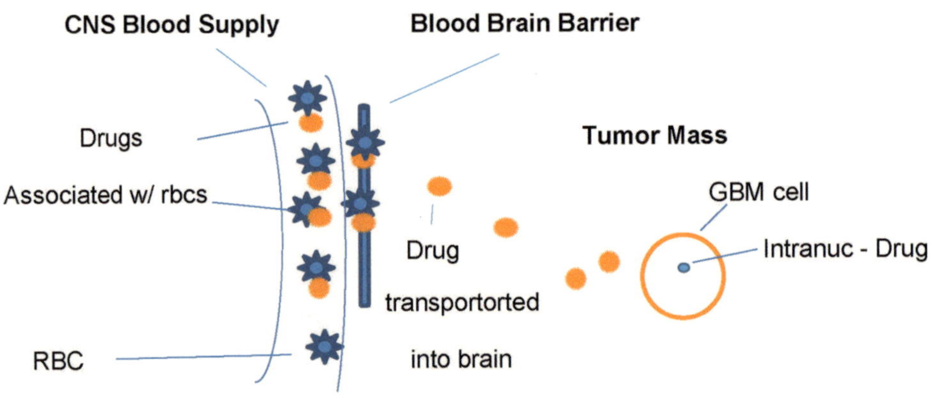

Figure 7.
Overview—Mechanism of action for DM-CHOC-PEN [2–6].

Cancer type	No. of subjects	DM-CHOC-PEN doses every 21 days (per kg)***	No. of responders (NED)	OS (OS ≥6 mo)
Glioblastoma*,**	11*,**	39, 85.8 or 98.7	2*,**	(6–13 mo.)*,**
Oligoastrocytoma*,**	2*,**	85.8 & 98.7	1**	3
Astrocytoma**	1**	85.8	1**	58 mo.

**Phase I.*
***Phase II.*
****Method of Treatment—DM-CHOC-PEN (mg/m²) was infused IV over 4 hr. every 21 days to each patient—aged 37–78 y/o [5, 17]; NED—no evidence of disease [5, 17].*

Table 1.
Primary brain tumor response to DM-CHOC-PEN therapy by cancer type-during phase I/II trials.

During the trials, tumor tissue from several patients that received the drug were obtained and analyzed. Adducts were identified that support the DNA sites that are alkylated by DM-CHOC- PEN and do not involve O^6-guanine sites, thus DM-CHOC-PEN should be active in most types of GBMs (**Figure 8**).

4.3 Immunotherapy targets

The principle challenge to the treatment of GBM, as exists for all tumors involving the CNS, is the difficulty to penetrate the blood brain barrier (BBB) and deliver drugs into the CNS and GBM [1]. In GBM, the BBB is weakened, allowing immune cells from the periphery to penetrate the CNS. However, GBM tends to selectively attract or turn immune cells that infiltrate the tumor into immune suppressive cells which lack anti-cancer activity [1].

Most immunotherapies target the reactivation of effector T-cells, which attack and eliminate cancer cells. But, in GBM, the effector T-cell infiltration is very low, secondary to the above inhibitory immune suppressive properties, and there is an abundance of immunosuppressive myeloid cells and a low concentration of cytotoxic cells [1]. Thus, developing immune modulators that prevent impairment of cytotoxic lymphocytes is of potential importance and could be useful alone or with cytotoxic agents [1].

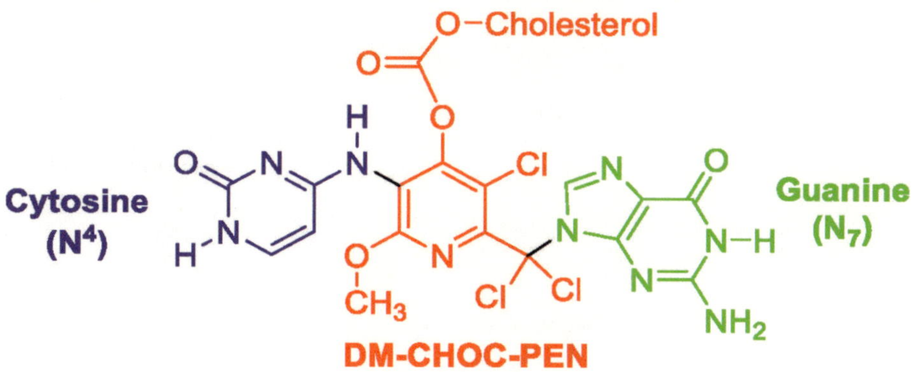

Figure 8.
An adduct has been identified in GBM tumor tissue obtained from patients post-DM-CHOC-PEN therapy.

4.4 Phenolic anti-glioblastoma compounds

Medical application of phenolic compounds is well documented through decades [18]. Current research trends are exploring the senotherapeutic activity of these agents [19–22]. The elevation of the presence of the senescent cells seems to be the central part of aging and age- related diseases including cancer [23]. There are increasing numbers of reports referring to the use of plant extracts that are phenolic compounds in ant-glioblastoma studies [24, 25].

Considering that targeted therapy for glioblastoma has had promising results *in vitro* monolayer cultures, the results from preclinical and clinical trials has been disappointing partly due to the poor blood brain barrier penetration. There currently is more emphasis on application of natural phenols that are able to penetrate the BBB as alternatives for glioblastoma treatment [26, 27].

Anti-glioblastoma activity has been investigated in depth for several phenols—curcumin, quercetin, catechins, and phloretin, to name a few [28–31]. In two-dimensional cell line tests, the above demonstrated that their IC50 values were ~ 50 μM concentration [32]. In addition, less than 2% of low molecular weight organic molecules crossed the BBB. For some phenolic compounds that cross the BBB a positive anti-cancer effect was observed [33]. However, the presence of phenolic compounds in the brain has been confirmed in only a few reports.

Figure 9 reviews natural phenols that have been extracted from plant purified and tested for anti-glioblastoma activity; majority of the phenols were glycosylated [34]. It has been well demonstrated that glycosylated organic compounds easily cross BBB [34, 35]. A perfect example of a glycosylated phenol that crosses the blood-brain barrier is curcumin oligosaccharide.

The IC50 value for curcumin after 24 hr. in a U87 cell culture was 10 μM and 13 μM for cultures with T98 cells [34]. However, in pre-clinical mice studies there was no detectable amount of curcumin in the brain or in T98 GBM cells after its intraperitoneal injection (IP). On the other hand, when curcumin gluco-oligosaccharide was injected I.V. to mice, 18 ng of curcumin per 1 g of brain tissue was determined. In addition, 5 days after the IP injection of the oligosaccharide into C57BL mice bearing intracerebral brain tumors, complete responses were observed [36].

This suggests that two-dimensional cell test results for anti-glioblastoma oligosaccharide conjugates can be translated to animal models. With this in mind phenolic

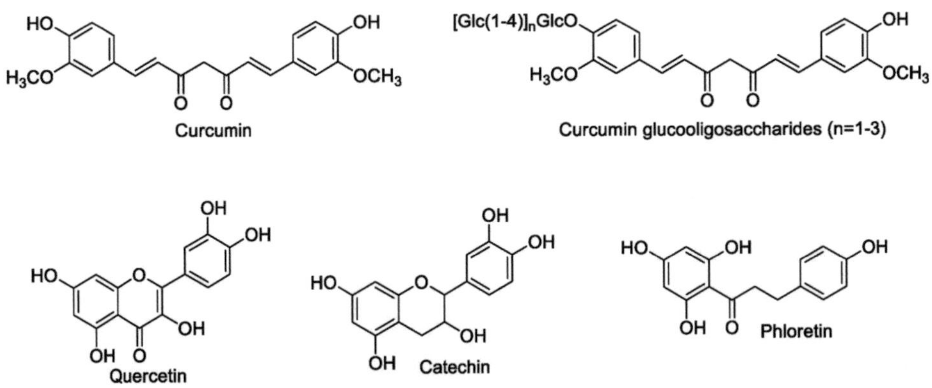

Figure 9.
Structures of naturally occurring anti-glioblastoma phenols.

Phenol	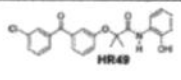	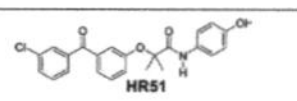	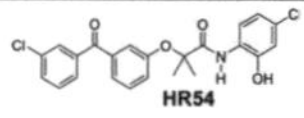
CV	0 ± 0.27	1.1 ± 1.42	1.89 ± 1.56
VLR	1 (logP = 5.49)	1 (logP = 5.49	1 (logP = 6.09)
BBB_Score	2.24/6 (37%)	2.24/6 (37%)	2.38/6 (40%)
CNS_ MPO	3.14/6 (52%)	3.14/6 (52%)	2.90/6 (48%)

*GBM cell line LN229 growing in culture was employed as the test system. Test compounds were evaluated in the 100 nanomolar—100 μM conc. Ranges VLR = violations Lipinski's 5 rule; CV = Cell viability (% of control) mean ± SD at 25 μM; VLR = violations Lipinski's 5 rule; BBB Score = Blood-brain barrier score [38]; CNS-MPO = central nervous system—multiparameter optimization [39]. *Fenofibric acid (2 microgm/mL) was used as a standard and demonstrated no activity in culture.*

Table 2.
Comparison of cell (LN229) viability and compute brain penetration ability for fenofibric acid phenols HR49, HR51, and HR54.*

derivatives of fenofibric acid are being evaluated in clinical trials to document their activity as anti-GBM agents [37].

A number of phenolic fenofibric acid derivative were synthesized and tested against the glioblastoma LN229 cell lines. There were numerous fenofibric acid derivatives that had IC50 values between 1 and 10 μM (see below).

Several of the derivatives are listed in **Table 2**. According to computational studies, a majority of these compounds have high lipophilicity (logP >5), but their probability of crossing the BBB was below 50%. Studies *in vivo* (mice) indicated that the phenols did cross the BBB and traces of the compounds were detected in the brain and GBM tissue [37]. The fenofibric acid phenols are believed to inhibit GBM proliferation *via* reducing metabolic activity (ATP production), resulting in apoptosis of GBM with cell death. This is very similar to the experiments that were performed with curcumin [32].

Thus, the development of prodrug glycosylated fenofibric phenols that inhibit GBM cellular replication appear to be a promising viable approach to penetrating the BBB and cytotoxic therapy *vs* GBM.

5. Conclusion

An attempt to review the chemistry, neuropharmacology and preliminary results—*in vitro* and *in vivo*—has been made. DM-CHOC-PEN has been studied in depth, as therapy for both metastatic and primary malignancies involving the CNS. The latter is a bi-functional alkylating agent as discussed in this paper. However, minimal information is available regarding cytotoxic mechanisms of action for the polyphenolic structures described herein. The positive responses observed and reported are support for continued studies with the poly phenols as well as initiation of a Phase III clinical trial with DM-CHOC-PEN in GBM.

Acknowledgements

Supported by—NCI/SBIR—R43/44CA132257 & NIH NIGMS 1 U54 GM104940.

Abbreviations

SRS	Stereo radiosurgery.
TMZ	Temozolamide.
DM-CHOC-PEN	4-demethyl-4-cholesteryloxycarbonylpenclomedine.

Author details

Lee Roy Morgan[1]*, Branko Jursic[2], Marcus Ware[3] and Roy S. Weiner[4]

1 DEKK-TEC, Inc., New Orleans, Louisiana, USA

2 Department of Chemistry, University of New Orleans, New Orleans, Louisiana, USA

3 Department of Oncology Neurosurgery, Ochsner Medical Center, New Orleans, Louisiana, USA

4 Department of Medicine, Section of Hematology and Medical Oncology, Tulane Medical Center, New Orleans, Louisiana, USA

*Address all correspondence to: lrm1579@aol.com

References

[1] Yun K. Researchers identify immunotherapy target to combat glioblastoma. Oncology Times. 2022;**18**:44. DOI: 10.1097/01.COT.0000831336.44021.26

[2] Morgan LR, Struck RF, Waud WR, LeBlanc B, Rodgers AH, Jursic BS. Carbonate and carbamate derivatives of 4-demethylpenclomedine as novel anticancer agents. Cancer Chemotherapy and Pharmacology. 2009;**64**:829-836. DOI: 10.1007/s00280-009-0933-9

[3] Morgan LR, Struck RF, Waud WR, Jursic BS, Serota D, Papagiannis C, et al. Carbonate and carbamate derivatives of 4-demethylpenclomedine as novel anticancer agents. Molecular Targets and Cancer Therapeutics. 2007;**6**:A280

[4] Morgan LR, Struck RF, Waud WR, Jursic BS, Serota D, Papagiannis C, et al. Carbonate and carbamate derivatives of 4-demethylpenclomedine as novel anticancer agents. Cancer Chemotherapy and Pharmacology. 2009;**64**:618-623

[5] Weiner RS, Friedlander P, Gordon C, Saenger Y, Ware RL, Mahmood T, et al. Results of phase II cancer clinical trials for 4-demethyl-4-cholesteryoxycarbo nylpenclomedine (DM-CHOC-PEN). Proceedings of the American Association for Cancer Research. 2016;**58**:236

[6] Weiner R, Ware M, Friedlander P, Gordon C, Saenger Y, Mahmood T, et al. A first-in-humans phase I cancer clinical trial for 4-demethyl-4-cholesteryloxycarbonyl-penclomedine (DM-CHOC-PEN) in humans. Cancer Research. 2013;**73**:73

[7] Struck RF, Tiwari A, Friedman HS, Keir S, Morgan LR, Waud WR. Acyl derivatives of demethylpenclomedine, an antitumor-active, non-neurotoxic metabolites of penclomedine. Cancer Chemotherapy and Pharmacology, 2001;**48**(1):47-52. DOI: 10.1007/s002800

[8] Srivenugopal KS, Yuan XH, Friedman HS, Ali-Osman F. Ubiquitination-dependent proteolysis of O^6-methylguanine-DNA methyltransferase in human and murine tumor cells following inactivation with O^6-benzylguanine or 1,3-bis(2-chloroethyl)-1-nitrosourea. Biochemistry. 1996;**35**:1328-1334

[9] Esteller M, Garcia-Foncillas J, Andion E, et al. Inactivation of the DNA-repair gene MGMT and the clinical response of gliomas to alkylating agents. New England Journal of Medicine. 2000;**343**:1350-1354

[10] Hegi ME, Diserens AC, Gorlia T, et al. MGMT gene silencing and benefit from temozolomide in glioblastoma. New England Journal of Medicine. 2005;**352**:997-1003. DOI: 10.1056/NEJMoa043331

[11] Paz MF, Yaya-Tur R, Rojas-Marcos I, et al. CpG island hypermethylation of the DNA repair enzyme methyltransferase predicts response to temozolomide in primary gliomas. Clinical Cancer Research. 2004;**10**:4933-4938. DOI: 10.1158/1078-0432.CCR-04-0392

[12] Belanich M, Pastor M, Randall T, et al. Retrospective study of the correlation between the DNA repair protein alkyl transferase and survival of brain tumor patients treated with carmustine. Cancer Research. 1996;**56**:783-788

[13] Idbaih A, Omuro A, Ducray F, Hoang-Xuan K. Molecular genetic markers as predictors of response to

chemotherapy in gliomas. Current Opinion in Oncology. 2007;**19**:606-611. DOI: 10.1097/CCO.0b013e3282f075f3

[14] Waud WR, Tiwari A, Schmid SM, Shih T-W, Strong JM, Hartman NR, et al. 4-Demethylpenclomedine, an antitumor-active, potentially non-metabolite of penclomedine. Cancer Research. 1997;**57**:815-817

[15] Jodrell DI, Bowman A, Stewart M, Dunlop N, French R, Mac Lellan A, et al. Dose-limiting neurotoxicity in a phase I study of penclomedine (NSC 388720, CRC 88-04), a synthetic alpha-picoline derivative, administered intravenously. British Journal of Cancer. 1998;**77**: 808-811. DOI: 10.1038/bjc.1998.131

[16] Morgan LR, Rodgers AH, Bastian G, Benes E, Waud WR, Jursic BS, et al. Comparative preclinical pharmacology and toxicology for 4-demethyl-4-cholesteryloxycarbonylpenclomedine (DM-CHOC-PEN): A potential neuro-alkylating agent for glioblastoma and metastatic cancers of the central nervous system. ECCO in European Journal of Cancer, Abst. 2011;**57**

[17] Morgan LR, Weiner RS, Ware ML, Bhandari M, P, Mahmood, T, Rodgers, and Friedlander. Early phase I results of 4-demethyl-4-cholesteryloxypenclomedine [DM-CHOC-PEN] in adolescent and young adult (AYA) subjects with advanced malignancies. Journal of Cancer Research Updates. 2018;7:75-78

[18] Tungmunnithum D, Thongboonyou A, Pholboon A, Yangsabai A. Flavonoids and other phenolic compounds from medicinal plants for pharmaceutical and medical aspects: An overview. Medical Overviews. 2018;**5**(3):93

[19] Li W, Qin L, Feng R, Hu G, Sun H, He Y, et al. Emerging senolytic agents derived from natural products. Mechanisms of Ageing and Development. 2019;**181**:1-6

[20] Zhu Y, Doornebal EJ, Pirtskhalava T, Giorgadze N, Wentworth M, Fuhrmann-Stroissnigg H, et al. New agents that target senescent cells: The flavone, fisetin, and the BCL-XL inhibitors, A1331852 and A1155463. Aging. 2017;**9**:955-963

[21] Xu Q, Fu Q, Li Z, et al. The flavonoid procyanidin C1 has senotherapeutic activity and increases lifespan in mice. Nature Metabolism. 2021;**3**:1706-1726

[22] Wang L, Lankhorst L, Bernards R. Exploiting senescence for the treatment of cancer. Nature Reviews Cancer. 2022;**37**:46-52

[23] ZvikasV, UrbanaviciuteI, BernotieneR, Kulakauskiene D, Morkunaite U, Balion Z, et al. Investigation of phenolic composition and anticancer properties of ethanolic extracts of japanese quince leaves. Food. 2020;**10**(1):8

[24] Vengoji R, Macha MA, Batra SK, Shonka NA. Natural products: A hope for glioblastoma patients. Oncotarget. 2018;**9**(31):221-222

[25] Gupta SV, Kizibash SH, Daniels DJ, Sarkaria JN. Editorial: Targeted therapies for glioblastoma—A critical appraisal. Frontiers in Oncology. 2019;**9**:1216

[26] Wang Y, Chen W, Shi Y, Yan C, Kong Z, Wang Y, et al. Imposing phase II and phase III clinical trials of targeted drugs for glioblastoma: Current status and Progress. Frontiers in Oncology. 2021;**11**:719

[27] Walker BC, Mittal S. Antitumor activity of curcumin in glioblastoma. International Journal of Molecular Sciences. 2020;**21**(24):943

[28] Kusaczuk M, Krętowski R, Naumowicz M, Stypułkowska A, Cechowska-Pasko M. A preliminary study of the effect of quercetin on cytotoxicity, apoptosis, and stress responses in glioblastoma cell lines. International Journal of Molecular Sciences. 2022;**23**(3):1345

[29] Cheng Z, Zhan Z, Han Y, Wang J, Wang Y, Chen X, et al. A review on anti-cancer effect of green tea catechins. Journal of Functional Foods. 2020;**74**:104

[30] Liu Y, Fan C, Pu L, et al. Phloretin induces cell cycle arrest and apoptosis of human glioblastoma cells through the generation of reactive oxygen species. Journal of Neurooncology. 2016;**128**:217-223

[31] Gersey ZC, Rodriguez GA, Barbarite E, et al. Curcumin decreases malignant characteristics of glioblastoma stem cells via induction of reactive oxygen species. BMC Cancer. 2017;**17**:99

[32] Velásquez-Jiménez D, Corella-Salazar DA, Zuñiga-Martínez BS, Domínguez-Avila JA, Montiel-Herrera M, Salazar-López NJ, et al. Phenolic compounds that cross the blood-brain barrier exert positive health effects as central nervous system antioxidants. Food & Function. 2021;**12**(21):10356-10369

[33] Zeiadeh I, Najjar A, Karaman R. Strategies for enhancing the permeation of CNS-active drugs through the blood-brain barrier: A review. Molecules. 2018;**23**(6):289

[34] Rebelo AL, Chevalier MT, Russo L, Pandit A. Role and therapeutic implications of protein glycosylation in neuroinflammation. Trends in Molecular Medicine. 2022;**28**(4):270-289

[35] Zoi V, Galani V, Vartholomatos E, Zacharopoulou N, Tsoumeleka E, Gkizas G, et al. Curcumin and radiotherapy exert synergistic anti-glioma effect *in vitro*. Biomedicine. 2021;**9**(11):1562

[36] Hamada H, Nakayama T, Shimoda K, et al. Curcumin oligosaccharides (gluco-oligosaccharides) penetrate the blood-brain barrier in mouse brain: Glycoside (polysaccharide) modification approach for brain drug delivery across the blood-brain barrier and tumor drug delivery. Natural Product Communications. 2020;**15**(11):1-4

[37] Stalinska J, Vittori C, Ingraham CH IV, et al. Anti-glioblastoma effects of phenolic variants of benzoylphenoxyacetamide (BPA) with high potential for blood brain barrier penetration. Scientific Reports. 2022;**12**:338

[38] Gupta M, Lee HJ, Barden CJ, Weaver DF. The blood-brain barrier (BBB) score. Journal of Medicinal Chemistry. 2019;**62**(21):982-983

[39] Wager TT, Hou X, Verhoest PR, Villalobos A. Central nervous system multiparameter optimization desirability: Application in drug discovery. ACS Chemical Neuroscience. 2016;**7**(6):767-775

Section 2

Treatment Targets

Chapter 8

A Role for Cardiac Glycosides in GBM Therapy

Yuchen Du, Xiao-Nan Li, Peiying Yang and Robert A. Newman

Abstract

There is a pressing need for new effective therapeutic strategies to treat glioblastoma (GBM). Cardiac glycoside compounds consisting of both cardenolides and bufadienolides have been shown to possess potent activity against GBM cell lines and in vivo GBM tumors. In addition, recent research has shown that certain cardiac glycoside compounds contribute to an additive and even synergistic manner with the standard of care GBM treatments such as radiotherapy and chemotherapy. Finally, the finding that cardiac glycosides may offer a unique role in the control of GBM stem cells offers hope for better therapeutic outcomes in treating this deadly form of brain cancer.

Keywords: cardenolides, bufadienolides, digoxin, oleandrin, *Nerium oleander*, PBI-05204, glioblastoma, radiotherapy, stem cells, Na,K-ATPase

1. Introduction

While basic and clinical research has led to better diagnostic techniques and therapeutics for the treatment of glioblastoma, unfortunately, these have translated into only a modest improvement in median survival for this disease due to a high rate of recurrence [1]. As median survival for most GBM patients from time of diagnosis is less than 15 months, the need for new therapeutic approaches is clear [1–3]. Recent studies have shown that both cardenolide and bufadienolides compounds may offer a new therapeutic strategy for the treatment of GBM either as standalone compounds or in combination with other therapeutic modalities such as radiotherapy or standard of care drugs such as temozolomide. One cardenolide compound, oleandrin, derived from *N. oleander*, has shown particular promise against human GBM tumors both in vitro and in vivo. Oleandrin is a good addition to radiotherapy and certain chemotherapeutic agents such as temozolomide. In addition, this molecule and extracts containing it, such as PBI-05204, have now been shown to provide valuable activity against GBM stem cells which, in large part, account for the treatment of resistance and disease recurrence.

2. Cardiac glycosides and GBM

Chemically, cardiac glycosides can be divided into two groups: cardenolides and bufadienolides. Bufadienolides include bufalin, gammabufotalin, marinobufagenin, and proscillaridin while common cardenolides include digoxin, digitoxin, ouabain, lanatoside C, and oleandrin [4, 5]. The action of members of both classes of compounds are known to have a role as therapeutic compounds for the treatment of congestive heart failure and, over the past decade, many of these compounds have also been reported to have the potential to treat a variety of human malignant diseases [6–9]. While high doses of cardenolides are frequently associated with cardiotoxicity, lower doses are still used for the treatment of congestive heart failure [10, 11]. In addition, low concentrations of selected cardenolides, such as oleandrin, are known to activate a precise signaling pathway or signalosome involving α-subunits of Na,K-ATPase and acting via Src-EGFR-Ras–Raf-extracellular signal-regulated kinase (ERK), Akt/Protein kinase (PK)B, and phosphoinositide 3-kinase (PI3K) to inhibit cell proliferation and survival [12, 13]. Proteomic profiling reveals upregulated PI3K-Akt–mTOR signaling across brain metastasis histology [14]. Given these are pivotal oncogenic factors for various malignancies, this represents an important new approach to the treatment of cancer. While the majority of published studies cite in vitro activity against key cancer cell lines, some, such as PBI-05204 (an extract of *N. oleander* containing oleandrin as a key active ingredient), have advanced to Phase I and II clinical trials for the treatment of patients with cancer [15, 16]. Importantly, constituents of both classes of cardiac glycoside compounds have shown promise as potential novel therapeutic agents for the treatment of GBM [17–28]. This is further supported by the result of our systematic repurposed drug screening to discover an effective therapeutic approach for the treatment of medulloblastoma. By applying a systemic biological approach including driver signaling network identification and drug functional network-based drug repositioning, we screened more than 1300 drug candidates. Among the 100 drugs predicted to be the most effective for the treatment of group 3 and 4 medulloblastoma, five cardiac glycosides including both cardenolides and bufadienolides were identified as having great potential to inhibit the growth of Group 3 and 4 medulloblastoma, which augments the therapeutic potential of cardiac glycosides in GBM [29].

2.1 Bufadienolides and GBM

Chansu is a traditional Chinese medicine and has been used for many years as a treatment for cancer. Bufalin, an active component of Chansu, is a naturally occurring compound classified as a bufadienolides and has been recognized as a specific inhibitor of Na, K-ATPase [21]. This compound has been shown to have antitumor activity against various cancers, such as liver, lung, intestinal, gastric, gynecological, and pancreatic [30]. Lan et al. point out that the sodium pump α-1 subunit of Na, K-ATPase regulates bufalin sensitivity of human glioblastoma cells through the p53 signaling pathway [20]. A novel observation by these researchers indicated that bufalin inhibits glioblastoma growth by promoting proteasomal degradation of the Na, K-ATPase α-1 subunit [31]. Additional mechanistic studies confirmed the important roles of Src and p53 signaling in mediating apoptosis. Importantly, bufalin inhibited the growth of glioma xenografts. The authors concluded that therapies targeting specific Na^+, K^+-ATPase α subunits such as α-1 and p53 signaling-mitochondrial apoptotic pathways may have the potential to treat gliomas [31].

A related bufadienolides compound, gamabufotalin, is another component of the traditional Chinese medicine Chansu and its pharmaceutical formula known as Huachansu. Yuan et al. have shown that gamabufotalin exhibited selective cytocidal effects against intractable cancer cells including glioblastoma, but minimal effects on normal peripheral blood mononuclear cells prepared from healthy volunteers [22]. Additionally, they also reported that gamabufotalin efficiently downregulated the percentage of $CD4^{+}CD25^{+}Foxp3^{+}$ regulatory T (Treg) cells, which have been considered to play a critical role in limiting antitumor immune response in the body and promoting immunological "ignorance' of cancer cells [32]. Recent research by Yuan et al. have shown that treatment of the human glioblastoma cell line U-87 with gamabufotalin produced downregulation of the expression of uPA, CA9, and upregulated the expression of TIMP3, all of which are associated with invasion/metastasis. They conclude that this molecule exhibits significant cytotoxicity against cancerous glial cells with high potency and selectivity through multiple cytotoxic signaling pathways [22].

A related bufadienolide, marinobufagenin (MBG), has also been reported to be able to inhibit glioma growth through its ability to bind to the sodium pump α-1 unit and interaction with the ERK signaling mediated mitochondrial apoptotic (MAPK/ERK) pathway [33]. MBG treatment of U87MG and U251 cells markedly inhibited α-1 subunit expression. The effect of MBG to inhibit U251 xenograft subcutaneous growth was also assessed. Mice were treated with MBG for 9 days after which tumor volume and weights were assessed. These determinations showed significant inhibition of tumor growth resulting from MBG treatment. In addition, immunohistochemical analysis of tumor tissue demonstrated a significant decrease in the activated form of p65. Taken together, the authors stated that their results indicate that MBG effectively inhibits glioma growth through ERK-mediated mitochondrial apoptotic pathways [33]. Furthermore, MBG was observed to inhibit activation of NF-κβ and expression of other proinflammatory mediators including iNOS, COX-2, TNF-α, and IL-6 suggesting anti-inflammatory activity.

Proscillaridin is a cardiac glycoside that is derived from plants of the genus Scilla and *Drimia maritima*. Denicolai et al. [28] used two human primary GBM stem cell lines (GSCs), GBM6 and GBM9 in addition to the regular GBM cells to investigate the relative potential of proscillaridin to inhibit cell growth both in vitro and in vivo. The chosen cell lines are interesting in that GBM6 cells are highly malignant whereas GBM9 cells exhibit a much lower migratory capability yet have a higher proliferation rate [28]. Proscillaridin A exerted both anti-proliferative and anti-migratory activities in these cell lines at a concentration of 0.05 μM. The authors stated that proscillaridin was more active than temozolomide which in their study did not affect the migration or proliferation rate of either GBM6 or GBM9 cells. Exploring likely mechanisms of action for proscillaridin, the authors reported that this compound induced concentration-dependent cytotoxicity through both an increase in GBM cell death and a G2/M cell phase arrest thereby impairing a GBM stem self-renewal capacity.

2.2 Cardenolides and GBM

2.2.1 Digoxin

Of all the known cardenolide compounds the most widely studied is digoxin which in the recent past was widely used for the treatment of atrial fibrillation. Its potential activity as a repurposed drug for the control of GBM, however, is less well-known. Papale et al. [34] have examined the potential role of digoxin in the control of adverse effects of GSCs. They hypothesized that GSCs express receptors that can bind alarmins released during necrosis, an event favoring GSCs migration. Alarmins are endogenous molecules that are constitutively available and released upon tissue damage and activate the immune system. Uncontrolled and excessive release of alarmins is believed to contribute to dysregulated processes seen in many inflammatory conditions such as tumorigenesis and tumor metastasis [35]. To investigate this hypothesis, GSC cell lines were kept under hypoxic conditions to determine the expression of hypoxic markers as well as receptors for advanced glycation end products. The authors reported that necrotic extracts increased migration, invasion, and cellular adhesion. Importantly, HIF-1α inhibition by digoxin prevented the response of GSCs to hypoxia. They concluded that inhibition of hypoxic pathways may represent a target for preventing brain invasion by glioblastoma stem cells [34]. Hypoxia and necrosis, with subsequent microenvironment inflammation, can be considered as two main features of growing GBM tumors and thus are believed to play a major role in determining the metastatic potential of GSCs in a tumor. The potential role of a cardenolide such as digoxin as an inhibitor of HIF-1α is intriguing as it may represent a novel means of inhibiting this master regulator in the complicated process of cellular adaptation to tumor microenvironments.

A related study of the role of hypoxia with regard to its potential to increase the expression of stem cell markers and promotion of clonogenicity of glioblastoma neurospheres was undertaken by Bar et al. [36]. They examined the effect of hypoxia on stem-like cells in glioblastoma using GBM-derived neurosphere cultures. When these were grown in 1% oxygen, HIF-1α protein levels increased dramatically as did mRNA encoding other hypoxic response genes, such as hypoxia-inducible gene-2, lysyl oxidase, and vascular endothelial growth factor. The rise in the stem-like fraction in GBM following hypoxia was paralleled by a two-fold increase in clonogenicity. The authors examined the potential of digoxin to prevent hypoxic-related events. They observed that this cardenolide suppressed HIF-1α protein expression, HIF-1α downstream targets, and slowed tumor growth in vivo. In addition, their data demonstrated that pretreatment with digoxin reduced GBM flank xenograft growth of hypoxic GBM cells. Daily intraperitoneal injections of digoxin were reported to have significantly inhibited the growth of established xenografts and suppressed the expression of vascular endothelial growth factors [36].

As stated earlier, we have shown that systemic in vivo treatment of patient-derived orthotopic xenograft (PDOX or orthotopic PDX) models of groups 3 (ICb-2555 MB) medulloblastoma that harbors c-Myc amplification and group 4 (ICb-1078 MB, that harbors an n-MYC amplification) medulloblastoma with digoxin, a member of cardiac glycoside approved for the treatment of heart failure, significantly prolonged animal survival times at plasma concentrations known to be tolerated in human. The antitumor effect of digoxin in medulloblastoma appears to be mediated by the down regulation of the Erk and Akt signaling pathway [29].

2.2.2 Digitoxin

Digitoxin is a cardiac glycoside similar in structure and effects to digoxin, though the effects are longer-lasting. This drug has been used to treat pain and inflammation associated with various diseases such as arthritis, AIDS, and atherosclerosis [23, 37, 38]. Studies have also shown that digitoxin induces growth inhibition and/or apoptosis of a variety of human cancer cells in vitro and in vivo [29]. Lee et al. examined the potential sensitizing effects of digitoxin and tumor necrosis factor-related ligand (TRAIL)-mediated apoptosis in human glioma cells [23]. TRAIL, a member of the tumor necrosis factor family, can bind to death receptors (DR4 or DR5) leading to oligomerization of the receptor's intracellular death domains and then to the recruitment of the adaptor molecule. Fas-associated death domain protein, and activation of caspases 3 and 8 [23]. However, an obstacle to effective therapy is the development of resistance to TRAIL by brain tumors. The research conducted by Lee et al. presented evidence that a combination of non-apoptosis inducing concentrations of digitoxin and TRAIL led to apoptosis of human glioma cells. Furthermore, they showed that the upregulation of DR5 expression and downregulation of the expression of survivin synergistically enhanced TRAIL-induced apoptosis by digitoxin in human glioma cells [23].

In a more recent article, researchers examined the sensitizing effects of digitoxin to TRAIL-induced apoptosis in GSCs cultured in vitro. They reported that the combination of TRAIL and digitoxin led to apoptosis of GSCs and an upregulation of DR5 expression in addition to down-regulation of surviving expression [24].

2.2.3 *Ouabain*

Ouabain, also known as g-strophanthin, is a plant-derived cardenolide that has in the past been used as an arrow poison in Africa. However, it has also been more traditionally used to treat hypotension, congestive heart failure, and some arrhythmias [39]. Interestingly, ouabain is also an endogenous molecule found in animals and humans during normal conditions and increases in concentration in response to high salt intake [40]. It has been reported that ouabain can activate multiple protein kinases such as MAPK, PKC, and phosphoinositide 3-kinase (PI3k)/Akt by binding to Na,K-ATPase [25] and that this is part of the anticancer mechanisms of this molecule. Yan et al. noted that some of these pathways are involved in p66hc phosphorylation [25] suggesting to them that ouabain-induced reactive oxygen species (ROS) was involved.

They examined the intracellular changes induced by ouabain in human glioblastoma cells and noted that prior reports of ouabain-induced mitochondrial membrane loss and elevated ROS production were associated with human cancer cell apoptosis. In a set of interesting experiments, these investigators showed that ROS was increased in glioblastoma cells exposed to ouabain, however, this was not due to calcium overload. Rather, it appears to be the result of p66Shc phosphorylation as part of the Src/Ras/ERK signal pathway [25].

Yang et al. also explored mechanisms of ouabain-mediated cell death of glioblastoma cells. Compared to untreated U-87MG cells, ouabain suppressed survival and attenuated cell motility in a concentration-dependent manner. In addition, they observed downregulation of p-Akt, mTOR, p-mTOR, and HIF-1α at low concentrations of ouabain. The authors suggest that these results indicate that ouabain exerted suppressive effects on tumor cell growth and motility, leading to cell death via regulating the intracellular Akt/mTOR signaling pathway and inhibiting the expression of HIF-1α in glioma cells [41].

2.2.4 *Lanatoside C*

Lanatoside C is an antiarrhythmic agent, a naturally occurring compound extracted from *Digitalis lanata*. Badr et al. reported that this cardenolide is a sensitizer of GBM cells to TRAIL-induced cell death partly by upregulation of the death receptor 5. This was evident in GBM cells in culture as well as in a GBM xenograft model in vivo [26]. Cells treated with lanatoside C showed necrotic cell morphology with the absence of caspase activation, low mitochondrial potential, and early intracellular ATP depletion. This suggests mitigation of apoptosis resistance by inducing an alternate cell death pathway. The combined treatment was highly effective as a low dose of lanatoside C sensitized GBM cells to TRAIL in culture killing over 90% of U87GBM cells, while it had no significant effect on primary fibroblasts [26]. The authors pointed out that to use the suggested combination of TRAIL with lanatoside C in vivo, there would have to be a means of delivering TRAIL intracerebrally.

In follow-up articles, the lab of Bakhos Tannous, PhD (Massachusetts General Hospital) used an adeno-associated virus (AAV) vector specifically designed for intracranial delivery of secreted, soluble tumor necrosis factor-related apoptosis-inducing ligand (sTRAIL) to GBM tumors in mice. They combined the AAV delivery vehicle with the TRAIL-sensitizing cardenolide, lanatoside C. This unique combination was applied to two different GBM models using human U87 glioma cells, primary patient-derived GBM neural spheres in culture and orthotopic GBM xenograft models in mice. The authors correctly point out that a major pitfall in testing new GBM therapeutics is the use of animal models that do not accurately recapitulate a phenocopy of the human tumor [42, 43]. Typical cell lines such as U87 form local tumors that do not invade the brain per se. Therefore, the investigators tested the AAV-sTRAIL and lanatoside C therapy using primary cells dissociated from GBM patient specimens and grown as stem-like neural spheres which invade the mouse brain upon intracranial injection which replicates that occurring in the original tumor [43]. Despite the ingenuity of this therapeutic approach both the single and multi-injection approach of sTRAIL combined with lanatoside C showed only a modest survival benefit with animals eventually succumbing to the disease.

2.2.5 UNBS1450

UNBS1450 is a hemi-synthetic cardenolide belonging to the cardiac steroid glycoside family. The molecule has been shown to induce apoptotic cell death in malignant cells. It inhibits NF-kβ transactivation and triggers apoptosis by cleavage of pro-caspases 8, 9, and 3/7, by decreasing expression of anti-apoptotic Mcl-1, and by recruitment of pro-apoptotic Bak and Bax proteins [44]. UNBS1450 has been tested in 58 distinct human cancer cell lines and displays antitumor effects similar to Taxol [45]. It has also been reported to be active on Taxol-resistance cell lines. Of particular interest was the observation that this semi-synthetic cardenolide demonstrated antiproliferative effects against three glioblastoma cell lines with a level of activity similar to vincristine but much greater than those displayed by temozolomide, tamoxifen, hydroxy-tamoxifen, lomustine, procarbazine, and carmustine [46, 47]. The ability of UNBS1450 to be especially effective against glioblastoma cell lines can be explained, in part, by the fact that U373-MG GBM cells express a higher level of Na, K-ATP α-1 subunits than normal cells which is a particular target for this molecule. Similar to other cardenolides, UNBS1450 also decreases the intracellular ATP concentration more markedly in glioblastoma cells than in normal cells [47]. The advanced feature of this compound is that it can inhibit three isoforms (α3β1, α2β1, and α1β1) with relatively higher efficiency (~6 to >200 times) than ouabain and digoxin [47]. While UNBS1450 was tested in clinical trials using a dose-intensification study to find the MTD, toxicity, and pharmacokinetic parameters of the molecule in patients with lymphoma, the clinical trials were unfortunately closed by the sponsor before reaching the MTD in patients [5].

2.2.6 Oleandrin

Oleandrin is a highly lipid-soluble cardenolide isolated from the plant *N. oleander* and has been used as a traditional herbal medicine due to its excellent pharmacological properties [38]. Like other cardenolides, oleandrin has been used for the treatment of congestive heart failure; however, more recently oleandrin has attracted attention due to its extensive anti-cancer and novel anti-viral effects. In vitro and in vivo investigations have shown that oleandrin possesses anticancer properties against several cancers including melanoma, leukemia, sarcoma, prostate, lung, pancreatic, and brain cancers [5–7, 12, 13, 17, 38]. Mechanisms underlying the anticancer activity of oleandrin include cell cycle arrest [48], altered membrane fluidity [49], modulation of cell signaling pathways (NF-kβ, JNK) [50], elevated Ca^{2+} and Na^{+} levels, decreased K^{+} levels inside the cell [51, 52], oxidative and mitochondrial stress [53], altered IL-8 levels [54], reduced expression of Rad51 [55], and decreased activation of fibroblast growth factor-2 [56]. Defined extracts of *N. oleander* containing this molecule (i.e., Anvirzel™ and PBI-05204) have undergone clinical trials in cancer patients where both the relative safety and pharmacokinetics of oleandrin were determined [15, 16, 57].

Of particular interest is the ability of oleandrin to act as a chemosensitizer for both chemotherapeutic and radiotherapeutic strategies. The development of resistance to drugs and radiotherapy is a major hurdle toward the effective treatment of cancer [58]. Oleandrin has been shown to reduce radiotherapy resistance in triple-negative breast cancer cells [59] and was also shown to sensitize human prostate cancer cells to radiotherapy [60]. It has also been indicated to exhibit significant antitumor effects in radiotherapy resistant MDA-MB231 cells which was reported to be due to inhibition of phosphor-STAT3, reduced levels of OCT3/4, β-catenin, and decreased MMP-9 activity [59]. These results have been suggested as important with respect to breast cancer invasion. Additionally, various studies have shown that oleandrin decreases tumor size and tumor development and inhibits cellular proliferation in human or murine glioma cells by increasing brain-derived neurotrophic factor (BDNF) levels, decreasing tumor infiltration, and reducing angiogenesis. It was also concluded that oleandrin can be used in adjuvant therapy with currently available chemotherapeutics such as temozolomide.

Oleandrin and extracts that contain this molecule may have unique abilities for the effective treatment of GBM. Digoxin is actively excluded from the brain via P-glycoprotein, yet oleandrin efficiently crosses the blood–brain barrier and inhibits P-glycoprotein expression [17, 61]. Lin et al. investigated 12 human tumor cell lines to explore pathways of tumor cell sensitivity to cardenolide compounds [62]. In vitro models of human glioma included HF U251 cells as well as native and modified melanoma BRO cells. A study by Lefranc and Kiss suggested that high expression of Na,K-ATPase α1 isoform in the presence of low α3 expression was associated with relative sensitivity to cardiac glycosides such as oleandrin, ouabain, and bufalin [63]. Other investigators, however, have found that the higher the Na, K-ATPase α3/α1 ratio, the greater the sensitivity to oleandrin [64].

Garofolo et al. examined the effects of oleandrin on glioma models in vivo [13]. They inoculated human glioma cells into mice and investigated the antitumor efficacy of oleandrin. Administration of this cardenolide reduced glioma growth and lowered cell proliferation. Furthermore, in a recent review of the potential of oleandrin to treat glioblastoma [17], the authors point out that oleandrin increases the cerebral levels of brain-derived neurotrophic factor (BDNF), decreases both microglia/macrophage infiltration and CD68 immunoreactivity in tumors, lowers astrogliosis in the tumoral penumbra, and attenuates glioma infiltration into healthy parenchymal tissue. In BDNF-knock out mice (bdnftm1Jae/J) and Trk-silenced glioma cells, the efficacy of oleandrin was diminished indicating a key role for BDNF in oleandrin's antitumor efficacy. Garofalo et al. [65] had previously shown that BDNF inhibited the chemotaxis of glioma cells by blocking the small G-protein RhoA through the truncated TrkB.T1 receptor and that BDNF infusion reduced glioma volume in mice. Additionally, oleandrin was also shown to enhance survival in glioma-implanted mice increasing the efficacy of temozolomide [13].

Colapietro et al. recently reported the efficacy of PBI-05204 (a defined extract of *N. oleander* containing oleandrin as a principle active ingredient) in inhibiting the growth of human glioblastoma. Their studies were designed to investigate the antitumor efficacy of this botanical drug against glioblastoma using both in vitro and in vivo cancer models as well as exploring its efficacy against glioblastoma stem cells. They reported that three human GBM cell lines, U87MG, U251, and T98G were inhibited by PBI-05204 in a concentration-dependent manner that was characterized by induction of apoptosis as evidenced by increased ANNEXIN V staining and caspase activities [66]. An important clue to the mechanisms of anti-glioma growth was the finding that the expression of proteins associated with both Akt and mTOR pathways was suppressed by PBI-05204 in all three cell lines. PBI-05204 significantly suppressed U87 spheroid formation and the expression of important stem cell markers such as SOX2, CD44, and CXCR4. Oral administration of PBI-05204 to nude mice resulted in a dose-dependent inhibition of U87MG, U251, and T98G xenograft growth. Additionally, PBI-05204 treated mice carrying U87-Luc cells as an orthotopic model exhibited significantly delayed onset of tumor progression and significantly increased overall survival. Immunohistochemical staining of xenograft tumor sections revealed declines in Ki67 and CD31 positively stained cells but increased TUNEL staining. Given the fact that PBI-05204 has already been in phase I and II clinical trials for cancer patients, the authors concluded that further examination of the role of PBI-05204 in GBM patients should be considered [66].

2.3 Combination therapies with cardiac glycoside compounds

Cardiac glycosides represent a class of compounds that work well together with both drugs and radiotherapy in models of GBM. This effective combination of therapeutic strategies has been shown for both bufadienolides and cardenolide compounds. With respect to bufalin, for example, Zhang et al. investigated the response of U251 and U87MG glioblastoma cell lines. Bufalin reduces cell proliferation in both cell lines and induced a G2/M cell cycle arrest [67]. They also observed that bufalin disrupted the mitochondrial membrane potential leading to reduced oxygen consumption and ATP production. In addition, homologous recombination efficacy, a measure of DNA repair, was reduced by ~40%. This was associated with increased γH2AX expression, a marker for the presence of DNA double-strand breaks. Bufalin was additive with radiation in the treatment of GBM cells in vitro. Cell death increased significantly under combination treatment compared to radiation treatment alone [67].

In a recent article, Colapietro et al. explored the role of PBI-05204 in models of human glioblastoma when combined with radiotherapy [58]. This study demonstrated that PBI-05204 treatment led to an increase *in vitro* the sensitivity of GBM cells to radiation in which the main mechanisms were the transition from autophagy to apoptosis, enhanced DNA damage, and reduced DNA repair after radiotherapy administration. The combination of PBI-05204 with radiotherapy was associated with reduced tumor progression as evidenced in both subcutaneous as well as orthotopic implanted GBM tumors. The authors state that, collectively, their results reveal that

PBI-05204 enhances antitumor activity of radiotherapy in preclinical/murine models of human GBM and again call for further exploration of the use of this botanical drug in combination therapies in clinical trials.

Cardiac glycoside compounds have also been reported to be able to add to the antitumor efficacy of chemotherapeutic compounds used to treat GBM. Gamabufotalin has been reported to promote temozolomide sensitivity in glioblastoma cells [68]. Both in vitro and in vivo studies were undertaken to examine mechanisms to explain gamabufotalin's ability to increase sensitivity of GBM to temozolomide. Studies revealed a negative feedback loop between ATPA3 (α3 subunit of Na,K-ATPase) and AQP4 (aquaporin 4, a 'water channel' protein molecule), which were predicted by molecular modeling and docking studies to interact with gamabufotalin. The role of AQP4 in GBM growth and proliferation is an interesting finding in light of other studies showing that AQP4 knock out could play a role in several neurodegenerative diseases. Lan et al. reported that AQP4 suppression could significantly promote temozolomide sensitivity with the result that gamabufotalin might mediate inhibition of GBM via regulation of the ATP1A3-AQP4 signaling pathway [69].

In unpublished studies, we have also explored the in vitro and in vivo effects of oleandrin when combined with both radiotherapy and temozolomide in human glioblastoma cell models. Our studies extend a potential role of oleandrin and extracts that contain this molecule (e.g., PBI-05204) in combination with radiotherapy [67]. As radiotherapy and temozolomide are considered 'standard of care' treatment for GBM, any extension of their relative efficacy and success in clinical outcomes is indeed welcomed. Our preliminary studies have indicated again that the combined use of oleandrin with radiotherapy and temozolomide inhibited autophagy in favor of apoptotic pathways, reduced expression of NF-κβ, and reduced cell survival mechanisms while inducing DNA damage by suppression of Rad51. The combined treatments led to an increase in disease-free survival in mice with orthotopically implanted GBM tumors compared to either temozolomide or oleandrin treatment alone. Additional confirmatory studies are needed and are presently underway.

Furthermore, to enhance the translational potential of the therapeutic activity of oleandrin and extracts containing this compound (PBI-05204) in GBM, we evaluated the anti-proliferative effect of oleandrin in primary GBM cells isolated from human GBM-derived intra-cerebral (IC) orthotopic PDX models. We treated the three primary human GBM cell lines, IC-3704, IC-4687, and IC-3752 with different doses of oleandrin (1–100 or 1–1000 nM) and tested cell viability at 72 hrs after treatment. As shown in **Figure 1**, oleandrin exposure significantly inhibited the growth of all three GBM cells in a dose-dependent manner, with comparable low median inhibitory concentrations (IC_{50}) of 8.57, 9.73, and 6.02 nM for IC-3704 (**Figure 1A**), IC-4687 (**Figure 1B**) and IC-3752 (**Figure 1C**), respectively. To further test the antitumor efficacy of oleandrin-containing extract (PBI-05204) on human GBM tumors, we evaluated the overall survival of mice bearing the human GBM-derived IC orthotopic PDX tumor. The IC-1406 GBM was established through direct injection of surgical tumor specimens into mouse cerebrum areas [70]. The tumor was collected from a patient with a diagnosis of Turcort's syndrome carrying a c.137G > T (p.546 l) in the PMS2 gene and this mutation was present in orthotopic tumors. The IC-1406 GBM cell orthotopic model was developed by injecting these particular cells (1×10^5) into the right cerebrum. Treatment with PBI-05204 (25 mg/kg, qd × 5 days) was started at 2 weeks post-tumor cell injection. Analysis of median survival times of mice bearing IC-1406 GBM tumor was significantly

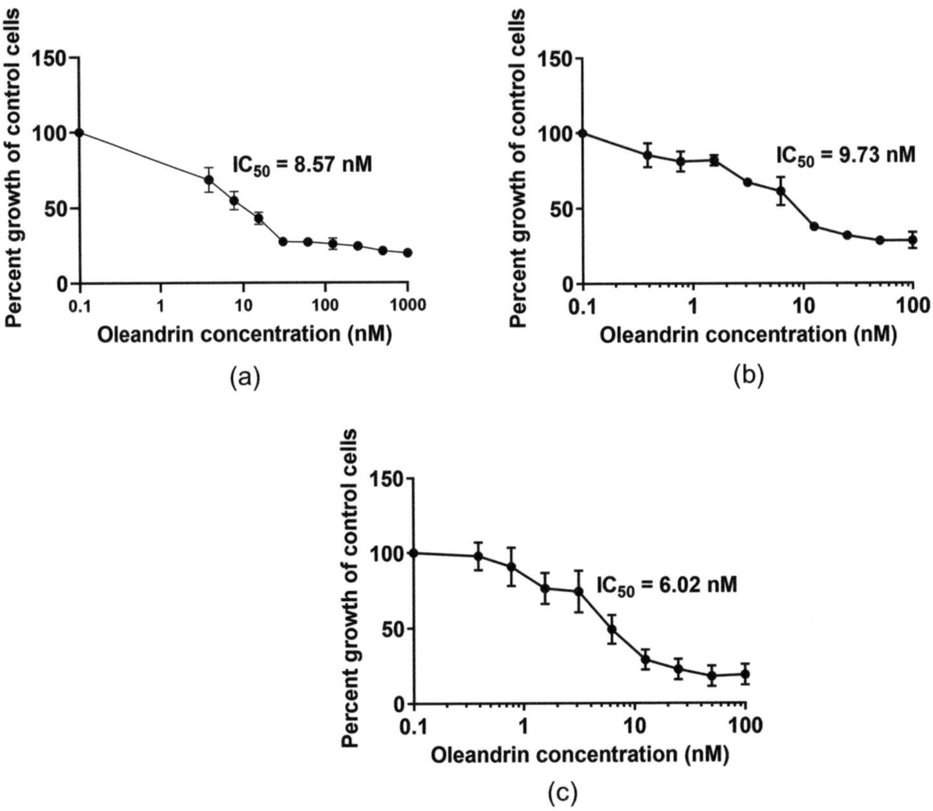

Figure 1.
Growth curves of human GBM cells derived from a human orthotopic PDX model. Primary cultured cells from IC-3704GBM (a), IC-4687GBM (b) and IC-3752GBM (c) cells (6×10^3) were plated and allowed to attach for overnight. They were then treated with oleandrin (1–100 nM) for 72 hrs. Cell proliferation was assessed by MTT assays. Data are presented as mean ± SD.

increased from 90 days in the control group to 122 days in the PBI-05204 treated group ($p < 0.006$) (**Figure 2A**), suggesting oleandrin and PBI-05204 exert strong antitumor efficacy in PDX derived GBM cells and their orthotopic model. While we had reported previously that PBI-05204 enhanced the antitumor efficacy of radiotherapy using established human GBM cell lines, such as U87MG, U251, and TG98 cell line mouse xenograft models, we then examined the possibility that PBI-05204 may have significant sensitizing effects on radiotherapy using a patient-derived orthotopic GBM PDX model IC-1128GBM [71]. As shown in **Figure 2B**, the combination of radiotherapy (XRT, 2 Gy × 5) and PBI-05204 resulted in a significant enhancement of overall survival compared to control or either single treatment modality alone. For example, the average overall survival of mice treated with PBI-05204 plus XRT was 158 days which was significantly longer than that in control mice (116 days, $p < 0.001$), PBI-05204 treated mice (118 days, $p < 0.001$), or XRT treated mice (144 days, $p = 0.022$), again suggesting PBI-05204 can enhance the antitumor efficacy of radiotherapy in GBM.

To understand the potential mechanisms involved in PBI-05204-elicited anti-tumor effects in the PDX derived GBM tumor, we examined the expression of cell cycle and apoptosis regulators as well as cell signaling proteins in tumor tissues collected from the IC-1406 PDX orthotopic model using Reverse Phase Proteomic

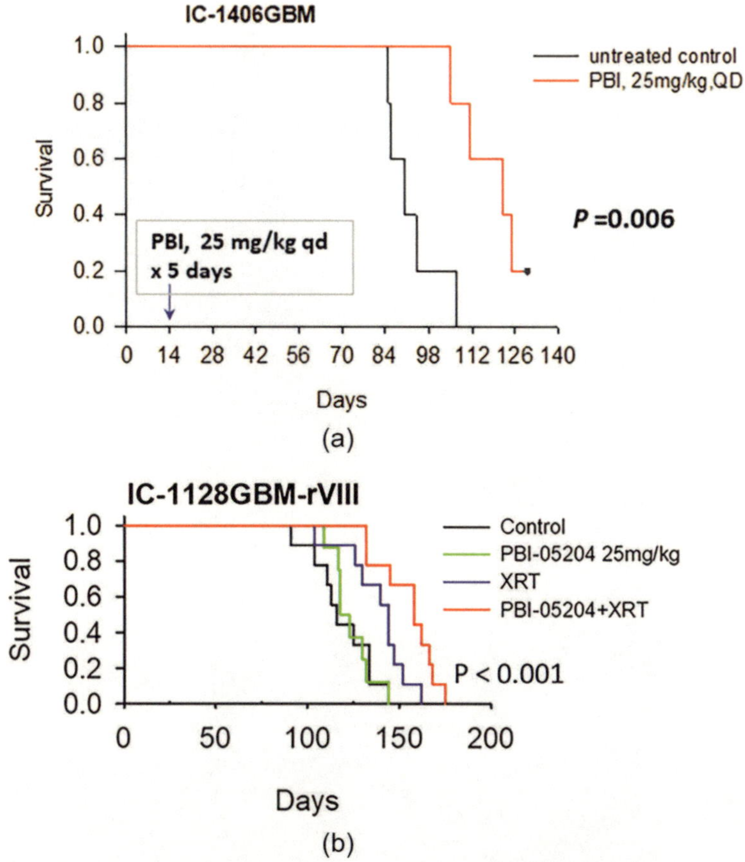

Figure 2.
Antitumor efficacy of PBI-05204 alone or in combination with radiotherapy in human GBM-derived intracerebral (IC) orthotopic PDX models. (a) Kaplan Meyer curves of mice bearing orthotopic PDX model of IC-1406 GBM treated with PBI-05204. (b) Kaplan Meyer curves of IC-1128 GBM derived PDX model at passage 8 (rVIII) after treatment with PBI-05204 (25 mg/kg), radiotherapy (XRT, 2 Gy/day × 5 days), or a combination of PBI-05204 and XRT.

Array (RPPA) analysis as performed by the Functional Proteomics Core Facility at The University of Texas MD Anderson Cancer Center. As shown in the Heatmap (**Figure 3A**), PBI-05204 treatment led to altered expression of several proteins associated with cell cycle, apoptosis, and oncogenic signaling pathway in the IC-1406 PDX model. Among these proteins, PBI-05204 BT significantly down-regulated SOX2 by 41%, an important stem cell marker presented in various cancer stem cells including GBM. Intriguingly, the abundance of tumor suppressor and negative regulator of PI3K/Akt pathway PTEN was significantly increased by PBI-05204 treatment by almost 2-fold. Consistent with this finding, the activity of a downstream target of PI3k/Akt pathways Ribosomal protein S6 was notably decreased by PBI-05204 evidenced by the phosphorylation of this protein was reduced in PBI-05204 treated tumor tissues compared to that of control mice (**Figure 3B**). These findings suggest that PBI-05204 can potentially inhibit the growth of GBM by upregulating PTEN and consequently downregulating the PI3K/Akt pathway and affecting cancer stem cells which were consistent with our previous study using the established human GBM cells.

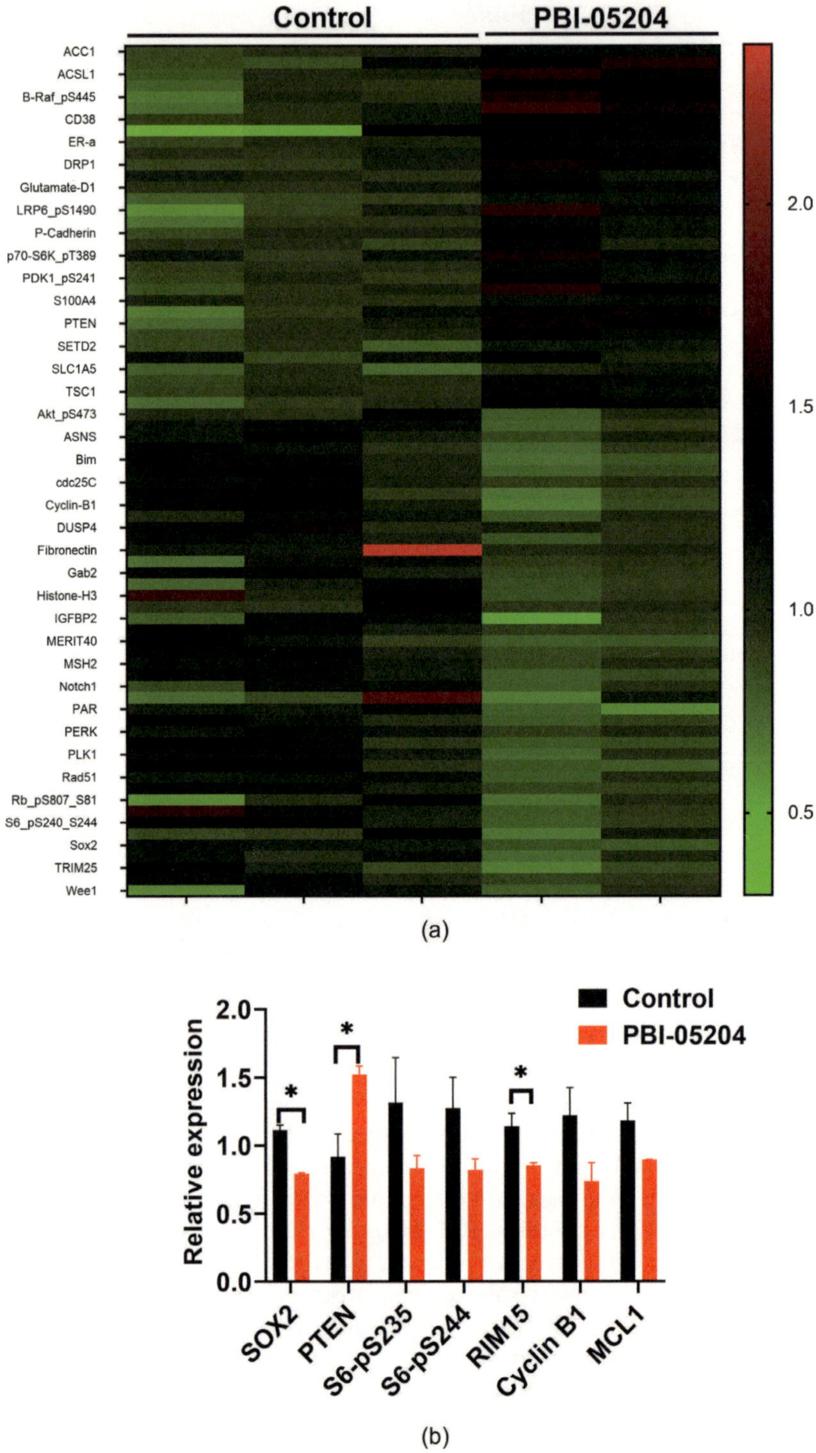

Figure 3.

*Proteomic analysis of tumor tissues derived from IC1406 PDX models by reverse phase proteomic Array (RPPA). (a) Heatmap of cell cycle regulating proteins and cell signaling proteins in PBI-05204 treated tumor tissues by RPPA. (b) Expression of cell cycle regulating proteins and cell signaling proteins showing about 20% changes following PBI-05204 treatment. Data are presented as mean ± SD. * $p < 0.05$ versus control.*

3. Cardiac glycosides and glioblastoma stem cells

Conventional treatment of GBM promotes a transient elimination of the tumor and, unfortunately, is almost always followed by tumor recurrence due to an increase in glioblastoma stem cell (GSC) populations [72]. It is believed that GSCs are the primary driving force behind GBM relapses. GSCs are typically resistant to further chemotherapeutic efforts and are typically resistant to additional radiotherapy [72]. To effectively eliminate GSCs, it is critical to target their essential functions and metabolism before effective strategies can be developed against them. While no single therapeutic modality has yet been shown to be completely effective against a heterogenous GSC population, recent studies have shown that cardiac glycosides may prove to have effective activity against GSCs and offer insights as to how they inhibit this specific cell population.

One important target that has been suggested as important for GSC proliferation is the hypoxia-inducible factor (HIF) family of transcriptional factors as they are master regulators of diverse cellular responses to hypoxic conditions. Among these, HIF1α plays a pivotal role in GBM survival, resistance, and invasion [73]. Nigim et al. [74] have reported a new orthotopic model of glioblastoma that recapitulates the hypoxic tumor environment of GBM tumors. This model is based on stem-like GBM cells that were isolated from a recurrent GBM. Their research demonstrates that digoxin is an effective inhibitor of HIF-1α expression and angiogenesis in vivo and provides survival benefits. Using the MGG123 model, the authors have shown that digoxin potently inhibits HIF-1α protein expression even after its induction with hypoxic conditions in vitro. Importantly, they also demonstrated digoxin-mediated HIF-1α silencing in orthotopic GBM xenografts. A related series of studies reported by Bar et al. demonstrated that digoxin also inhibits the growth of cultured GBM cells and flank GBM xenografts with concomitant reduction of HIF-1α and CD133 levels [36]. Thus, digoxin, and perhaps related cardiac glycosides, may effectively target HIF-1α, an important target against GSCs.

Proscillaridin A was shown to have cytotoxic and exhibit anti-migratory properties on GBM cell lines including stem-like cells, but not on healthy neural cells [28]. Berges et al. disclosed a novel pathway by which proscillaridin A and digoxin modulate microtubule network functioning in GBM and stem-like cells [27]. They found that at low concentrations proscillaridin A induced an alteration of microtubule dynamic instability. This was the result of GSK3β activation following the binding of proscillaridin binding to Na, K-ATPase, leading, in turn, to EB1 phosphorylation and subsequent inhibition of cell migration. They conclude that cardiac glycosides at low concentrations mimic the anti-migratory and cytotoxic effects of microtubule inhibiting drugs although they bind to Na, K-ATPase, and not directly to tubulin. As such, cardiac glycosides may represent an alternative treatment strategy and potent candidates for drug repositioning.

Many articles have cited the importance of cardiac glycosides targeting certain alpha subunits (e.g., α1 and/or α3) of Na,K-ATPase to combat the proliferation of glioblastoma cells, Li et al. [75] have indicated that targeting the β2 subunit of Na,K-ATPase represents a new approach to induce glioblastoma cell apoptosis through elevation of intracellular Ca^{2+}. The β-subunit is a glycoprotein involved in the structural maturation of Na,K-ATPase, and regulates enzyme stability, α-subunit activity, and cell adhesion processes. They point out that selectively targeting the β2 subunit that is not expressed in the heart might avoid cardiotoxicity. In contrast, the β2 subunit is more highly expressed in glioblastoma stem-like cells than in GBM cells. Its down-regulation selectively induces apoptosis in GSCs and is associated with significant inhibition of tumor growth in vivo.

Our own research has recently reported the effect of a defined extract of *Nerium oleander* containing oleandrin (PBI-05204) against human glioblastoma models and its ability to modulate GSC cell-renewal properties [67]. Three human GBM cell lines, U87MG, U251, and T98 associated with Akt and mTOR pathways were inhibited by PBI-05204 in a concentration-dependent manner that was characterized by induction of apoptosis as evidenced by increased ANNEXIN V staining and caspase activities. PBI-05204 significantly suppressed U87 spheroid formation and the expression of important stem cell markers such as SOX2, CD44, and CXCR4. Additionally, we also reported that when PBI-05204 was added to the irradiated GBM cells, it enhanced the antitumor efficacy of radiation in both GBM cells and their relevant animal models as well as significantly reducing the stemness of GBM cells. This was believed due to the down-regulation of CD44 and stro-1, an important mesenchymal stem cell marker in U87MG cells [58].

4. Conclusions

Cardenolide and bufadienolides compounds as well as semi-synthetic cardiac glycoside compounds such as UNBS1450 have now been shown to have potent activity against GBM cell lines as well as established in vivo tumor models. These compounds have been reported to have multiple mechanisms of action which are, in many cases, unique from those of conventional chemotherapeutic agents already approved as the standard of care drugs for GBM. It would thus appear that the combination of cardenolide or bufadienolides compounds with approved radiotherapy and chemotherapy (i.e., temozolomide) approaches to the treatment of GBM is an option worth exploring. Additionally, some cardenolides, such as oleandrin, are capable of crossing the blood–brain barrier and residing there in the brain (up to 24 hrs) longer than that in plasma providing an advantage of these compounds for the treatment of GBM. Finally, considering cognitive impairment is one of the major toxicities of radiotherapy and that some of these compounds, including neriifolin, oleandrin, and others, have been shown to exert neuroprotective effects [76], these compounds might not only be able to slow down the growth of GBM, but also provide a benefit assisting in the repair of radiation-induced damage to injured neurons. Some cardenolide compounds such as PBI-05204 containing oleandrin have already been through both Phase I and II clinical trials in cancer patients. Exciting new research has now clearly shown that this class of compounds also has potent activity in effectively reducing GBM stem cell populations known to be an important reason for the progression of disease after initial surgery and other therapeutic strategies have been performed.

Acknowledgements

The authors are grateful for the financial support of Phoenix Biotechnology, Inc.

Conflict of interest

Robert A. Newman is the Chief Science Officer for Phoenix Biotechnology, Inc.; Peiying Yang is a consultant for Phoenix Biotechnology, Inc. All other authors claim no conflict of interest.

DOI: http://dx.doi.org/10.5772/intechopen.105022

Author details

Yuchen Du[1], Xiao-Nan Li[1], Peiying Yang[2] and Robert A. Newman[3]*

1 Northwestern University Feinberg School of Medicine and Ann and Robert H. Lurie Children's Hospital of Chicago, Chicago, IL, USA

2 University of Texas MD Anderson Cancer Center, Houston, TX, USA

3 Phoenix Biotechnology, Inc., San Antonio, TX, USA

*Address all correspondence to: newmanscientificconsulting@gmail.com

References

[1] Kamiya-Matsuoka C, Gilbert MR. Treating recurrent glioblastoma: An update. CNS Oncology. 2015;**4**(2): 91-104. DOI: 10.2217/cns.14.55

[2] Janjua TI, Rewatkar P, Ahmed-Cox A, Saeed I, Mansfeld FM, Kulshreshtha R, et al. Frontiers in the treatment of glioblastoma: Past, present and emerging. Advanced Drug Delivery Reviews. 2021;**171**:108-138. DOI: 10.1016/j.addr.2021.01.012

[3] Wu W, Klockow JL, Zhang M, Lafortune F, Chang E, Jin L, et al. Glioblastoma multiforme (GBM): An overview of current therapies and mechanisms of resistance. Pharmacological Research. 2021;**171**:105780. DOI: 10.1016/j.phrs.2021.105780

[4] Bejček J, Jurášek M, Spiwok V, Rimpelová S. *Quo vadis* cardiac glycoside research? Toxins (Basel). 2021;**13**(5):344. DOI: 10.3390/toxins13050344

[5] Reddy D, Kumavath R, Barh D, Azevedo V, Ghosh P. Anticancer and antiviral properties of cardiac glycosides: A review to explore the mechanism of actions. Molecules. 2020;**25**(16):3596. DOI: 10.3390/molecules25163596

[6] Slingerland M, Cerella C, Guchelaar HJ, Diederich M, Gelderblom H. Cardiac glycosides in cancer therapy: From preclinical investigations towards clinical trials. Investigational New Drugs. 2013;**31**(4):1087-1094. DOI: 10.1007/s10637-013-9984-1

[7] Bejček J, Spiwok V, Kmoníčková E, Rimpelová S. Na^+/K^+-ATPase revisited: On its mechanism of action, role in cancer, and activity modulation. Molecules. 2021;**26**(7):1905. DOI: 10.3390/molecules26071905

[8] Diederich M, Muller F, Cerella C. Cardiac glycosides: From molecular targets to immunogenic cell death. Biochemical Pharmacology. 2017;**125**: 1-11. DOI: 10.1016/j.bcp.2016.08.017

[9] Menger L, Vacchelli E, Adjemian S, Martins I, Ma Y, Shen S, et al. Cardiac glycosides exert anticancer effects by inducing immunogenic cell death. Science Translational Medicine. 2012;**4**(143):143ra99. DOI: 10.1126/scitranslmed.3003807

[10] Kelly RA. Cardiac glycosides and congestive heart failure. American Journal of Cardiology. 1990;**65**(10):10E-16E

[11] Marcus FI. The use of digitalis for the treatment of congestive heart failure: A tale of its decline and resurrection. Cardiovascular Drugs and Therapy. 1989;**3**(4):473-476

[12] Kanwal N, Rasul A, Hussain G, Anwar H, Shah MA, Sarfraz I, et al. Oleandrin: A bioactive phytochemical and potential cancer killer via multiple cellular signaling pathways. Food and Chemical Toxicology. 2020;**143**:111570. DOI: 10.1016/j.fct.2020.111570

[13] Garofalo S, Grimaldi A, Chece G, Porzia A, Morrone S, Mainiero F, et al. The glycoside oleandrin reduces glioma growth with direct and indirect effects on tumor cells. The Journal of Neuroscience. 2017;**37**(14):3926-3939. DOI: 10.1523/JNEUROSCI.2296-16.2017

[14] Decker MW, Pelleymounter MA, Gallagher M. Effects of training on a spatial memory task on high affinity choline uptake in hippocampus and cortex in young adult and aged rats. The Journal of Neuroscience. 1988;**1**:90-99

[15] Hong DS, Henary H, Falchook GS, Naing A, Fu S, Moulder S, et al. First-in-human study of PBI-05204, an oleander-derived inhibitor of akt, FGF-2, Nf-κB and p70s6k, in patients with advanced solid tumors. Investigational New Drugs. 2014;**32**(6):1204-1212. DOI: 10.1007/s10637-014-0127-0

[16] Roth MT, Cardin DB, Borazanci EH, Steinbach M, Picozzi VJ, Rosemury A, et al. A Phase II, Single-Arm, Open-Label, Bayesian Adaptive Efficacy and Safety Study of PBI-05204 in Patients with Stage IV Metastatic Pancreatic Adenocarcinoma. The Oncologist. 2020;**25**(10):e1446-e1450. DOI: 10.1634/theoncologist.2020-0440

[17] Elmaci İ, Alturfan EE, Cengiz S, Ozpinar A, Altinoz MA. Neuroprotective and tumoricidal activities of cardiac glycosides. Could oleandrin be a new weapon against stroke and glioblastoma? The International Journal of Neuroscience. 2018;**128**(9):865-877. DOI: 10.1080/00207454.2018.1435540

[18] Chen D, Song M, Mohamad O, Yu SP. Inhibition of Na+/K+-ATPase induces hybrid cell death and enhanced sensitivity to chemotherapy in human glioblastoma cells. BMC Cancer. 2014;**14**:716. DOI: 10.1186/1471-2407-14-716

[19] Karpova L, Eva A, Kirch U, Boldyrev A, Scheiner-Bobis G. Sodium pump alpha1 and alpha3 subunit isoforms mediate distinct responses to ouabain and are both essential for survival of human neuroblastoma. The FEBS Journal. 2010;**277**(8):1853-1860. DOI: 10.1111/j.1742-4658.2010.07602.x

[20] Lan YL, Zou YJ, Lou JC, Xing JS, Wang X, Zou S, et al. The sodium pump α1 subunit regulates bufalin sensitivity of human glioblastoma cells through the p53 signaling pathway. Cell Biology and Toxicology. 2019;**35**(6):521-539. DOI: 10.1007/s10565-019-09462-y

[21] Lan YL, Wang X, Lou JC, Xing JS, Yu ZL, Wang H, et al. Bufalin inhibits glioblastoma growth by promoting proteasomal degradation of the Na^+/K^+-ATPase α1 subunit. Biomedicine & Pharmacotherapy. 2018;**103**:204-215. DOI: 10.1016/j.biopha.2018.04.030

[22] Yuan B, Shimada R, Xu K, Han L, Si N, Zhao H, et al. Multiple cytotoxic effects of gamabufotalin against human glioblastoma cell line U-87. Chemico-Biological Interactions. 2019;**314**:108849. DOI: 10.1016/j.cbi.2019.108849

[23] Lee DH, Lee CS, Kim DW, Ae JE, Lee TH. Digitoxin sensitizes glioma cells to TRAIL-mediated apoptosis by upregulation of death receptor 5 and downregulation of survivin. Anti-Cancer Drugs. 2014;**25**(1):44-52

[24] Shang Z, Zhang L. Digitoxin increases sensitivity of glioma stem cells to TRAIL-mediated apoptosis. Neuroscience Letters. 2017;**653**:19-24. DOI: 10.1016/j.neulet.2017.05.019

[25] Yan X, Liang F, Li D, Zheng J. Ouabain elicits human glioblastoma cells apoptosis by generating reactive oxygen species in ERK-p66SHC-dependent pathway. Molecular and Cellular Biochemistry. 2015;**398**(1-2):95-104. DOI: 10.1007/s11010-014-2208-y

[26] Badr CE, Wurdinger T, Nilsson J, Niers JM, Whalen M, Degterev A, et al. Lanatoside C sensitizes glioblastoma cells to tumor necrosis factor-related apoptosis-inducing ligand and induces an alternative cell death pathway. Neuro-Oncology. 2011;**13**(11):1213-1224. DOI: 10.1093/neuonc/nor067

[27] Berges R, Denicolai E, TchoghandjianA, Baeza-KalleeN, HonoreS,

Figarella-Branger D, et al. Proscillaridin A exerts anti-tumor effects through GSK3β activation and alteration of microtubule dynamics in glioblastoma. Cell Death & Disease. 2018;**9**(10):984. DOI: 10.1038/s41419-018-1018-7

[28] Denicolaï E, Baeza-Kallee N, Tchoghandjian A, Carré M, Colin C, Jiglaire CJ, et al. Proscillaridin A is cytotoxic for glioblastoma cell lines and controls tumor xenograft growth in vivo. Oncotarget. 2014;**5**(21):10934-10948. DOI: 10.18632/oncotarget.2541

[29] Huang L, Garrett Injac S, Cui K, Braun F, Lin Q, Du Y, et al. Systems biology-based drug repositioning identifies digoxin as a potential therapy for groups 3 and 4 medulloblastoma. Science Translational Medicine. 2018;**10**(464):eaat0150

[30] Takai N, Kira N, Ishii T, Yoshida T, Nishida M, Nishida Y, et al. Bufalin, a traditional oriental medicine, induces apoptosis in human cancer cells. Asian Pacific Journal of Cancer Prevention. 2012;**13**(1):399-402. DOI: 10.7314/apjcp.2012.13.1.399

[31] Lan YL, Lou JC, Jiang XW, Wang X, Xing JS, Li S, et al. A research update on the anticancer effects of bufalin and its derivatives. Oncology Letters. 2019;**17**(4):3635-3640. DOI: 10.3892/ol.2019.10062

[32] Yuan B, He J, Kisoh K, Hayashi H, Tanaka S, Si N, et al. Effects of active bufadienolide compounds on human cancer cells and CD4+CD25+Foxp3+ regulatory T cells in mitogen-activated human peripheral blood mononuclear cells. Oncology Reports. 2016;**36**(3):1377-1384. DOI: 10.3892/or.2016.4946

[33] Lan YL, Wang X, Lou JC, Xing JS, Zou S, Yu ZL, et al. Marinobufagenin inhibits glioma growth through sodium pump α1 subunit and ERK signaling-mediated mitochondrial apoptotic pathway. Cancer Medicine. 2018;**7**(5):2034-2047. DOI: 10.1002/cam4.1469

[34] Papale M, Buccarelli M, Mollinari C, Russo MA, Pallini R, Ricci-Vitiani L, et al. Hypoxia, inflammation and necrosis as determinants of glioblastoma cancer stem cells progression. International Journal of Molecular Sciences. 2020;**21**(8):2660. DOI: 10.3390/ijms21082660

[35] Chan JK, Roth J, Oppenheim JJ, Tracey KJ, Vogl T, Feldmann M, et al. Alarmins: Awaiting a clinical response. The Journal of Clinical Investigation. 2012;**122**(8):2711-2719. DOI: 10.1172/JCI62423

[36] Bar EE, Lin A, Mahairaki V, Matsui W, Eberhart CG. Hypoxia increases the expression of stem-cell markers and promotes clonogenicity in glioblastoma neurospheres. The American Journal of Pathology. 2010;**177**(3):1491-1502. DOI: 10.2353/ajpath.2010.091021

[37] López-Lázaro M. Digitoxin as an anticancer agent with selectivity for cancer cells: Possible mechanisms involved. Expert Opinion on Therapeutic Targets. 2007;**11**(8):1043-1053. DOI: 10.1517/14728222.11.8.1043

[38] Newman RA, Yang P, Pawlus AD, Block KI. Cardiac glycosides as novel cancer therapeutic agents. Molecular Interventions. 2008;**8**(1):36-49. DOI: 10.1124/mi.8.1.8

[39] Wu J, Li D, Du L, Baldawi M, Gable ME, Askari A, et al. Ouabain prevents pathological cardiac hypertrophy and heart failure through activation of phosphoinositide 3-kinase

α in mouse. Cell & Bioscience. 2015;**5**:64. DOI: 10.1186/s13578-015-0053-7

[40] Pavlovic D. Endogenous cardiotonic steroids and cardiovascular disease, where to next? Cell Calcium. 2020;**86**:102156. DOI: 10.1016/j.ceca.2019.102156

[41] Yang XS, Xu ZW, Yi TL, Xu RC, Li J, Zhang WB, et al. Ouabain suppresses the growth and migration abilities of glioma U-87MG cells through inhibiting the Akt/mTOR signaling pathway and downregulating the expression of HIF-1α. Molecular Medicine Reports. 2018;**17**(4):5595-5600. DOI: 10.3892/mmr.2018.8587

[42] Crommentuijn MH, Maguire CA, Niers JM, Vandertop WP, Badr CE, Würdinger T, et al. Intracranial AAV-sTRAIL combined with lanatoside C prolongs survival in an orthotopic xenograft mouse model of invasive glioblastoma. Molecular Oncology. 2016;**10**(4):625-634. DOI: 10.1016/j.molonc.2015.11.011

[43] Crommentuijn MH, Kantar R, Noske DP, Vandertop WP, Badr CE, Würdinger T, et al. Systemically administered AAV9-sTRAIL combats invasive glioblastoma in a patient-derived orthotopic xenograft model. Molecular Therapeutics Oncolytics. 2016;**3**:16017. DOI: 10.1038/mto.2016.17

[44] Cerella C, Muller F, Gaigneaux A, Radogna F, Viry E, Chateauvieux S, et al. Early downregulation of Mcl-1 regulates apoptosis triggered by cardiac glycoside UNBS1450. Cell Death & Disease. 2015;**6**(6):e1782. DOI: 10.1038/cddis.2015.134

[45] Juncker T, Cerella C, Teiten MH, Morceau F, Schumacher M, Ghelfi J, et al. UNBS1450, a steroid cardiac glycoside inducing apoptotic cell death in human leukemia cells. Biochemical Pharmacology. 2011;**81**(1):13-23. DOI: 10.1016/j.bcp.2010.08.025

[46] Lefranc F, Mijatovic T, Kondo Y, Sauvage S, Roland I, Debeir O, et al. Targeting the alpha 1 subunit of the sodium pump to combat glioblastoma cells. Neurosurgery. 2008;**62**(1):211-221

[47] Lefranc F, Kiss R. The sodium pump alpha1 subunit as a potential target to combat apoptosis-resistant glioblastomas. Neoplasia. 2008;**10**(3):198-206. DOI: 10.1593/neo.07928

[48] Newman RA, Kondo Y, Yokoyama T, Cartwright C, Chan D, Johansen M, et al. Autophagic cell death of human pancreatic tumor cells mediated by oleandrin, a lipid-soluble cardiac glycoside. Integrative Cancer Therapies. 2007;**6**(4):354-364. DOI: 10.1177/1534735407309623

[49] Raghavendra PB, Sreenivasan Y, Manna SK. Oleandrin induces apoptosis in human, but not in murine cells: Dephosphorylation of Akt, expression of FasL, and alteration of membrane fluidity. Molecular Immunology. 2007;**44**(9):2292-2302. DOI: 10.1016/j.molimm.2006.11.009

[50] Manna SK, Sah NK, Newman RA, Cisneros A, Aggarwal BB. Oleandrin suppresses activation of nuclear transcription factor-kappaB, activator protein-1, and c-Jun NH2-terminal kinase. Cancer Research. 2000;**60**(14):3838-3847

[51] McConkey DJ, Lin Y, Nutt LK, Ozel HZ, Newman RA. Cardiac glycosides stimulate Ca^{2+} increases and apoptosis in androgen-independent, metastatic human prostate adenocarcinoma cells. Cancer Research. 2000;**60**(14):3807-3812

[52] Poindexter BJ, Feng W, Dasgupta A, Bick RJ. Oleandrin produces changes in intracellular calcium levels in isolated cardiomyocytes: A real-time fluorescence imaging study comparing adult to neonatal cardiomyocytes. Journal of Toxicology and Environmental Health. Part A. 2007;**70**(6):568-574. DOI: 10.1080/15287390600882408

[53] Newman RA, Yang P, Hittelman WN, Lu T, Ho DH, Ni D, et al. Oleandrin-mediated oxidative stress in human melanoma cells. Journal of Experimental Therapeutics & Oncology. 2006;**5**(3):167-181

[54] Raviprakash N, Manna SK. Short-term exposure to oleandrin enhances responses to IL-8 by increasing cell surface IL-8 receptors. British Journal of Pharmacology. 2014;**171**(14):3339-3351. DOI: 10.1111/bph.12493

[55] Bao Z, Tian B, Wang X, Feng H, Liang Y, Chen Z, et al. Oleandrin induces DNA damage responses in cancer cells by suppressing the expression of Rad51. Oncotarget. 2016;**7**(37):59572-59579. DOI: 10.18632/oncotarget.10726

[56] Smith JA, Madden T, Vijjeswarapu M, Newman RA. Inhibition of export of fibroblast growth factor-2 (FGF-2) from the prostate cancer cell lines PC3 and DU145 by Anvirzel and its cardiac glycoside component, oleandrin. Biochemical Pharmacology. 2001;**62**(4):469-472. DOI: 10.1016/s0006-2952(01)00690-6

[57] Mekhail T, Kaur H, Ganapathi R, Budd GT, Elson P, Bukowski RM. Phase 1 trial of Anvirzel in patients with refractory solid tumors. Investigational New Drugs. 2006;**24**(5):423-427. DOI: 10.1007/s10637-006-7772-x

[58] Colapietro A, Yang P, Rossetti A, Mancini A, Vitale F, Chakraborty S, et al. The botanical drug PBI-05204, a supercritical CO_2 extract of nerium oleander, is synergistic with radiotherapy in models of human glioblastoma. Frontiers in Pharmacology. 2022;**13**:852941. DOI: 10.3389/fphar.2022.852941

[59] Ko YS, Rugira T, Jin H, Park SW, Kim HJ. Oleandrin and its derivative Odoroside A, both cardiac glycosides, exhibit anticancer effects by inhibiting invasion via suppressing the STAT-3 signaling pathway. International Journal of Molecular Sciences. 2018;**19**(11):3350. DOI: 10.3390/ijms19113350

[60] Nasu S, Milas L, Kawabe S, Raju U, Newman R. Enhancement of radiotherapy by oleandrin is a caspase-3 dependent process. Cancer Letters. 2002;**185**(2):145-151. DOI: 10.1016/s0304-3835(02)00263-x

[61] Ni D, Madden TL, Johansen M, Felix E, Ho DH, Newman RA. Murine pharmacokinetics and metabolism of oleandrin, a cytotoxic component of Nerium oleander. Journal of Experimental Therapeutics & Oncology. 2002;**2**(5):278-285. DOI: 10.1046/j.1359-4117.2002.01052.x

[62] Lin Y, Ho DH, Newman RA. Human tumor cell sensitivity to oleandrin is dependent on relative expression of Na+, K+ -ATPase subunits. Journal of Experimental Therapeutics & Oncology. 2010;**8**(4):271-286

[63] Mijatovic T, Dufrasne F, Kiss R. Cardiotonic steroids-mediated targeting of the Na(+)/K(+)-ATPase to combat chemoresistant cancers. Current Medicinal Chemistry. 2012;**19**(5):627-646. DOI: 10.2174/092986712798992075

[64] Yang P, Cartwright C, Efuet E, Hamilton SR, Wistuba II, Menter D, et al. Cellular location and expression of Na^+, K^+ -ATPase α subunits affect the anti-proliferative activity of oleandrin. Molecular Carcinogenesis. 2014;**53**(4):253-263. DOI: 10.1002/mc.21968

[65] Garofalo S, D'Alessandro G, Chece G, Brau F, Maggi L, Rosa A, et al. Enriched environment reduces glioma growth through immune and non-immune mechanisms in mice. Nature Communications. 2015;**6**:6623. DOI: 10.1038/ncomms7623

[66] Colapietro A, Yang P, Rossetti A, Mancini A, Vitale F, Martellucci S, et al. The botanical drug PBI-05204, a supercritical CO_2 extract of nerium oleander, inhibits growth of human glioblastoma, reduces Akt/mTOR activities, and modulates GSC cell-renewal properties. Frontiers in Pharmacology. 2020;**11**:552428. DOI: 10.3389/fphar.2020.552428

[67] Zhang X, Huang Q, Wang X, Xu Y, Xu R, Han M, et al. Bufalin enhances radiosensitivity of glioblastoma by suppressing mitochondrial function and DNA damage repair. Biomedicine & Pharmacotherapy. 2017;**94**:627-635. DOI: 10.1016/j.biopha.2017.07.136

[68] Lan YL, Chen C, Wang X, Lou JC, Xing JS, Zou S, et al. Gamabufotalin induces a negative feedback loop connecting ATP1A3 expression and the AQP4 pathway to promote temozolomide sensitivity in glioblastoma cells by targeting the amino acid Thr794. Cell Proliferation. 2020;**53**(1):e12732. DOI: 10.1111/cpr.12732

[69] Lan YL, Wang X, Lou JC, Ma XC, Zhang B. The potential roles of aquaporin 4 in malignant gliomas. Oncotarget. 2017;**8**(19):32345-32355. DOI: 10.18632/oncotarget.16017

[70] Liu Z, Zhao X, Mao H, Baxter PA, Huang Y, Yu L, et al. Intravenous injection of oncolytic picornavirus SVV-001 prolongs animal survival in a panel of primary tumor-based orthotopic xenograft mouse models of pediatric glioma. Neuro-Oncology. 2013;**9**:1173-1185. DOI: 10.1093/neuonc/not065

[71] Shu Q, Wong KK, Su JM, Adesina AM, Yu LT, Tsang YT, et al. Direct orthotopic transplantation of fresh surgical specimen preserves CD133+ tumor cells in clinically relevant mouse models of medulloblastoma and glioma. Stem Cells. 2008;**26**(6):1414-1424. DOI: 10.1634/stemcells.2007-1009

[72] Lathia JD, Mack SC, Mulkearns-Hubert EE, Valentim CL, Rich JN. Cancer stem cells in glioblastoma. Genes & Development. 2015;**29**(12):1203-1217. DOI: 10.1101/gad.261982.115

[73] Lee DH, Cheul OS, Giles AJ, Jung J, Gilbert MR, Park DM. Cardiac glycosides suppress the maintenance of stemness and malignancy via inhibiting HIF-1α in human glioma stem cells. Oncotarget. 2017;**8**(25):40233-40245. DOI: 10.18632/oncotarget.16714

[74] Nigim F, Cavanaugh J, Patel AP, Curry WT Jr, Esaki S, Kasper EM, et al. Targeting hypoxia-inducible factor 1α in a new orthotopic model of glioblastoma recapitulating the hypoxic tumor microenvironment. Journal of Neuropathology and Experimental Neurology. 2015;**74**(7):710-722. DOI: 10.1097/NEN.0000000000000210

[75] Li S, Dai Z, Yang D, Li W, Dai H, Sun B, et al. Targeting β2 subunit of Na^+/K^+-ATPase induces glioblastoma cell apoptosis through elevation of intracellular Ca^2. American Journal of Cancer Research. 2019;**9**(6): 1293-1308

[76] Wang JKT, Portbury S, Thomas MB, Barney S, Ricca DJ, Morris DL, et al. Cardiacglycosidesprovideneuroprotection against ischemic stroke: Discovery by a brain slice-based compound screening platform. Proceedings of the National Academy of Sciences of the United States of America. 2006;**103**(27):10461-10466. DOI: 10.1073/pnas.0600930103

Chapter 9

Potential Role of Cancer Stem Cells in Glioblastoma: A Therapeutic Aspect

Meenakshi Tiwari, Lokendra Kumar Sharma and Ajit Kumar Saxena

Abstract

High-grade glioma (HGG) such as glioblastoma multiforme (GBM) is an aggressive brain tumor that is still associated with poor prognosis. With the discovery and advancement in understanding of cancer stem cells (CSC) in glioma, these cells have emerged as seed cells for tumor growth and recurrence and appear as a potential target for therapeutics. Glioma stem cells (GSCs) demonstrate capacity of self-renewal, proliferation, and differentiation into multiple cell types and can contribute to tumor heterogeneity. Their role is established in tumorigenesis, metastasis, chemo- and radio-resistance and appears as a major cause for tumor recurrence. Thus, targeting GSCs by various therapeutics may improve effectiveness of the drugs in use alone or in combination to significantly improve patient survival outcome in GBM cases. In this chapter, we have discussed various mechanisms that drive GSC including signaling pathways and tumor microenvironment. We have also discussed the mechanism behind resistance of GSCs toward therapeutics and the pathways that can be targeted to improve the outcome of the patients.

Keywords: Glioblastoma multiforme, cancer stem cells, glioma stem cells, signaling pathways, chemotherapeutics, tumor microenvironment, resistance to therapy

1. Introduction

Glioblastoma multiforme (GBM), classified as grade IV glioma, is highly invasive, heterogeneous, and malignant primary brain tumor. It accounts for ~57% of all gliomas and ~ 48% of all primary malignant central nervous system (CNS) tumors [1, 2]. Such tumors are associated with poor quality of life of the patient due to progressive decline in neurologic function, thus making a huge impact on the patients, care givers, and their families. The standard treatment includes multimodal approach involving maximal surgical resection followed by radiotherapy, systemic therapy (chemotherapy, targeted therapy), and supportive care; however, long-term survival is exceptional. Despite the treatment, these tumors regrow and that too with aggressive phenotype, which worsen the symptoms leading to prognosis with average overall survival time < 14.6 months for primary GBM patients and < 6.9 months for recurrent

GBM patients [3]. Understanding the molecular mechanism involved in therapeutic resistance and tumor regrowth despite standard treatment is imperative.

In this regard, researchers have identified existence of cancer stem cells (CSCs) in a variety of cancers that play crucial role in tumor initiation, maintenance, resistance to therapy, recurrence, metastasis, and generation of more aggressive phenotype [4]. These properties of CSC are manifested by their potential to self-renew, proliferate, ability to differentiate in multiple phenotypes, plasticity, quiescence, and dormancy. It is suggested that these CSCs originate either from normal stem cells that were already present in tissue or can be generated from dedifferentiation of somatic cells from bulk of tumor. Based on the properties of CSCs, they pose not only a barrier for anticancer therapy but also are responsible for recurrence into more aggressive phenotype. Various researchers have shown that CSC escape anticancer therapy due to their ability to enter dormancy, plasticity, renewal, and regrowth into heterogeneous group of tumor cells. Of interest, recent evidences have suggested that these CSCs are further enriched in response to standard radio-chemotherapy, which may be responsible for tumor regrowth and aggressive phenotype. These enriched CSCs might be result from the existing population of CSCs that evades the therapy or as per recent evidences, can be generated from non-CSCs from the bulk of tumor in response to therapy. Of note, CSCs have been identified in HGG cases also known as glioma stem cells (GSCs) that contribute to tumor heterogeneity and resistance to therapies, thus a major contributor of tumor recurrence. These GSCs are considered as a potential therapeutic target, therefore understanding the molecular pathways that drive GSCs becomes imperative [5]. In this book chapter, we have discussed about the properties of cancer stem cells, cell surface markers, signaling pathways, and mechanism of resistance to therapies and ways by which these pathways can be targeted using different chemotherapeutic agents.

2. Biology of cancer stem cells

Stem cells are specialized cells present in our body that possess properties such as capacity to self-renew, proliferate, and differentiate into multiple cell types. This quality of self-renewal along with associated signaling pathways is shared between both stem cells and cancer stem cells with added feature of oncogenicity in CSCs. The most common pathways that drive multipotency and self-renewal of stem cells include the Notch, Sonic hedgehog (Shh), and Wnt signaling pathways [4]. Due to activation of oncogenic pathways, CSCs can give rise to tumor mass consisting of heterogeneous cell population. Initially, Bonnet and Dick characterized CSCs in acute myeloid leukemia as leukemia-initiating cell that possessed properties of leukemia stem cell [6]. Later, such cells were also identified in a variety of solid tumors, including prostate [7], colon [8], lung [9], ovarian [10], and brain [11] tumors. It is hypothesized that CSCs are the seed of a tumor that are responsible for tumorigenesis by initiation, maintenance, propagation, resistance to therapy, recurrence as well as progression of the tumor [12].

3. Glioma stem cells

In brain tumors, presence of CSC has been identified and characterized by various groups and are defined as GSCs or glioma initiating cells [11]. When cultured, these cells grown into neurospheres that constitute of cells that express SC markers including Nestin and CD133. When these cells are injected into nude mice, they lead to tumor formation due to their SC properties [13]. To add further, various groups have utilized properties of stem cells that are present in brain predominantly in subventricular zone (SVZ) to initiate tumor by exposure to chemicals (ethylnitrosourea) or viruses (avian sarcoma virus) in animals that strongly support the importance of stem cells in tumor formation [7, 14, 15]. These cells contribute to tumor heterogeneity and plasticity and have shown resistance to therapies and thus have emerged as a major contributor of tumor recurrence [5, 16, 17]. These CSCs are also influenced by micro environmental conditions such as nutrient deprivation, hypoxia, pH, vasculature, radiation, and chemotherapeutic treatment (explained in detail in coming sections) [16–19].

Several putative GSC surface markers, such as CD133, CD15, and CD44, and GSC transcription factors, such as SRY-box transcription factor 2 (SOX2), octamer-binding transcription factor 4 (OCT4), and NANOG, have been discovered [20, 21]. However, before its clinical implication, higher sensitivity and specificity of these GSC markers need to be established [21, 22].

4. Major signaling pathways that drive glioma stem cells

In order to maintain stemness properties, GSCs depend upon number of signaling pathways that also support them to sustain under adverse conditions during tumorigenesis [23–25]. To understand the process of stemness in GSC, the signaling pathways that are also a part of normal neuronal stem cells are discussed. These pathways mainly include Notch, bone morphogenic proteins (BMPs), NF-κB, Wnt, epidermal growth factor (EGF), and Shh that determine the property of stemness.

4.1 Notch signaling

Notch signaling pathway is crucial in developmental process and plays a major role during embryonic development. This pathway regulates cellular proliferation, differentiation, apoptosis, and cell lineage decisions. In GSCs, Notch signaling pathways are highly active, which in turn maintain stemness by inhibiting differentiation. Notch signaling is also involved in oncogenic transformation. It has been identified that inhibition of Notch signaling decreases oncogenic potential of GSCs [26, 27].

4.2 Bone morphogenetic proteins (BMPs)

BMP group of molecules belongs to the transforming growth factor-β (TGF-β) superfamily of proteins. BMPs plays role during embryogenesis, development as well as adult tissue homeostasis. It interacts with different signaling molecules including Wnt/β-catenin, basic helix-loop-helix (bHLH), and hypoxia-inducible factor-1α (HIF-1α) to regulate different processes in all the body organs [28, 29]. BMPs have been identified to regulate the niche as well as stem cells residing within. Besides normal functions, BMPs are also involved in tumorigenesis where BMP2 and BMP4 have emerged as key players. It is identified that dysregulation of the BMP pathway results in sustained cell transformation in stem cells and their niche. BMP signaling pathways are also involved in regulation of cellular proliferation, differentiation, and apoptosis in NSCs. NSCs are differentiated to astroglial lineage via Wnt-mediated

BMP signaling [30] and antagonist of BMP can inhibit differentiation of GSCs and maintains its self-renewal and tumorigenic potential [31]. Further, it was demonstrated that delivery of BMP4 can inhibit brain tumor growth in in vivo system and decreased the rate of mortality [32].

4.3 Wnt/β-catenin signaling

Wnt/β-catenin signaling is a highly conserved pathway that regulates cellular proliferation, differentiation, migration, genetic stability, apoptosis, and stem cell renewal. This pathway also regulates NSC expansion and promotes astroglial lineage differentiation during neural development [33, 34]. In GSC, *β*-catenin regulates proliferation and differentiation and dysregulated Wnt signaling leads to tumor growth [35–37]. *β*-Catenin interacts with FoxM1 to regulate the transcription of various oncogeneic genes such as c-Myc that leads to gliomagenesis [38, 39].

4.4 Epidermal growth factor receptor (EGFR) signaling

The EGFR pathway is one of the most crucial pathways involved in cellular processes including proliferation, differentiation, migration, and apoptosis in a variety of cells including stem cells. Dysregulation of this pathway has been linked to cancer. Critical role of EGFR has been identified in NSCs as well [40–42]. In GSC EGFR works through activation of *β*-catenin pathway and promotes self-renewal capacity of GSC and induction of tumorigenic potential [43].

4.5 Sonic hedgehog (Shh) signaling

The Shh signaling pathway is crucial for proper embryonic development as it governs tissue polarity, patterning maintenance, cellular proliferation, intercellular communication, and differentiation [44, 45]. Persistent Shh pathway signaling has been observed in the subventricular zone of adult brain where it plays a critical role in regional specification and maintenance of NSCs [46]. Aberrant regulation of the Shh pathway due to mutation has been identified to cause tumorigenesis in a wide variety of cancer tissues including gliomas and GSCs. This pathway is highly active in GSCs where it regulates stemness genes and thus maintains self-renewal of GSC and promotes tumorigenesis and inhibition of Shh signaling reduces both stemness as well as *in vivo* tumorigenicity by induction of autophagic cell death [47].

5. Pathways that contributing to resistance of glioma stem cells toward therapies that lead to tumor regrowth

Resistance of CSCs toward therapies resulting in their enrichment and regrowth of tumor due to proliferation of these cells has been suggested by various researchers [48–50]. In HGG, despite the effectiveness of TMZ in removing the bulk tumor cells, regrowth with a more aggressive phenotype is inevitable, and researchers have identified critical role of CSCs in such regrowth. For instance, in HGG, treatment with therapeutic doses of temozolomide (TMZ) leads to expansion of GSCs pool in both patient-derived and established glioma cell lines. Such expansions are reported not only due to enrichment and proliferation of existing CSCs but also due to interconversion between differentiated tumor cells and GSCs [18]. Similarly, bevacizumab (VEGF antibody) although reduces GBM tumor growth, it is followed by tumor regrowth where the role of autocrine signaling through the VEGF-VEGFR2-Neuropilin-1 (NRP1) axis leads to enrichment of active VEGFR2 GSC subset in human GBM cells [51]. It is evident that the therapeutics evoke enrichment of CSCs involving multiple mechanisms. Thus, understanding various ways by which CSCs escape the radio- and chemotherapy, more effective treatment modalities can be developed. Broadly, in CSCs various different mechanism such as epithelial-mesenchymal transition (EMT), multiple drug resistance (MDR) dormancy, tumor environment contribute to resistance toward therapeutics and other adverse conditions faced by them in tumor microenvironment and are discussed as follows.

5.1 DNA repair systems

GSCs possess better DNA repair capacity as compared with bulk tumor cells [52]. These cells express higher levels of DNA repair enzymes such as O6-methylguanine-methyltransferase (MGMT), which are responsible for therapy resistance against DNA alkylating agents such as TMZ [53–56]. However, there are contradictory studies that also suggest that TMZ resistance in GSCs is independent of MGMT status and alternate pathways might be involved [57, 58]. Further, preferential expression of DNA checkpoint kinases 1 (Chk1) and 2 (Chk2) lead to more efficient repair of DNA damage in CD133-positive glioma cells than CD133-negative glioma cells [54]. Other transcriptional regulators such as BMI, DNA-PK, poly (ADP-ribose) polymerase-1, hnRNP U, and histone H1, which play a role in DNA double-strand break repair, are highly expressed in CD133-positive GBM cells and play pivotal role in GSCs' functions [59, 60].

5.2 Epithelial-mesenchymal transition (EMT)

EMT involves phenotypic changes in cells from epithelial to mesenchymal type involving high expression of markers such as N-cadherin and vimentin under various physiological as well as pathological conditions including cancer [61]. Interestingly, CSCs also share the EMT-like cell features [62], and it is believed that the link between EMT and CSCs might be responsible for cancer drug resistance acquisition and plasticity resulting in cancer cells transformation into the malignant cells and *vice versa* [63]. Circulating tumor cells from patients with metastasis co-express markers of EMT as well as CSCs. Further, induction of EMT confers stem-like features in cancer cells [64, 65]. Various regulators of EMT have been identified that regulate stemness. ZEB1 is one such regulator of EMT that regulates stemness and chemoresistance induction by regulating MGMT via miR-200c and c-MYB in malignant glioma [66]. Therefore, a strong association of EMT and CSCs has been identified that provides not only resistance but also promotes metastasis [67].

5.3 Dormancy of CSCs

As the understanding of CSC biology has improved, it has been identified that CSCs can exist in proliferative or dormant state. Dormant CSCs maintain a low metabolic activity, however, show similarities with the normal proliferative counterpart in terms of stemness and other signaling pathways. For instance, dormant stem cells are low in metabolic activity that preferentially utilize the glycolytic pathway and produce low levels of levels of reactive oxygen species (ROS) [68]. However, these dormant/quiescent cells demonstrate high plasticity and can be reactivated to reenter proliferative stage and lead to tumor formation. Such dormant cells are also chemoresistant due to their dormant nature; interestingly, proliferative CSC can also enter dormancy in response to chemotherapeutics agents. In GBM, existence of a relatively quiescent subset of GSCs has been observed, which is responsible for maintaining the long-term tumor growth and responsible for recurrence by entering into highly proliferative cells upon receiving proper signals [69].

5.4 Anti-apoptosis

Various anti-apoptotic protein such as B-cell lymphoma-2 (BCL-2), BCL2 like 1 (BCL2L1), myeloid cell leukemia-1, MCL1 and BCL-xL are highly expressed in GSCs than differentiated bulk tumor cells. These proteins not only play role in GSCs maintenance but also provide survival advantage to these cells against various chemotherapeutic agents [70]. Other mediator of GSCs resistance includes BMI1, a GSC-enriched protein that inhibits p53-mediated apoptosis against TMZ [71]. Inhibition of such anti-apoptotic pathways can increase sensitivity of GSCs against different therapeutic agents.

5.5 Multidrug resistance

Stem cells express higher levels of several ATP-binding cassette (ABC) transporters resulting in efflux ability for various antineoplastic drugs [72]. In GSCs, increased *ABCG1* expression has been documented in the side population cells in flow cytometry that present the GSC phenotype [73]. Further, multidrug resistance 1 (*MDR1*) overexpression was reported higher in $CD133^+$ GSCs than $CD133^-$ bulk tumor cells [74]. *ABCG2/BCRP* and *ABCB1/MDR1* overexpression in GSCs has also been correlated with resistance of GSCs to chemotherapeutic drugs and use of an ABC transporter inhibitor, such as verapamil, can help in increasing sensitivity of GSCs toward chemotherapeutic agents such as temozolomide, doxorubicin, and mitoxantrone in GSCs [75]. Similarly, methylation of ABC transporter *ABCG2/BCRP* promoter by melatonin (*N*-acetyl-5-methoxytryptamine) promotes toxic effect of TMZ on GSCs [75]. Interestingly, treatment with chemotherapeutic agents can further increase expression of these MDR proteins conferring resistance to these cells against chemotherapeutic agents [76]. Thus, inhibition of drug efflux proteins such as MDR proteins appears as a potential target for increasing sensitivity of GSCs toward various chemotherapeutic agents [75, 77].

5.6 Metabolism

GSCs show metabolic adaptations to survive adverse conditions of tumor microenvironment that includes low pH, hypoxia, and low nutrient supply; at the same time they proliferate at a high rate to maintain their stemness [16, 17]. Majority of GSCs rely on glucose uptake via high-affinity glucose transporter 3 (GLUT3) to provide carbon source for nucleotide biosynthesis for rapid proliferating cells along with high energy demands [78–80]. These cells also highly express glutamine synthetase as compared with differentiated glioma cells for higher glutamine uptake, which acts as preferential source for *de-novo* purine biosynthesis [81]. Further studies demonstrate that in therapy-resistant GSCs expression of glucose uptake associated genes is downregulated, and they preferentially use fatty acids as a major ATP source [82].

Additionally, slow-cycling GSCs rely on oxidative phosphorylation and lipid metabolism than fast-cycling GSCs which prefer glycolysis [83]. These anabolic advantages of GSCs may contribute to their chemoresistant phenotype and can be targeted to improve sensitivity of GBM treatment.

5.7 Autophagy

Autophagy is a catabolic pathway which is a cellular stress response under physiological as well as pathological conditions. This pathways acts by removal of damaged macromolecules such as proteins, nucleic acid, and lipids and recycles them for cellular processes and thus promotes cell survival; however, defect or dysregulation of such pathway may lead to cell death [84]. Role of autophagy is well established in a variety of cancers including GBM where it can play a role in cell survival or cell death [84, 85]. Autophagy also contributes to the maintenance of stemness characteristics of GSCs as well as provides chemoresistance to CSC against therapeutic agents [19, 86]. Inhibition of autophagy sensitizes GSCs towards a variety of therapeutic agents [19, 87–89]. Interestingly, other studies demonstrated that induction of autophagy by mammalian target of rapamycin (mTOR) inhibitors as well as curcumin-induced autophagy shows anti proliferative effect, induces differentiation and also improves sensitivity of GSC towards DNA damaging agents [90–92]. Together, these results suggest that GSCs require a balanced level of autophagy, too much or too little can significantly affect their stemness potential and resistance toward therapeutics. Further, role of autophagy has also been shown to support motility/migration capacity of GSCs [93]. However, role of autophagy in suppression of the self-renewal ability and tumorigenicity of GSCs has also been demonstrated where autophagy mediates Notch1 degradation [94]. Thus, role of autophagy in GSCs is crucial for maintenance of stemness as well as chemotherapeutic agents; targeting such pathway appears as a p These cells also highly express glutamine synthetase otential strategy to make the existing treatment more effective.

5.8 Extrinsic chemoresistance

Besides the signaling pathways and genetic signature of GSCs, extracellular environment also called as microenvironment in which these cells resides also plays crucial role in its functions and determines response towards therapeutic agents [95]. It has been identified that GSCs reside in inner tumor mass where rapid growth and high energy requirement of these cells along with neovasculature result in hypoxic conditions as well as low pH [29, 96]. These adverse conditions further promote expression of GSC markers and associated phenotype [97]. Various hypoxia and acidic pH-induced genes such as hypoxia-inducible factor (HIF) 1 and 2alpha and vascular endothelial growth factor (VEGF) are highly expressed in GSCs that contribute to GSC functions [98, 99]. It has been shown that in GSCs Notch signaling and MGMT expression are also regulated by HIF-1α, resulting in GSC stemness and also resistance toward TMZ [100, 101]. Further, hypoxic GSCs release extracellular vesicles that deliver HIF-1α induced miR-30b-3p that further activates STAT3 pathway and promotes TMZ resistance [102]. Further, it has been identified that TMZ increases the GSC pool in non-GSC subpopulations, indicating that non-GSC shows plasticity and can be converted to GSCs that might be responsible for resistance as well as regrowth of the tumor [18, 19]. Together, these findings suggest that *stemness* of GSCs may be regulated by tumor microenvironment as well as cellular plasticity; TMZ can stimulate the dedifferentiation of non-GSCs, which might contribute to resistance and recurrence after therapy [18, 19].

5.9 Role of Notch and sonic hedgehog pathways in mediating chemoresistance

Various signaling pathways such as Notch and SHH are active in GSCs compared with bulk tumor cells [103]. Further, in response to TMZ treatment of GSCs from primary GBM cells resulted in upregulation of *NOTCH 1*, *NCOR2*, *HES1*, *HES5*, and *GLI1* genes, suggesting resistance of these cells and increase in the population of such stem cells in glioma, which could be reversed by inhibitors of Notch or SHH inhibitors [104]. Epithelial-mesenchymal transition (EMT) mediates GBM chemoresistance. Another fact contributing to resistance of GSCs is the potential of epithelial-mesenchymal transition. It has been shown that EMT mediator gene *ZEB1 can* regulate *stemness* and *SOX2* and OLIG2 in gliomas [105].

6. Strategies targeting glioma stem cells

Despite extensive research in oncology, the target is being missed leading to recurrence in a variety of high-grade tumors including malignant gliomas. With advancement in understanding of GSCs and its capacity of initiation, progression, resistance as well as recurrence of tumor, they appear as most promising target to treat cancers such as HGG. The drugs that can target GSC are being developed using multiple strategist including molecular targeting, autophagy inhibition, drug repositioning, and indirect targeting of GSC niches [17, 21, 106].

6.1 Targeting GSC markers and related signaling pathways

GSCs are regulated by various pathways involving differential expression of epidermal growth factor receptor (EGFR), Notch1, sonic hedgehog (Shh), and STAT3, as well as related signaling pathways.

As discussed earlier, CD133 is the most well-characterized cell surface marker for GSCs, which has become a potential target for antibody-based therapy. Different immunotherapeutic approaches such use of synthetic monoclonal antibody, dual-antigen T cell engager, and chimeric antigen receptor (CAR) T cell have been utilized to target CD133+ GSCs. RW03 (anti-CD133 antibody) targets self-renewal ability of GSCs without effecting its proliferative capacity and could be a promising strategy in targeting GSCs [107]. Further, photothermal therapy has also shown selective efficacy in diminishing CD133-positive cells both *in-vitro* and *in-vivo* [108].

EGFR, a receptor tyrosine kinase, which is highly expressed in GSCs, is crucial for its survival, self-renewal, and tumorigenicity. Of importance, EGFR variant III (EGFRvIII) mutation is most commonly detectable (25–33%) in GBM cases [109]. Thus, EGFR inhibition becomes a potential target to inhibit GSCs proliferation, self-renewal, and induction of apoptosis [110]. EGFR inhibition in fact enhanced chemo- and radio-sensitivity of human glioma CSCs. Various reversible and irreversible inhibits of EGFR are available that can bind EGFR alone or along with its co-receptor HER2 [111, 112]. First-generation EGFR TKIs include gefitinib and erlotinib that can reversibly bind EGFR along with HER2; however, less than 20% of patients presented a response to these treatments [112, 113]. Irreversible inhibitor of EGFR, osimertinib, has shown efficiency in crossing the blood-brain barrier (BBB) and significantly inhibits GBM tumorigenesis *in-vivo* [114]. It has also entered phase II clinical studies [115, 116], however, has shown to be marginally effective, which could be due to heterogeneity of GBM [117, 118]. Further, combined treatment of antibodies against EGFRvIII and CD133 showed higher effectivity in elimination of GSCs compared with the antibody against either EGFRvIII or CD133 [111].

Various signaling pathways such as Notch and SHH are active in GSCs compared with bulk tumor cells [114]. Further, in response to TMZ treatment of GSCs from primary GBM cells resulted in upregulation of *NOTCH 1*, *NCOR2*, *HES1*, *HES5*, and *GLI1* genes, suggesting resistance of these cells and increase in the population of such stem cells in glioma, which could be reversed by inhibitors of Notch or SHH inhibitors [118]. Notch1 signaling that contributes to regulation of GSC can be blocked by γ-secretase inhibitor [119]. RO4929097, a γ-secretase inhibitor, reduces the viability of GSCs [120]. Further, Notch1 also regulates VEGF activity in GSCs, and co-inhibition of Notch1 and VEGF have shown synergistic effects in GBM [121]; however, their combined inhibition (RO4929097 with bevacizumab) in phase I clinical trial did not show much improvement in overall survival (OS) and progression-free survival (PFS) in GBM cases [122]. Other studies also identify the role of γ-secretase inhibitor, N-[N-(3, 5-difluorophenacetyl-L-alanyl)]-S-phenylglycine t-butyl ester (DAPT) in improving TMZ sensitivity [123].

Shh/Gli signaling that regulates GSCs cell proliferation, stem cell fate determination, and differentiation has also appeared as potential target for GSCs therapeutics [124]. Inhibition of hedgehog pathway by LDE225 induces autophagic cell death in GSCs with higher sensitivity of CD133-positive cells than CD133-negative cells [125]. LDE225 inhibits expression and nuclear translocation of Gli proteins, a transcriptional effectors of the Shh signaling pathway [126]. Casein kinase 2 (CK2) is another target to inhibit Shh/Gli signaling via transcriptional activation of β-catenin [127] and inhibition of CK2 by, CX-4945 (silmitasertib), reduces MGMT expression and sensitized tumor cells to TMZ [128].

Signal transducer and activator of transcription 3 (STAT3) that regulates multiple processes such as cell cycle and survival, regulation, immune response, and differentiation, tumorigenic transformation has also been implicated in GSC maintenance [129, 130]. Resveratrol (RV), a polyphenol present in grapes, a tumor preventive agent targets STAT3 signaling. In glioma, RV has shown antineoplastic actions by apoptosis induction and improving radio sensitivity of GSCs CD133+ cell population along with reducing of tumorigenic potential. Furthermore, RV also modulates Wnt signaling pathway and EMT activators, thereby regulating stemness of GSCs and reducing cellular motility [131, 132]. Another molecule that inhibits STAT pathway is WP1066, which is an analog of the natural product caffeic acid benzyl ester and targets GSCs. This molecule has shown promising results in clinical trial for patients with recurrent malignant glioma [133]. Other STAT3 inhibitors, STX-0119 and WP1066 have shown ability to suppress GSC proliferation *in-vitro*; however, inhibition of tumor growth in subcutaneous xenograft model of GSCs was shown only by STX-0119. STX-0119 further demonstrated ability to downregulate expression of GSCs markers [134]. Another small-molecule STAT3 inhibitor, ODZ10117, also decreased the stem cell properties of GSCs and reduced tumor growth in vivo [130].

6.2 Targeting tumor microenvironment

GSCs are localized in specific niches, which have been identified as protective microenvironments in GBM. Five types of GSC niches have been identified where different cell types exists and have specific singling pathways: peri-vascular, peri-arteriolar, peri-hypoxic, peri-immune, and extracellular matrix out of which peri-vascular niche is the most frequently described GSC [135]. GSC microenvironment lacks organizations and has compromised BBB, higher levels of hypoxia, and excessive angiogenesis making it a target for anti-angiogenic therapy [136, 137].

6.3 Drugs targeting metabolic pathways

Drug repositioning also called as repurpose drugs is a growing concept that explores pre-existing a well-established drug to treat diseases aside from the intended ones. This concept results in lowering the overall developmental cost, time and risk assessments, as the efficacy and safety of the original drug have already been well accessed and approved by regulatory authorities [138]. In case of GSCs, repurpose drugs are being tested and have shown encouraging results. Especially, anti-diabetes drugs have been most well studied with promising results in GSCs targeting. Metformin, successfully used for type 2 diabetes mellitus, has entered phase I clinical trial for GBM in combination with TMZ [139]. Metformin preferentially acts in GSCs by inhibiting Akt activation and also induces conversion on GSCs to non-GSCs [140, 141]. Similarly glimepiride, another anti-diabetes drug, impairs GSCs by targeting glycolytic flux and increases its radio sensitivity to GBM [142]. Further, more repurpose drugs need to be identified that can effectively target GSCs along with its associated mechanism before it can be used in clinical application [138].

6.4 Targeting autophagy pathways

Autophagy is a cellular stress response, which can either promote survival or cell death. Our laboratory along with others has identified that autophagy is required for maintenance of GSCs and also plays a role in resistance of GSCs toward chemotherapy [19, 142, 143]. Targeting autophagy by commonly used agent chloroquine (CQ), which blocks the fusion of autophagosomes with lysosomes, has been shown to inhibit GSCs as well as sensitized them toward chemotherapeutic agents [19, 144]. This drug has also entered multiple clinical trials as an adjuvant treatment for GBM; where its antitumor effects of CQ are not limited to GSCs [145]. Further, combination of autophagy inhibitors with radiation effectively induced apoptosis and inhibited tumorosphere formation in GSCs [146, 147]. More selective autophagy inhibitor NSC185058, antagonist of autophagy-related 4B, inhibits tumorigenic potential of GSCs and enhances GBM sensitivity to radiotherapy in xenograft mouse models [148].

7. Conclusions and future directions

Treatment of HGG remains challenging. With identification of GSCs and their properties to resist treatment and repopulate the original tumor, a big momentum has been created in the development of novel therapeutics. Such therapeutic will involve a combination of drugs that controls the bulk tumor mass along with CSCs-directed agents. It has been identified that GSCs are responsible for tumorigenesis, therapeutic resistance, and tumor recurrence, and thus GSC-targeting drugs are being developed for improvement of treatment regime. These GSCs can survive cancer treatment by activating multiple mechanisms such as EMT, signaling pathways to regulate self-renewal, its interaction with tumor microenvironment, higher expression of drug transporters or detoxification proteins, plasticity, autophagy induction, anti-apoptotic mechanism, induction of dormant phenotype, and many others to overcome the toxic effects of therapeutics. With knowledge of these pathways, anticancer therapeutics are targeted against GSCs, which includes directing specific and pathways that regulate GSCs and protect them from therapeutic stress. Such GSC-directed drugs can be combined with agents that are currently in use to achieve better survival rates of cancer patients.

Identification of bioactive products and their molecular mechanisms that can modulate GSCs needs to be incorporated in treatment regime of HGG patients. With recent advancements in the field of high-throughput screening and genetic and epigenetic signatures, specific targeted drugs that can target bulk tumor with minimal generation of induced GSCs along with combination of drug that can target GSCs can be developed. Furthermore, tumor microenvironment that significantly regulates GSCs is also a potential target to prevent rate of dedifferentiation. It is important to consider that current therapeutic can result in conversion of non-GSC to GSCs; therefore, newer drugs or combinations need to be developed that can prevent this detrimental conversion. More stringent strategies involving GSC-targeted therapy along with glioma molecular subtypes need to be designed for selective and effective clinical trials.

However, most therapeutic agents have failed to be approved for clinical application or during clinical trials due to lack of understanding of the underlying mechanisms or failure to consider individual characteristics of the tumor. Further investigation of the molecular pathways that drive GSCs and make them resistant to therapies along with subtype-specific pathways of GSCs is required. Such studies will significantly improve not only the understanding of disease but will also direct the development of highly specific drugs with minimal side effects along with improved patient outcome.

Acknowledgements

The authors would like to acknowledge the funding support from Department of Biotechnology Bio-CARe grant, Govt. of India (BT/P19357/BIC/101/927/2016 to M.T.) and Intramural Research Grant by SGPGIMS (PGI/DIR/RC/36/2021) to LKS.

Conflict of interest

The authors declare that they have no conflict of interest.

Author details

Meenakshi Tiwari[1*], Lokendra Kumar Sharma[2] and Ajit Kumar Saxena[1]

1 Department of Pathology/Lab Medicine, All India Institute of Medical Sciences-Patna, Patna, Bihar, India

2 Department of Molecular Medicine and Biotechnology, Sanjay Gandhi Post Graduate Institute of Medical Sciences, Lucknow, Uttar Pradesh, India

*Address all correspondence to: meenakshimani79@yahoo.co.in; drmeenakshit@aiimspatna.org

References

[1] Dolecek TA, Propp JM, Stroup NE, Kruchko C. CBTRUS statistical report: Primary brain and central nervous system tumors diagnosed in the United States in 2005-2009 [published correction appears in Neuro Oncol. 2013 May;15(5):646-7]. Neuro-Oncology. 2012;**14**(Suppl 5):v1-v49. DOI: 10.1093/neuonc/nos218

[2] Davis ME. Glioblastoma: Overview of disease and treatment. Clinical Journal of Oncology Nursing. 2016;**20**(5 Suppl):S2-S8. DOI: 10.1188/16.CJON.S1.2-8

[3] Hanif F, Muzaffar K, Perveen K, Malhi SM, Simjee SU. Glioblastoma Multiforme: A review of its epidemiology and pathogenesis through clinical presentation and treatment. Asian Pacific Journal of Cancer Prevention. 2017;**18**(1):3-9. Published 2017 Jan 1. DOI: 10.22034/APJCP.2017.18.1.3

[4] Reya T, Morrison SJ, Clarke MF, Weissman IL. Stem cells, cancer, and cancer stem cells. Nature. 2001;**414**(6859):105-111. DOI: 10.1038/35102167

[5] Kang H, Lee H, Kim D, et al. Targeting glioblastoma stem cells to overcome Chemoresistance: An overview of current therapeutic strategies. Biomedicine. 2022;**10**(6):1308. Published 2022 Jun 2. DOI: 10.3390/biomedicines10061308

[6] Bonnet D, Dick JE. Human acute myeloid leukemia is organized as a hierarchy that originates from a primitive hematopoietic cell. Nature Medicine. 1997;**3**(7):730-737. DOI: 10.1038/nm0797-730

[7] Collins AT, Berry PA, Hyde C, Stower MJ, Maitland NJ. Prospective identification of tumorigenic prostate cancer stem cells. Cancer Research. 2005;**65**(23):10946-10951. DOI: 10.1158/0008-5472.CAN-05-2018

[8] Ricci-Vitiani L, Lombardi DG, Pilozzi E, et al. Identification and expansion of human colon-cancer-initiating cells. Nature. 2007;**445**(7123):111-115. DOI: 10.1038/nature05384

[9] Kim CF, Jackson EL, Woolfenden AE, et al. Identification of bronchioalveolar stem cells in normal lung and lung cancer. Cell. 2005;**121**(6):823-835. DOI: 10.1016/j.cell.2005.03.032

[10] Zhang S, Balch C, Chan MW, et al. Identification and characterization of ovarian cancer-initiating cells from primary human tumors. Cancer Research. 2008;**68**(11):4311-4320. DOI: 10.1158/0008-5472.CAN-08-0364

[11] Singh SK, Clarke ID, Terasaki M, et al. Identification of a cancer stem cell in human brain tumors. Cancer Research. 2003;**63**(18):5821-5828

[12] Sundar SJ, Hsieh JK, Manjila S, Lathia JD, Sloan A. The role of cancer stem cells in glioblastoma. Neurosurgical Focus. 2014;**37**(6):E6. DOI: 10.3171/2014.9.FOCUS14494

[13] Yuan X, Curtin J, Xiong Y, et al. Isolation of cancer stem cells from adult glioblastoma multiforme. Oncogene. 2004;**23**(58):9392-9400. DOI: 10.1038/sj.onc.1208311

[14] Copeland DD, Bigner DD. The role of the subependymal plate in avian sarcoma virus brain tumor induction: Comparison of incipient tumors in neonatal and adult rats. Acta Neuropathologica.

1977;**38**(1):1-6. DOI: 10.1007/BF00691268

[15] Vick NA, Lin MJ, Bigner DD. The role of the subependymal plate in glial tumorigenesis. Acta Neuropathologica. 1977;**40**(1):63-71. DOI: 10.1007/BF00688574

[16] Gimple RC, Bhargava S, Dixit D, Rich JN. Glioblastoma stem cells: Lessons from the tumor hierarchy in a lethal cancer. Genes & Development. 2019;**33**(11-12):591-609. DOI: 10.1101/gad.324301.119

[17] Rodriguez SMB, Staicu GA, Sevastre AS, et al. Glioblastoma stem cells-useful tools in the Battle against cancer. International Journal of Molecular Sciences. 2022;**23**(9):4602. Published 2022 Apr 21. DOI: 10.3390/ijms23094602

[18] Auffinger B, Tobias AL, Han Y, et al. Conversion of differentiated cancer cells into cancer stem-like cells in a glioblastoma model after primary chemotherapy. Cell Death and Differentiation. 2014;**21**(7):1119-1131. DOI: 10.1038/cdd.2014.31

[19] Abbas S, Singh SK, Saxena AK, Tiwari S, Sharma LK, Tiwari M. Role of autophagy in regulation of glioma stem cells population during therapeutic stress. Journal of Stem Cells & Regenerative Medicine. 2020;**16**(2):80-89. Published 2020 Dec 11. DOI: 10.46582/jsrm.1602012

[20] Suvà ML, Tirosh I. The glioma stem cell model in the era of single-cell genomics. Cancer Cell. 2020;**37**(5):630-636. DOI: 10.1016/j.ccell.2020.04.001

[21] Tang X, Zuo C, Fang P, et al. Targeting glioblastoma stem cells: A review on biomarkers, signal pathways and targeted therapy. Frontiers in Oncology. 2021;**11**:701291. Published 2021 Jul 8. DOI: 10.3389/fonc.2021.701291

[22] Saygin C, Matei D, Majeti R, Reizes O, Lathia JD. Targeting cancer Stemness in the clinic: From hype to Hope. Cell Stem Cell. 2019;**24**(1):25-40. DOI: 10.1016/j.stem.2018.11.017

[23] Hemmati HD, Nakano I, Lazareff JA, et al. Cancerous stem cells can arise from pediatric brain tumors. Proceedings of the National Academy of Sciences of the United States of America. 2003;**100**(25):15178-15183. DOI: 10.1073/pnas.2036535100

[24] Rich JN, Eyler CE. Cancer stem cells in brain tumor biology. Cold Spring Harbor Symposia on Quantitative Biology. 2008;**73**:411-420. DOI: 10.1101/sqb.2008.73.060

[25] Vescovi AL, Galli R, Reynolds BA. Brain tumour stem cells. Nature Reviews. Cancer. 2006;**6**(6):425-436. DOI: 10.1038/nrc1889

[26] Kanamori M, Kawaguchi T, Nigro JM, et al. Contribution of Notch signaling activation to human glioblastoma multiforme. Journal of Neurosurgery. 2007;**106**(3):417-427. DOI: 10.3171/jns.2007.106.3.417

[27] Purow BW, Haque RM, Noel MW, et al. Expression of Notch-1 and its ligands, Delta-like-1 and Jagged-1, is critical for glioma cell survival and proliferation. Cancer Research. 2005;**65**(6):2353-2363. DOI: 10.1158/0008-5472.CAN-04-1890

[28] Kurooka H, Nakahiro T, Mori K, Sano K, Yokota Y. BMP signaling is responsible for serum-induced Id2 expression. Biochemical and

Biophysical Research Communications. 2012;**420**(2):281-287. DOI: 10.1016/j.bbrc.2012.02.150

[29] Pistollato F, Chen HL, Rood BR, et al. Hypoxia and HIF1alpha repress the differentiative effects of BMPs in high-grade glioma. Stem Cells. 2009;**27**(1):7-17. DOI: 10.1634/stemcells.2008-0402

[30] Kasai M, Satoh K, Akiyama T. Wnt signaling regulates the sequential onset of neurogenesis and gliogenesis via induction of BMPs. Genes to Cells. 2005;**10**(8):777-783. DOI: 10.1111/j.1365-2443.2005.00876.x

[31] Yan K, Wu Q, Yan DH, et al. Glioma cancer stem cells secrete Gremlin1 to promote their maintenance within the tumor hierarchy. Genes & Development. 2014;**28**(10):1085-1100. DOI: 10.1101/gad.235515.113

[32] Piccirillo SG, Reynolds BA, Zanetti N, et al. Bone morphogenetic proteins inhibit the tumorigenic potential of human brain tumour-initiating cells. Nature. 2006;**444**(7120):761-765. DOI: 10.1038/nature05349

[33] Paina S, Garzotto D, DeMarchis S, et al. Wnt5a is a transcriptional target of dlx homeogenes and promotes differentiation of interneuron progenitors in vitro and in vivo. The Journal of Neuroscience. 2011;**31**(7):2675-2687. DOI: 10.1523/JNEUROSCI.3110-10.2011

[34] Pei Y, Brun SN, Markant SL, et al. WNT signaling increases proliferation and impairs differentiation of stem cells in the developing cerebellum. Development. 2012;**139**(10):1724-1733. DOI: 10.1242/dev.050104

[35] Grigoryan T, Wend P, Klaus A, Birchmeier W. Deciphering the function of canonical Wnt signals in development and disease: Conditional loss- and gain-of-function mutations of beta-catenin in mice. Genes & Development. 2008;**22**(17):2308-2341. DOI: 10.1101/gad.1686208

[36] Hatten ME, Roussel MF. Development and cancer of the cerebellum. Trends in Neurosciences. 2011;**34**(3):134-142. DOI: 10.1016/j.tins.2011.01.002

[37] Munji RN, Choe Y, Li G, Siegenthaler JA, Pleasure SJ. Wnt signaling regulates neuronal differentiation of cortical intermediate progenitors. The Journal of Neuroscience. 2011;**31**(5):1676-1687. DOI: 10.1523/JNEUROSCI.5404-10.2011

[38] Bowman A, Nusse R. Location, location, location: FoxM1 mediates β-catenin nuclear translocation and promotes glioma tumorigenesis. Cancer Cell. 2011;**20**(4):415-416. DOI: 10.1016/j.ccr.2011.10.003

[39] Zhang N, Wei P, Gong A, et al. FoxM1 promotes β-catenin nuclear localization and controls Wnt target-gene expression and glioma tumorigenesis. Cancer Cell. 2011;**20**(4):427-442. DOI: 10.1016/j.ccr.2011.08.016

[40] Ayuso-Sacido A, Moliterno JA, Kratovac S, et al. Activated EGFR signaling increases proliferation, survival, and migration and blocks neuronal differentiation in post-natal neural stem cells. Journal of Neuro-Oncology. 2010;**97**(3):323-337. DOI: 10.1007/s11060-009-0035-x

[41] Wong RW. Transgenic and knock-out mice for deciphering the roles of EGFR ligands. Cellular and Molecular Life Sciences. 2003;**60**(1):113-118. DOI: 10.1007/s000180300007

[42] Ayuso-Sacido A, Graham C, Greenfield JP, Boockvar JA. The duality of epidermal growth factor receptor (EGFR) signaling and neural stem cell phenotype: Cell enhancer or cell transformer? Current Stem Cell Research & Therapy. 2006;**1**(3):387-394. DOI: 10.2174/157488806778226849

[43] Yang W, Xia Y, Ji H, et al. Nuclear PKM2 regulates β-catenin transactivation upon EGFR activation [published correction appears in nature. 2017 Sep 20]. Nature. 2011;**480**(7375):118-122. DOI: 10.1038/nature10598

[44] Agarwala S, Sanders TA, Ragsdale CW. Sonic hedgehog control of size and shape in midbrain pattern formation. Science. 2001;**291**(5511): 2147-2150. DOI: 10.1126/science.1058624

[45] Roelink H, Porter JA, Chiang C, et al. Floor plate and motor neuron induction by different concentrations of the amino-terminal cleavage product of sonic hedgehog autoproteolysis. Cell. 1995;**81**(3):445-455. DOI: 10.1016/0092-8674(95)90397-6

[46] Ihrie RA, Shah JK, Harwell CC, et al. Persistent sonic hedgehog signaling in adult brain determines neural stem cell positional identity. Neuron. 2011;**71**(2):250-262. DOI: 10.1016/j.neuron.2011.05.018

[47] Clement V, Sanchez P, de Tribolet N, Radovanovic I, Ruiz i Altaba A. HEDGEHOG-GLI1 signaling regulates human glioma growth, cancer stem cell self-renewal, and tumorigenicity [published correction appears in Curr Biol. 2007 Jan 23;17(2):192]. Current Biology. 2007;**17**(2):165-172. DOI: 10.1016/j.cub.2006.11.033

[48] Dean M, Fojo T, Bates S. Tumour stem cells and drug resistance. Nature Reviews. Cancer. 2005;**5**(4):275-284. DOI: 10.1038/nrc1590

[49] Visvader JE, Lindeman GJ. Cancer stem cells in solid tumours: Accumulating evidence and unresolved questions. Nature Reviews. Cancer. 2008;**8**(10):755-768. DOI: 10.1038/nrc2499

[50] Alison MR, Lim SM, Nicholson LJ. Cancer stem cells: Problems for therapy? [published correction appears in J Pathol. 2012 Feb;226(3):e1]. The Journal of Pathology. 2011;**223**(2):147-161. DOI: 10.1002/path.2793

[51] Hamerlik P, Lathia JD, Rasmussen R, et al. Autocrine VEGF-VEGFR2-Neuropilin-1 signaling promotes glioma stem-like cell viability and tumor growth. The Journal of Experimental Medicine. 2012;**209**(3):507-520. DOI: 10.1084/jem.20111424

[52] Ropolo M, Daga A, Griffero F, et al. Comparative analysis of DNA repair in stem and nonstem glioma cell cultures. Molecular Cancer Research. 2009;**7**(3):383-392. DOI: 10.1158/1541-7786.MCR-08-0409

[53] Liu G, Yuan X, Zeng Z, et al. Analysis of gene expression and chemoresistance of CD133+ cancer stem cells in glioblastoma. Molecular Cancer. 2006;**5**:67. Published 2006 Dec 2. DOI: 10.1186/1476-4598-5-67

[54] Bao S, Wu Q, McLendon RE, et al. Glioma stem cells promote radioresistance by preferential activation of the DNA damage response. Nature. 2006;**444**(7120):756-760. DOI: 10.1038/nature05236

[55] Pistollato F, Abbadi S, Rampazzo E, et al. Intratumoral hypoxic gradient drives stem cells distribution and MGMT

expression in glioblastoma. Stem Cells. 2010;**28**(5):851-862. DOI: 10.1002/stem.415

[56] Gong X, Schwartz PH, Linskey ME, Bota DA. Neural stem/progenitors and glioma stem-like cells have differential sensitivity to chemotherapy. Neurology. 2011;**76**(13):1126-1134. DOI: 10.1212/WNL.0b013e318212a89f

[57] Beier D, Röhrl S, Pillai DR, et al. Temozolomide preferentially depletes cancer stem cells in glioblastoma. Cancer Research. 2008;**68**(14):5706-5715. DOI: 10.1158/0008-5472.CAN-07-6878

[58] Blough MD, Westgate MR, Beauchamp D, et al. Sensitivity to temozolomide in brain tumor initiating cells. Neuro-Oncology. 2010;**12**(7):756-760. DOI: 10.1093/neuonc/noq032

[59] Abdouh M, Facchino S, Chatoo W, Balasingam V, Ferreira J, Bernier G. BMI1 sustains human glioblastoma multiforme stem cell renewal. The Journal of Neuroscience. 2009;**29**(28):8884-8896. DOI: 10.1523/JNEUROSCI.0968-09.2009

[60] Facchino S, Abdouh M, Chatoo W, Bernier G. BMI1 confers radioresistance to normal and cancerous neural stem cells through recruitment of the DNA damage response machinery. The Journal of Neuroscience. 2010;**30**(30):10096-10111. DOI: 10.1523/JNEUROSCI.1634-10.2010

[61] Noh MG, Oh SJ, Ahn EJ, et al. Prognostic significance of E-cadherin and N-cadherin expression in gliomas. BMC Cancer. 2017;**17**(1):583. Published 2017 Aug 29. DOI: 10.1186/s12885-017-3591-z

[62] Shibue T, Weinberg RA. EMT, CSCs, and drug resistance: The mechanistic link and clinical implications. Nature Reviews. Clinical Oncology. 2017;**14**(10):611-629. DOI: 10.1038/nrclinonc.2017.44

[63] Loret N, Denys H, Tummers P, Berx G. The role of epithelial-to-mesenchymal plasticity in ovarian cancer progression and therapy resistance. Cancers (Basel). 2019;**11**(6):838. Published 2019 Jun 17. DOI: 10.3390/cancers11060838

[64] Puisieux A, Brabletz T, Caramel J. Oncogenic roles of EMT-inducing transcription factors. Nature Cell Biology. 2014;**16**(6):488-494. DOI: 10.1038/ncb2976

[65] Mani SA, Guo W, Liao MJ, et al. The epithelial-mesenchymal transition generates cells with properties of stem cells. Cell. 2008;**133**(4):704-715. DOI: 10.1016/j.cell.2008.03.027

[66] Siebzehnrubl FA, Silver DJ, Tugertimur B, et al. The ZEB1 pathway links glioblastoma initiation, invasion and chemoresistance. EMBO Molecular Medicine. 2013;**5**(8):1196-1212. DOI: 10.1002/emmm.201302827

[67] Polyak K, Weinberg RA. Transitions between epithelial and mesenchymal states: Acquisition of malignant and stem cell traits. Nature Reviews. Cancer. 2009;**9**(4):265-273. DOI: 10.1038/nrc2620

[68] Chen W, Dong J, Haiech J, Kilhoffer MC, Zeniou M. Cancer stem cell quiescence and plasticity as major challenges in cancer therapy. Stem Cells International. 2016;**2016**:1740936. DOI: 10.1155/2016/1740936

[69] Chen J, Li Y, Yu TS, et al. A restricted cell population propagates glioblastoma growth after chemotherapy. Nature. 2012;**488**(7412):522-526. DOI: 10.1038/nature11287

[70] Fanfone D, Idbaih A, Mammi J, Gabut M, Ichim G. Profiling anti-apoptotic BCL-xL protein expression in glioblastoma Tumorspheres. Cancers (Basel). 2020;**12**(10):2853. Published 2020 Oct 2. DOI: 10.3390/cancers12102853

[71] Alajez NM, Shi W, Hui AB, et al. Targeted depletion of BMI1 sensitizes tumor cells to P53-mediated apoptosis in response to radiation therapy. Cell Death and Differentiation. 2009;**16**(11):1469-1479. DOI: 10.1038/cdd.2009.85

[72] Begicevic RR, Falasca M. ABC transporters in cancer stem cells: Beyond chemoresistance. International Journal of Molecular Sciences. 2017;**18**(11):2362. Published 2017 Nov 8. DOI: 10.3390/ijms18112362

[73] Chua C, Zaiden N, Chong KH, et al. Characterization of a side population of astrocytoma cells in response to temozolomide. Journal of Neurosurgery. 2008;**109**(5):856-866. DOI: 10.3171/JNS/2008/109/11/0856

[74] Yamada K, Tso J, Ye F, et al. Essential gene pathways for glioblastoma stem cells: Clinical implications for prevention of tumor recurrence. Cancers (Basel). 2011;**3**(2):1975-1995. Published 2011 Apr 18. DOI: 10.3390/cancers3021975

[75] Martín V, Sanchez-Sanchez AM, Herrera F, et al. Melatonin-induced methylation of the ABCG2/BCRP promoter as a novel mechanism to overcome multidrug resistance in brain tumour stem cells. British Journal of Cancer. 2013;**108**(10):2005-2012. DOI: 10.1038/bjc.2013.188

[76] Nakai E, Park K, Yawata T, et al. Enhanced MDR1 expression and chemoresistance of cancer stem cells derived from glioblastoma. Cancer Investigation. 2009;**27**(9):901-908. DOI: 10.3109/07357900801946679

[77] Tivnan A, Zakaria Z, O'Leary C, et al. Inhibition of multidrug resistance protein 1 (MRP1) improves chemotherapy drug response in primary and recurrent glioblastoma multiforme. Frontiers in Neuroscience. 2015;**9**:218. Published 2015 Jun 16. DOI: 10.3389/fnins.2015.00218

[78] Flavahan WA, Wu Q, Hitomi M, et al. Brain tumor initiating cells adapt to restricted nutrition through preferential glucose uptake. Nature Neuroscience. 2013;**16**(10):1373-1382. DOI: 10.1038/nn.3510

[79] Kang H, Lee S, Kim K, et al. Downregulated CLIP3 induces radioresistance by enhancing stemness and glycolytic flux in glioblastoma. Journal of Experimental & Clinical Cancer Research. 2021;**40**(1):282. Published 2021 Sep 6. DOI: 10.1186/s13046-021-02077-4

[80] Wang X, Yang K, Xie Q, et al. Purine synthesis promotes maintenance of brain tumor initiating cells in glioma. Nature Neuroscience. 2017;**20**(5):661-673. DOI: 10.1038/nn.4537

[81] Tardito S, Oudin A, Ahmed SU, et al. Glutamine synthetase activity fuels nucleotide biosynthesis and supports growth of glutamine-restricted glioblastoma. Nature Cell Biology. 2015;**17**(12):1556-1568. DOI: 10.1038/ncb3272

[82] Ye F, Zhang Y, Liu Y, et al. Protective properties of radio-chemoresistant glioblastoma stem cell clones are associated with metabolic adaptation to reduced glucose dependence. PLoS One. 2013;**8**(11):e80397. Published 2013 Nov 18. DOI: 10.1371/journal.pone.0080397

[83] Hoang-Minh LB, Siebzehnrubl FA, Yang C, et al. Infiltrative and drug-resistant slow-cycling cells support metabolic heterogeneity in glioblastoma. The EMBO Journal. 2018;**37**(23):e98772. DOI: 10.15252/embj.201798772

[84] White E. Deconvoluting the context-dependent role for autophagy in cancer. Nature Reviews. Cancer. 2012;**12**(6): 401-410. Published 2012 Apr 26. DOI: 10.1038/nrc3262

[85] Yang K, Niu L, Bai Y, Le W. Glioblastoma: Targeting the autophagy in tumorigenesis. Brain Research Bulletin. 2019;**153**:334-340. DOI: 10.1016/j.brainresbull.2019.09.012

[86] Ryskalin L, Gaglione A, Limanaqi F, et al. The autophagy status of cancer stem cells in Gliobastoma Multiforme: From cancer promotion to therapeutic strategies. International Journal of Molecular Sciences. 2019;**20**(15):3824. Published 2019 Aug 5. DOI: 10.3390/ijms20153824

[87] Taylor MA, Das BC, Ray SK. Targeting autophagy for combating chemoresistance and radioresistance in glioblastoma. Apoptosis. 2018;**23**(11-12):563-575. DOI: 10.1007/s10495-018-1480-9

[88] Golden EB, Cho HY, Jahanian A, et al. Chloroquine enhances temozolomide cytotoxicity in malignant gliomas by blocking autophagy. Neurosurgical Focus. 2014;**37**(6):E12. DOI: 10.3171/2014.9.FOCUS14504

[89] Dolma S, Selvadurai HJ, Lan X, et al. Inhibition of dopamine receptor D4 impedes Autophagic flux, proliferation, and survival of glioblastoma stem cells. Cancer Cell. 2016;**29**(6):859-873. DOI: 10.1016/j.ccell.2016.05.002

[90] Zhuang WZ, Long LM, Ji WJ, Liang ZQ. Rapamycin induces differentiation of glioma stem/progenitor cells by activating autophagy. Chinese Journal of Cancer. 2011;**30**(10):712-720. DOI: 10.5732/cjc.011.10234

[91] Zhuang W, Li B, Long L, Chen L, Huang Q, Liang Z. Induction of autophagy promotes differentiation of glioma-initiating cells and their radiosensitivity. International Journal of Cancer. 2011;**129**(11):2720-2731. DOI: 10.1002/ijc.25975

[92] Zhuang W, Long L, Zheng B, et al. Curcumin promotes differentiation of glioma-initiating cells by inducing autophagy. Cancer Science. 2012;**103**(4):684-690. DOI: 10.1111/j.1349-7006.2011.02198.x

[93] Galavotti S, Bartesaghi S, Faccenda D, et al. The autophagy-associated factors DRAM1 and p62 regulate cell migration and invasion in glioblastoma stem cells. Oncogene. 2013;**32**(6):699-712. DOI: 10.1038/onc.2012.111

[94] Tao Z, Li T, Ma H, et al. Autophagy suppresses self-renewal ability and tumorigenicity of glioma-initiating cells and promotes Notch1 degradation. Cell Death & Disease. 2018;**9**(11):1063. Published 2018 Oct 18. DOI: 10.1038/s41419-018-0957-3

[95] Beier D, Schulz JB, Beier CP. Chemoresistance of glioblastoma cancer stem cells--much more complex than expected. Molecular Cancer. 2011;**10**:128. Published 2011 Oct 11. DOI: 10.1186/1476-4598-10-128

[96] Monteiro AR, Hill R, Pilkington GJ, Madureira PA. The role of hypoxia in glioblastoma invasion. Cell. 2017;**6**(4):45. Published 2017 Nov 22. DOI: 10.3390/cells6040045

[97] Colwell N, Larion M, Giles AJ, et al. Hypoxia in the glioblastoma microenvironment: Shaping the phenotype of cancer stem-like cells. Neuro-Oncology. 2017;**19**(7):887-896. DOI: 10.1093/neuonc/now258

[98] Li Z, Bao S, Wu Q, et al. Hypoxia-inducible factors regulate tumorigenic capacity of glioma stem cells. Cancer Cell. 2009;**15**(6):501-513. DOI: 10.1016/j.ccr.2009.03.018

[99] Hjelmeland AB, Wu Q, Heddleston JM, et al. Acidic stress promotes a glioma stem cell phenotype. Cell Death and Differentiation. 2011;**18**(5):829-840. DOI: 10.1038/cdd.2010.150

[100] Qiang L, Wu T, Zhang HW, et al. HIF-1α is critical for hypoxia-mediated maintenance of glioblastoma stem cells by activating Notch signaling pathway. Cell Death and Differentiation. 2012;**19**(2):284-294. DOI: 10.1038/cdd.2011.95

[101] Persano L, Pistollato F, Rampazzo E, et al. BMP2 sensitizes glioblastoma stem-like cells to Temozolomide by affecting HIF-1α stability and MGMT expression. Cell Death & Disease. 2012;**3**(10):e412. Published 2012 Oct 18. DOI: 10.1038/cddis.2012.153

[102] Yin J, Ge X, Shi Z, et al. Extracellular vesicles derived from hypoxic glioma stem-like cells confer temozolomide resistance on glioblastoma by delivering miR-30b-3p. Theranostics. 2021;**11**(4):1763-1779. Published 2021 Jan 1. DOI: 10.7150/thno.47057

[103] Cochrane CR, Szczepny A, Watkins DN, Cain JE. Hedgehog signaling in the maintenance of cancer stem cells. Cancers (Basel). 2015;**7**(3):1554-1585. Published 2015 Aug 11. DOI: 10.3390/cancers7030851

[104] Ulasov IV, Nandi S, Dey M, Sonabend AM, Lesniak MS. Inhibition of sonic hedgehog and Notch pathways enhances sensitivity of CD133(+) glioma stem cells to temozolomide therapy. Molecular Medicine. 2011;**17**(1-2, 112):103. DOI: 10.2119/molmed.2010.00062

[105] Wellner U, Schubert J, Burk UC, et al. The EMT-activator ZEB1 promotes tumorigenicity by repressing stemness-inhibiting microRNAs. Nature Cell Biology. 2009;**11**(12):1487-1495. DOI: 10.1038/ncb1998

[106] Alves ALV, Gomes INF, Carloni AC, et al. Role of glioblastoma stem cells in cancer therapeutic resistance: A perspective on antineoplastic agents from natural sources and chemical derivatives. Stem Cell Research & Therapy. 2021;**12**(1):206. Published 2021 Mar 24. DOI: 10.1186/s13287-021-02231-x

[107] Piper K, DePledge L, Karsy M, Cobbs C. Glioma stem cells as immunotherapeutic targets: Advancements and challenges. Front. Oncologia. 2021;**11**:615704. Published 2021 Feb 24. DOI: 10.3389/fonc.2021.615704

[108] Wang CH, Chiou SH, Chou CP, Chen YC, Huang YJ, Peng CA. Photothermolysis of glioblastoma stem-like cells targeted by carbon nanotubes conjugated with CD133 monoclonal antibody. Nanomedicine. 2011;**7**(1):69-79. DOI: 10.1016/j.nano.2010.06.010

[109] Aldape KD, Ballman K, Furth A, et al. Immunohistochemical detection of EGFRvIII in high malignancy grade astrocytomas and evaluation of prognostic significance. Journal of Neuropathology and Experimental Neurology. 2004;**63**(7):700-707. DOI: 10.1093/jnen/63.7.700

[110] Pang LY, Saunders L, Argyle DJ. Epidermal growth factor receptor activity is elevated in glioma cancer stem cells and is required to maintain chemotherapy and radiation resistance. Oncotarget. 2017;**8**(42):72494-72512. Published 2017 Aug 3. DOI: 10.18632/oncotarget.19868

[111] Emlet DR, Gupta P, Holgado-Madruga M, et al. Targeting a glioblastoma cancer stem-cell population defined by EGF receptor variant III. Cancer Research. 2014;**74**(4):1238-1249. DOI: 10.1158/0008-5472.CAN-13-1407

[112] Karachaliou N, Fernandez-Bruno M, Bracht JWP, Rosell R. EGFR first- and second-generation TKIs-there is still place for them in EGFR-mutant NSCLC patients. Translational Cancer Research. 2019;**8**(Suppl. 1):S23-S47. DOI: 10.21037/tcr.2018.10.06

[113] Sharma SV, Bell DW, Settleman J, Haber DA. Epidermal growth factor receptor mutations in lung cancer. Nature Reviews. Cancer. 2007;**7**(3):169-181. DOI: 10.1038/nrc2088

[114] Liu X, Chen X, Shi L, et al. The third-generation EGFR inhibitor AZD9291 overcomes primary resistance by continuously blocking ERK signaling in glioblastoma. Journal of Experimental & Clinical Cancer Research. 2019;**38**(1):219. Published 2019 May 23. DOI: 10.1186/s13046-019-1235-7

[115] Colclough N, Chen K, Johnström P, et al. Preclinical comparison of the blood-brain barrier permeability of Osimertinib with other EGFR TKIs. Clinical Cancer Research. 2021;**27**(1):189-201. DOI: 10.1158/1078-0432.CCR-19-1871

[116] Peled N, Kian W, Inbar E, et al. Osimertinib in advanced EGFR-mutant lung adenocarcinoma with asymptomatic brain metastases: An open-label, 3-arm, phase II pilot study. Neurooncoly Advances. 2021;**4**(1):vdab188. Published 2021 Dec 27. DOI: 10.1093/noajnl/vdab188

[117] Cardona AF, Jaramillo-Velásquez D, Ruiz-Patiño A, et al. Efficacy of osimertinib plus bevacizumab in glioblastoma patients with simultaneous EGFR amplification and EGFRvIII mutation. Journal of Neuro-Oncology. 2021;**154**(3):353-364. DOI: 10.1007/s11060-021-03834-3

[118] Makhlin I, Salinas RD, Zhang D, et al. Clinical activity of the EGFR tyrosine kinase inhibitor osimertinib in EGFR-mutant glioblastoma. CNS. Oncologia. 2019;**8**(3):CNS43. DOI: 10.2217/cns-2019-0014

[119] Fan X, Khaki L, Zhu TS, et al. NOTCH pathway blockade depletes CD133-positive glioblastoma cells and inhibits growth of tumor neurospheres and xenografts. Stem Cells. 2010;**28**(1):5-16. DOI: 10.1002/stem.254

[120] Saito N, Fu J, Zheng S, et al. A high Notch pathway activation predicts response to γ secretase inhibitors in proneural subtype of glioma tumor-initiating cells. Stem Cells. 2014;**32**(1):301-312. DOI: 10.1002/stem.1528

[121] Saito N, Aoki K, Hirai N, et al. Effect of Notch expression in glioma stem cells on therapeutic response to chemo-radiotherapy in recurrent glioblastoma. Brain Tumor Pathology. 2015;**32**(3):176-183. DOI: 10.1007/s10014-015-0215-7

[122] Pan E, Supko JG, Kaley TJ, et al. Phase I study of RO4929097 with bevacizumab in patients with recurrent malignant glioma. Journal of Neuro-Oncology. 2016;**130**(3):571-579. DOI: 10.1007/s11060-016-2263-1

[123] Gilbert CA, Daou MC, Moser RP, Ross AH. Gamma-secretase inhibitors enhance temozolomide treatment of human gliomas by inhibiting neurosphere repopulation and xenograft recurrence. Cancer Research. 2010;**70**(17):6870-6879. DOI: 10.1158/0008-5472.CAN-10-1378

[124] Liebelt BD, Shingu T, Zhou X, Ren J, Shin SA, Hu J. Glioma stem cells: Signaling, microenvironment, and therapy. Stem Cells International. 2016;**2016**:7849890. DOI: 10.1155/2016/7849890

[125] Torrisi F, Alberghina C, Lo Furno D, et al. Connexin 43 and sonic hedgehog pathway interplay in glioblastoma cell proliferation and migration. Biology (Basel). 2021;**10**(8):767. Published 2021 Aug 12. DOI: 10.3390/biology10080767

[126] Fu J, Rodova M, Nanta R, et al. NPV-LDE-225 (Erismodegib) inhibits epithelial mesenchymal transition and self-renewal of glioblastoma initiating cells by regulating miR-21, miR-128, and miR-200. Neuro-Oncology. 2013;**15**(6):691-706. DOI: 10.1093/neuonc/not011

[127] Nitta RT, Gholamin S, Feroze AH, et al. Casein kinase 2α regulates glioblastoma brain tumor-initiating cell growth through the β-catenin pathway. Oncogene. 2015;**34**(28):3688-3699. DOI: 10.1038/onc.2014.299

[128] Nitta RT, Bolin S, Luo E, et al. Casein kinase 2 inhibition sensitizes medulloblastoma to temozolomide [published correction appears in oncogene. 2019 Oct 28;]. Oncogene. 2019;**38**(42):6867-6879. DOI: 10.1038/s41388-019-0927-y

[129] Sai K, Wang S, Balasubramaniyan V, et al. Induction of cell-cycle arrest and apoptosis in glioblastoma stem-like cells by WP1193, a novel small molecule inhibitor of the JAK2/STAT3 pathway. Journal of Neuro-Oncology. 2012;**107**(3):487-501. DOI: 10.1007/s11060-011-0786-z

[130] Kim BH, Lee H, Park CG, et al. STAT3 inhibitor ODZ10117 suppresses glioblastoma malignancy and prolongs survival in a glioblastoma xenograft model. Cell. 2020;**9**(3):722. Published 2020 Mar 15. DOI: 10.3390/cells9030722

[131] Yang YP, Chang YL, Huang PI, et al. Resveratrol suppresses tumorigenicity and enhances radiosensitivity in primary glioblastoma tumor initiating cells by inhibiting the STAT3 axis. Journal of Cellular Physiology. 2012;**227**(3):976-993. DOI: 10.1002/jcp.22806

[132] Cilibrasi C, Riva G, Romano G, et al. Resveratrol impairs glioma stem cells proliferation and motility by modulating the Wnt signaling pathway. PLoS One. 2017;**12**(1):e0169854. Published 2017 Jan 12. DOI: 10.1371/journal.pone.0169854

[133] Groot J, Ott M, Wei J, et al. A first-in-human phase I trial of the oral p-STAT3 inhibitor WP1066 in patients with recurrent malignant glioma. CNS. Oncologia. 2022;**11**(2):CNS87. DOI: 10.2217/cns-2022-0005

[134] Ashizawa T, Miyata H, Iizuka A, et al. Effect of the STAT3 inhibitor STX-0119 on the proliferation of cancer stem-like cells derived from recurrent glioblastoma. International Journal of Oncology. 2013;**43**(1):219-227. DOI: 10.3892/ijo.2013.1916

[135] Aderetti DA, Hira VVV, Molenaar RJ, van Noorden CJF. The hypoxic peri-arteriolar glioma stem cell niche, an integrated concept of five types of niches in human glioblastoma. Biochimica Et Biophysica Acta. Reviews on Cancer. 2018;**1869**(2):346-354. DOI: 10.1016/j.bbcan.2018.04.008

[136] Reardon DA, Turner S, Peters KB, et al. A review of VEGF/VEGFR-targeted therapeutics for recurrent glioblastoma. Journal of the National Comprehensive Cancer Network. 2011;**9**(4):414-427. DOI: 10.6004/jnccn.2011.0038

[137] Ameratunga M, Pavlakis N, Wheeler H, Grant R, Simes J, Khasraw M. Anti-angiogenic therapy for high-grade glioma. Cochrane Database of Systematic Reviews. 2018;**11**(11):CD008218. Published 2018 Nov 22. DOI: 10.1002/14651858.CD008218.pub4

[138] Alomari S, Zhang I, Hernandez A, et al. Drug repurposing for glioblastoma and current advances in drug delivery-a comprehensive review of the literature. Biomolecules. 2021;**11**(12):1870. Published 2021 Dec 13. DOI: 10.3390/biom11121870

[139] Maraka S, Groves MD, Mammoser AG, et al. Phase 1 lead-in to a phase 2 factorial study of temozolomide plus memantine, mefloquine, and metformin as postradiation adjuvant therapy for newly diagnosed glioblastoma [published correction appears in Cancer. 2019 Apr 15;125(8):1387]. Cancer. 2019;**125**(3):424-433. DOI: 10.1002/cncr.31811

[140] Sato A, Sunayama J, Okada M, et al. Glioma-initiating cell elimination by metformin activation of FOXO3 via AMPK. Stem Cells Translational Medicine. 2012;**1**(11):811-824. DOI: 10.5966/sctm.2012-0058

[141] Würth R, Pattarozzi A, Gatti M, et al. Metformin selectively affects human glioblastoma tumor-initiating cell viability: A role for metformin-induced inhibition of Akt. Cell Cycle. 2013;**12**(1):145-156. DOI: 10.4161/cc.23050

[142] Kim W, Lee S, Seo D, et al. Cellular stress responses in radiotherapy. Cell. 2019;**8**(9):1105. Published 2019 Sep 18. DOI: 10.3390/cells8091105

[143] Feng F, Zhang M, Yang C, Heng X, Wu X. The dual roles of autophagy in gliomagenesis and clinical therapy strategies based on autophagic regulation mechanisms. Biomedicine & Pharmacotherapy. 2019;**120**:109441. DOI: 10.1016/j.biopha.2019.109441

[144] Jia B, Xue Y, Yan X, et al. Autophagy inhibitor chloroquine induces apoptosis of cholangiocarcinoma cells via endoplasmic reticulum stress. Oncology Letters. 2018;**16**(3):3509-3516. DOI: 10.3892/ol.2018.9131

[145] Verbaanderd C, Maes H, Schaaf MB, et al. Repurposing drugs in oncology (ReDO)-chloroquine and hydroxychloroquine as anti-cancer agents. Ecancermedicalscience. 2017;**11**:781. Published 2017 Nov 23. DOI: 10.3332/ecancer.2017.781

[146] Firat E, Weyerbrock A, Gaedicke S, Grosu AL, Niedermann G. Chloroquine or chloroquine-PI3K/Akt pathway inhibitor combinations strongly promote γ-irradiation-induced cell death in primary stem-like glioma cells. PLoS One. 2012;**7**(10):e47357. DOI: 10.1371/journal.pone.0047357

[147] Lomonaco SL, Finniss S, Xiang C, et al. The induction of autophagy by gamma-radiation contributes to the radioresistance of glioma stem cells. International Journal of Cancer. 2009;**125**(3):717-722. DOI: 10.1002/ijc.24402

[148] Huang T, Kim CK, Alvarez AA, et al. MST4 phosphorylation of ATG4B regulates Autophagic activity, Tumorigenicity, and Radioresistance in glioblastoma. Cancer Cell. 2017;**32**(6):840-855.e8. DOI: 10.1016/j.ccell.2017.11.005

Chapter 10

A Story of Immunization with Autologous IFN-γ Secreting Glioma Cells in Patients with Glioblastoma Multiforme is Safe and Prolongs Both Overall and Progress Free Survival

Leif G. Salford, Peter Siesjö, Gunnar Skagerberg, Anna Rydelius, Catharina Blennow, Åsa Lilja, Bertil Rolf Ragnar Persson, Susanne Strömblad, Edward Visse and Bengt Widegren

Abstract

The study was a non-randomized controlled phase I-II trial to study were to ascertain the safety, feasibility and efficacy of immunotherapy with autologous IFN-γ transfected tumour cells in patients with glioblastoma multiforme. Autologous tumour cells harvested during surgery were cultured and transduced with the human IFN-γ gene. Irradiated cells were administered as intradermal immunizations every third week. Endpoints for safety were records of toxicity and adverse events, for feasibility the per cent of treated patients out of eligible patients and time to treatment and for clinical efficacy overall survival (OS) and progress free survival (PFS). Eight eligible patients, between 50 and 69 years, were immunized between 8 and 14 times after treatment with surgery and radiotherapy without adverse events or toxicity. Neurological status and quality of life were unchanged during immunotherapy. The immunized patients had a significantly ($p < 0.05$) longer median overall survival (488 days, 16.1 months than a matched control group of nine patients treated with only surgery and radiotherapy (271 days, 9.0 months). The prolongation of survival was also significant compared to all GBM treated at the same institution during the same period and published control groups within the same age cohort.

Keywords: brain tumour, clinical trial, interferon-gamma, immunotherapy, translational

1. Introduction

The most aggressive primary brain tumour, glioblastoma multiforme (GBM) [1], is the most therapy-resistant human tumour. The mean survival time after diagnosis for patients with GBM had been approximately a year for more than 30 years when our study was performed, despite advances in surgery and radiotherapy. Consequently, very few patients survive the disease [2].

By the use of combined radiotherapy and chemotherapy with temozolomide, Stupp et al. demonstrated a small but significant increase in mean survival time from 12.1 to 14.3 months [3]. Unlike most other tumours, there is a considerable age-related impact on the survival of patients with GBM, where patients under the age of 50 years have more prolonged survival than those over the age of 50 [4, 5]. The mechanisms behind this are not precise, and both diverse biologies of the tumours in patients of different ages and senescence of the immune system have been proposed [6, 7]. The importance of immune reactivity against tumours has been highlighted by several reports, demonstrating a clear correlation between the numbers of tumour infiltrating lymphocytes and the prognosis of survival in patients with various neoplastic diseases [8, 9].

Glioblastomas induce profound immune suppression by several proposed mechanisms, such as releasing immunosuppressive substances, such as prostaglandin E2 (PGE2) and interleukin-10 (IL-10). It also releases growth factor-beta (TGF-α) [10, 11], which up-regulate apoptotic ligands such as programmed death receptor 1-ligand (PD1-L) [12] and induction of regulatory T cells [13].

Experimental intracranial tumour models report successful immunotherapy results [14, 15]. In addition, several investigators have reported promising preliminary results of clinical immunotherapy in patients with glioblastoma multiforme [16–18]. However, the results have been difficult to interpret due to heterogeneity of patients regarding age, the extent of resection and additional therapy.

We have previously reported successful immunotherapy against rodent brain tumours using autologous tumour cells secreting the cytokines IFN-γ, IL-7, nor expressing the adhesion molecule B7-1, where immunizations with IFN-γ secreting tumour cells were the most potent treatment [19, 20]. In our models, the proportion of CD8+ T-cells and NK cells of tumour-infiltrating leukocytes from immunized animals was larger than in tumours from control immunized animals [21].

Here we report the result of those experiments translated into a clinical trial of patients diagnosed with GBM aged 50–69 years. The study's goal was to ascertain whether immunization with transduced autologous tumour cells secreting IFN-γ; was feasible, safe for the patients and could show any evidence of clinical responses.

2. Material and methods

2.1 Study design

We designed this study as a phase I-II, non-randomized, therapeutic, exploratory, controlled study. Endpoints for feasibility were the number of treated patients out of eligible patients and the time from surgery to the start of immunizations. Endpoints for safety were records of toxicity and adverse reactions. Immune responses became monitored with immunohistochemistry of skin biopsies from the vaccination sites. Overall survival (OS) and progression-free survival (PFS) set the endpoints for clinical responses.

2.2 Patients

The study was performed with the permission of the Swedish Medical Products Agency and with the acceptance of the Local Ethical Board of the University of Lund. All patients gave their written consent to participate in the study. The patients were recruited from glioma cases referred to the Department of Neurosurgery at Lund University Hospital during 2000–2004. It is to be noted that temozolomide or other chemotherapeutic drugs were not included in the normal therapy in this age cohort at the time of the study. All patients were recruited before the inclusion of temozolomide in the regular treatment of glioma.

A. Inclusion criteria:

- Only patients from the Southern Swedish referral area (which includes 1.6 million people) were eligible for the protocol.
- PAD: Astrocytoma grade IV, (WHO) = Glioblastoma Multiforme.
- Age 50–69 years.
- >80% resection of tumour volume.
- Patient's written consent.
- Karnofsky performance score ≥70 preoperatively.
- Radiotherapy (RT) only other treatment after surgery.

B. Exclusion criteria:

- Severe systemic disease.
- Autoimmune disease.
- Psychiatric illness.
- Deviation (major) from protocol.

C. Patient recruitment

Group	No.	<80% resection	Not GBM	Other reason for exclusion
Treated	8	0	0	0
Control	9	0	0	0
Excluded	11	5	5	1
All	*28*	*5*	*5*	*1*

GBM, glioblastoma multiforme.

Table 1.
Criteria of inclusion, exclusion, and recruitment of patients.

2.3 Provisional and definite inclusion of patients

Patients with a confirmed diagnosis of GBM according to WHO-criteria [1] and whose first postoperative MRI revealed the resection to comprise 80% or more of the preoperative tumour volume were provisionally included in the study. The tentatively included patients whose tumour cells did not exhibit in vitro growth sufficient enough for transduction and immunization or where the cells could not be transfected appropriately constituted the control group. **Table 1** show criteria for inclusion (A), exclusion (B) and patient recruitment (C).

2.4 Preoperative investigations

Preoperatively the patients were examined with MRI, including diffusion- and perfusion sequences [22]. In addition, preoperatively and postoperatively, the patients were also evaluated by neurological (NIHSS) and quality of life (QOL) assessments (SF 36).

2.5 Surgical treatment

Temozolomide or other chemotherapeutic drugs were not included in the normal therapy in this age cohort at the time of the study. Tumour resection was performed using standard neurosurgical techniques, frequently applying neuro-navigation and ultrasonic aspiration. Viable tumour tissue was harvested for histopathological diagnosis and for culturing in vitro.

Based on clinical experience and judgment, repeated surgery was considered and performed as needed for diagnostic or palliative purposes throughout the study.

2.6 Postoperative treatment

All patients received irradiation treatment of the brain (58 Gy in 29 fractions) commencing within five weeks from surgery. Steroids were administered when symptoms occurred after tumour recurrence. No patients received steroids during the immunization period.

2.7 Postoperative investigations

Postoperative MRI as above was performed within 48 hours after surgery before immunization was started and at every second immunization. At the same time, patients were evaluated preoperatively with *National Institutes of Health Stroke Scale* (NIHSS) and *Short-Form Health Survey* (SF-36).

2.8 Cell culture

Tumour tissue obtained at surgery was cultured in vitro and regularly karyotyped until the cells exhibited an abnormal karyotype. Then the cultivated cells were transduced using an adenoviral vector carrying the IFN-γ Human gene as well as the gene for the Green Fluorescent Protein and subsequently irradiated with 100 Gy to prevent a further growth in vivo [23, 24].

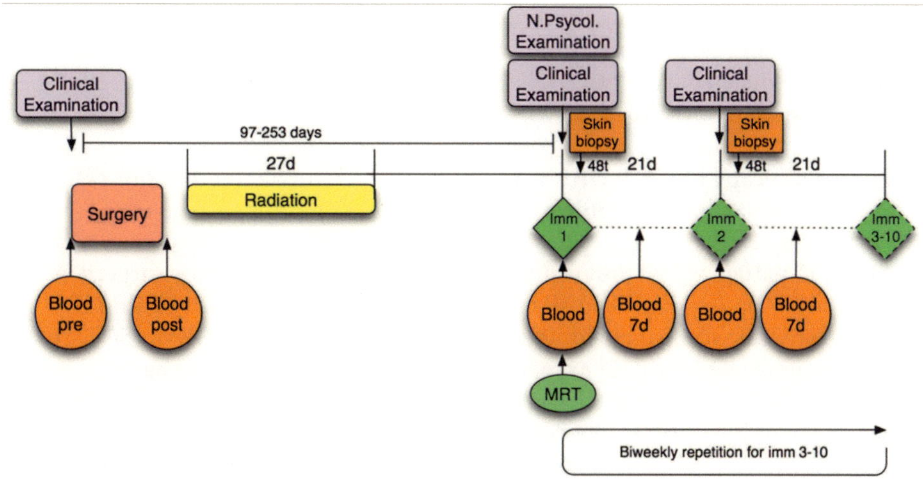

Figure 1.
Timeline of immunization and monitoring procedures.

2.9 Immunization procedure

The patients included in the study received intradermal injections of their own irradiated and transfected cultured tumour cells at five sites in the upper arm at alternating sides every third week. The immunizations were repeated up to fourteen times or until the patient deteriorated and required steroids to alleviate symptoms. **Figure 1** shows the immunization and monitoring procedures.

2.10 Histopathological studies

Besides establishing the WHO diagnosis at the first surgery, further histopathological investigations were performed in some surgical specimens and in material obtained at autopsy in some patients [25].

3. Results

3.1 Immunotherapy of GBM with autologous IFN-γ transfected tumour cells is safe

There could be a potential danger of evoking immune responses against normal CNS cells or inducing an inflammatory response that might spread to the regular brain after immunotherapy utilizing autologous tumour cells. However, we did not observe any major side effects or toxicity after immunizations.

The induction of autoimmune responses would most definitively have influenced the patients' neurologic status. Neurological and cognitive grades were evaluated with the NIH Stroke Scale (NHSS) and no deterioration before tumour recurrence were recorded during immunizations in any patient (data not shown). Neither did postoperative MRI investigations show any inflammatory changes around the resection cavity nor in surrounding brain tissue [22].

Apart from achieving prolonged survival, a novel therapy also aims at maintaining or improving the quality of life (QOL) of the treated patients. Assessment of QOL by SF-36 did not reveal any deterioration during immunizations. However, there was a tendency to short-term memory deficits in some of the treated patients (data not shown). Nevertheless, overall the patients in the study experienced an increase in QOL during period of the treatment.

3.2 Immunotherapy of GBM with autologous IFN-γ transfected tumour cells is feasible in 45% of the eligible patients

In total 28 patients were provisionally included in the study before surgery. After surgery, only 17 patients fulfilled all criteria of inclusion in the study (**Table 1**).

Eleven patients were excluded - due to another diagnosis than GBM, (5/11), insufficient tumour resection (5/11) or major psychiatric illness (1/11) (**Table 1**).

In nine of the 17 included patients, malignant cells were successfully cultured in vitro and became transduced as described above. One of these patients underwent six immunizations but was excluded from the study due to incomplete resection at review (**Table 1**). Thus finally, the treatment group in the study consisted of eight immunized patients with detailed information shown in **Table 2**. It was possible to vaccinate 8/17(45%) of eligible patients with GBM and 8/23(35%) of patients diagnosed with GBM.

The control group consisted of the remaining nine patients (**Table 2**). In the treatment group, patients became vaccinated between 8 and 14 times. Additional immunizations

No.	Age	Sex	Imm*	Tumour location	OS	PFS
Treated patients						
1	52	M	10+4	Right occipital	800	433
2	53	F	10	Left frontal	639	286
3	59	F	10	Left temporal	582	353
4	63	F	8	Left frontal	313	239
5	64	F	10	Left frontal	758	666
6	66	M	8	Left frontal	366	239
7	68	F	10	Left frontal	354	161
8	68	M	8	Left frontal	394	253
Control patients						
1	50	M	—	Right frontal	461	161
2	55	M	—	Right frontal	414	185
3	55	F	—	Left frontal	173	110
4	55	F	—	Left temporal	505	263
5	57	M	—	Left parietal	515	169
6	58	F	—	Right parietal	155	102
7	61	M	—	Right occipital	245	46
8	62	F	—	Left frontal	271	96
9	69	F	—	Left occipital	188	7

F, female; M, male; Imm, number of immunizations; OS, overall survival days; PFS, progress free survival days.*

Table 2.
Individual patient data of treated and control groups.

	Treated	Matched control	Other Ctrl
Number of patients	8	9	90
Female	5	5	45
Female %	63	57	50
Male	3	4	45
Male %	37	43	50
Age (mean)	62	58	61
Age (STDV)	6	5	6
Age (range)	53–68	50–69	50–69
% resection (mean)	94	86	NA
% resection (range)	90–99	80–97	NA
Time to imm (mean)	154	—	NA
Time to imm (range)	97–253	—	NA
Secondary surgery (n)	7	8	NA
Secondary surgery (pat)	6	7	NA
Radiotherapy	Y	Y	Y
Chemotherapy	N	N	N
OS (mean) days	525 (17.4*)	325 (10.8*)	262 (9.0*)
OS (median) days	488 (16.3*)	271 (9.0*)	193 (6.4*)
OS (range) days	313–800	155–515	38#-962
PFS (mean) days	306 (10.1*)	151 (5.0*)	NA
PFS (median) days	267 (8.8*)	161 (5.3*)	NA
PFS (range) days	99–617	76–240	NA

Other ctrl, all patients with the diagnosis of GBM between 50 and 70 years of age treated during 2000–2003 (2 years) at our institution except the treated and matched control patients involved in the study; OS, overall survival; PFS, progress free survival
**Months*
#Patients surviving less than 30 days postoperatively were excluded due to presumed surgical mortality.

Table 3.
Group data of treated and matched control of the study and as well as other controls.

were given depending on the availability of cells and patient status, although the protocol stipulated a minimum of four immunizations (**Table 3**). One patient received four additional immunizations after special approval from the Medical Products Agency. In conclusion, the immunization procedure was feasible in 45% of eligible patients.

3.3 Immunotherapy of GBM with autologous IFN-γ transfected tumour cells prolongs survival

The eight treated patients had a significantly prolonged overall median survival (488 days, 16.3 months) compared to the control group (288 days, 9.0 months) (**Figure 2** and **Table 3**). There was also a significantly longer progress-free survival in the treated group (**Table 3**). No noteworthy differences between the groups appeared regarding age, gender, or repeated surgery (**Table 3**).

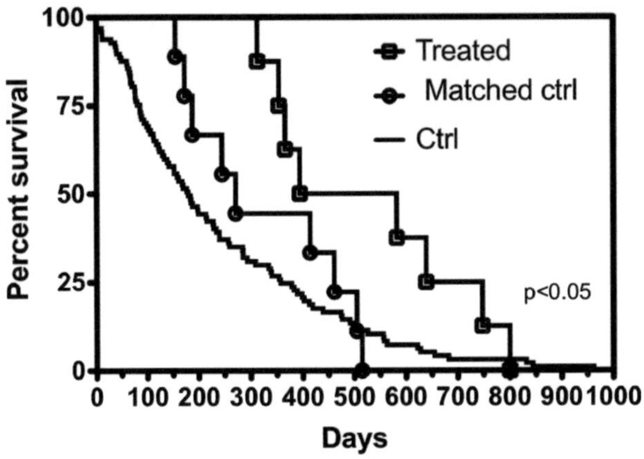

Figure 2.
Kaplan-Maier graph showing overall survival of immunized matched and non-matched control patients. The survival was analysed with the logrank test, the p value depicted refers to comparison between immunized and matched control patients.

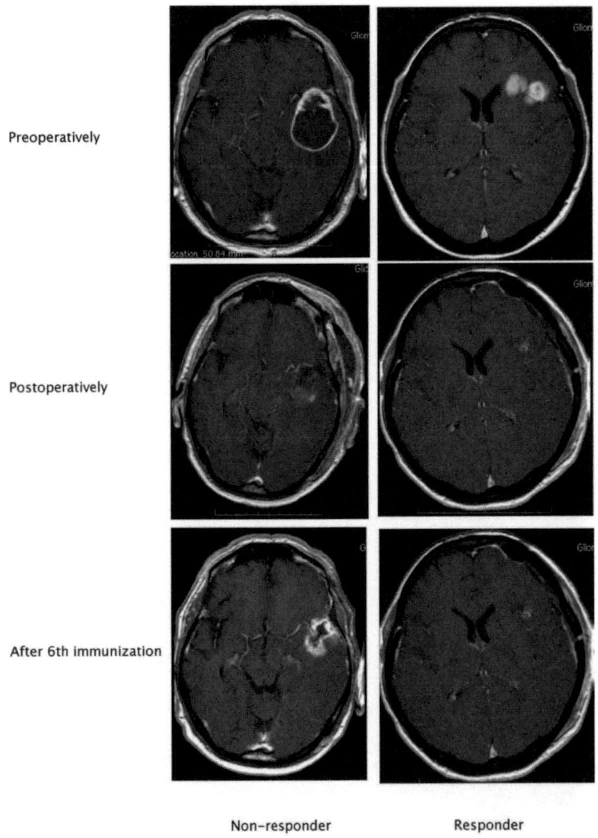

Figure 3.
Representative MRI (T1 with gadolinium) images from nonresponding and responding patients preoperatively, postoperatively and at the sixth immunization. The postoperative image of the non-responding patient shows a dense area, which constituted a haemorrhage also seen on non-gadolinium enhanced images (not shown).

Serial MR examinations showed no or stable contrast-enhancing areas in the responding patients and progressing towards contrast-enhancing areas in non-responding patients during immunizations (**Figure 3**). To rule out selection bias, we compared the matched control group with all patients treated at the same institution (all patients 50–69 years during 2000–2003 minus treated and matched control groups, $n = 91$). The data given in **Table 3** show no significant differences between the survival times of the matched control group and the other control group, which indicate no apparent selection bias.

There was also a clear indication that age was a prognostic factor apart from immunotherapy. Non-immunized patients aged 50–59 years survived 12.2 months, and immunized patients survived 22.2 months while non-immunized patients in the group aged 60–69 years survived 7.7 months, and vaccinated patients survived 14.3 months. Of the non-immunized patients, 0/9 survived >18 months, while 4/8 of the vaccinated patients survived >18 months and 2/8 >24 months. However, the study and control groups were too small to conduct more detailed statistics as COX regression analysis. In summary, the immunized group of patients had a prolonged overall survival (7.3 months compared to matched controls and 9.9 months compared to unmatched controls) that was not previously reported for patients with GBM over 50 years.

Figure 4 shows the survival results from nine vaccinated patients and 11 patients treated with surgery only, and subsequent radiotherapy presented at the World Federation of Neuro-Oncology and the European Neuro-Oncology Association in Edinburgh, Scotland. Post-diagnosis survival in nine glioma patients treated with vaccination was 14.3 months, which is significant ($P < 0.02$) longer compared to the 9.6 months of 11 patients normally treated with surgery only, and subsequent radiotherapy [26, 27].

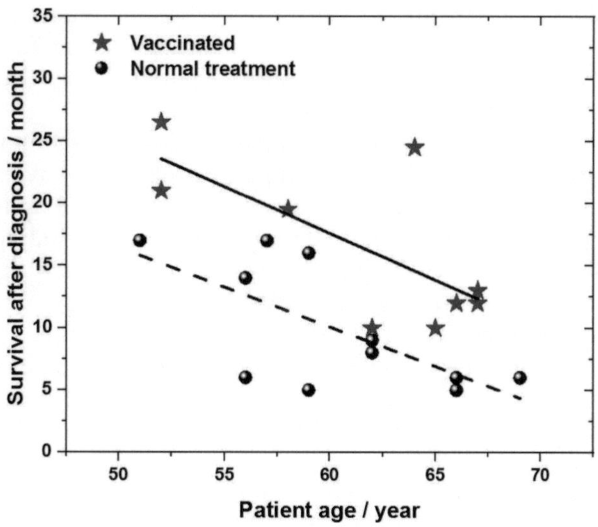

Figure 4.
Post-diagnosis survival in nine glioma patients treated with vaccination and 11 patients normally treated with surgery and subsequent radiotherapy alone. Regression equations: Survival vaccinated (month) = 62(±18) – 0.75(±0.29)·Age(a) Survival normally treated (month) = 46(±12) – 0.64(±0.23)·Age(a) (dashed line).

4. Discussion

Based on our experimental results, we have treated eight patients with the diagnosis of GBM using immunizations with autologous tumour cells transfected with the human IFN-γ gene and compared them to 9 untreated but otherwise identically treated patients. Immunotherapy of malignant primary CNS tumours is no novelty, and the different therapeutic modalities attempted in general immunotherapy has also been utilized in trials of immunotherapy of these tumours with limited results [28, 29].

Promising results have been reported from several clinical trials based on immune therapy against high-grade gliomas:

- the Victory trial utilizing the EGFRvIII peptide conjugated with keyhole limpet hemocyanin (KLH) combined with autologous dendritic cells for immunization [30],
- the use of protein extracts from tumours in combination with autologous dendritic cells [16, 17, 31, 32],
- the use of cultured autologous GBM cells irradiated and infected with Newcastle Disease Virus before immunization [18] and
- the use of immunizations with tumour cells transfected with the sense for TGF-ß [33].

We chose to select the patients within a defined age cohort and within an outlined resection volume to rule out confounding factors. Although under discussion, recent reports have indicated that the extent of resection of high-grade gliomas is a prognostic factor and therefore, we excluded patients with a resection less than 80% of the preoperative volume [34]. Other reports of immunotherapy of high-grade gliomas have claimed a higher success rate of a culture of explanted tumour biopsies than we have found [18, 32, 33] Although several putative tumour markers for glioblastoma multiforme have been proposed [35], there are no ubiquitous ones that can be used for the identification of tumour cells in culture.

Unlike other investigators, who have used panels of associated tumour markers, we have utilized karyotyping to detect tumour cells in cultures to avoid contamination of non-tumour cells [24]. This procedure may have excluded tumour cells with a near-normal karyotype, but it has reduced the probability of including contaminating non-tumour cells in the vaccine. The prognosis for patients with malignant primary CNS tumours varies depending on grade and type of tumour, age, performance status at diagnosis, and expression pattern of different proteins and genes [34, 36, 37]. Even within the entity of GBM, the survival range is extensive, and a major impact of age and performance status at diagnosis has been demonstrated. This makes the interpretation of results from clinical studies difficult when patients of different ages and grades of tumour are included.

In some of the studies published on immunotherapy of patients with primary malignant brain tumours, younger patients and also patients with the diagnosis of anaplastic astrocytoma have been included. The latter group has a substantially longer expected survival than patients with GBM, and therefore, it is hard to evaluate the actual effect of immunotherapy in some of these studies [18, 33, 38] The reported mean survival rates for treated patients with GBM in these studies were 700, 462 and 931 days with mean ages 49, 50, and 44 years respectively. In the report by Steiner et al., the survivals of individual patients were stated and the median survival of patients 50–69 was 500 days (range 252–868). Although the current patient group is too small for statistical sub-analysis, both age and immunotherapy were strongly indicated as independent predictors of increased survival (data not shown).

Additional patients have received immunizations after adjuvant temozolomide and radiotherapy followed by 4–6 cycles of temozolomide, and one other patient, not included in this study, aged 57, who received this therapy had an overall survival of 24,5 months. This is a preliminary indication that immunizations might be feasible in this setting, and another case of concurrent immunotherapy and administration of temozolomide has been reported [39]. DTH reactions in the skin at the immunization sites were recorded in all patients, but there was no correlation with overall survival (data not shown).

Analysis of peripheral blood, before and during the vaccinations, has shown signs of immune activation. Recombinant antibody micro-array technology [40] has been used to perform differential plasma protein profiling of the non-immunized and immunized GMB patients and of age-matched healthy controls from this study [41]. We have previously reported that in one patient who was re-operated on during immunizations and in the patients re-operated on after the cessation of immunizations, a transient influx of T cells into the tumour tissue could be observed [25]. This indicates that the same pattern of a lymphocyte influx as observed in our experimental model indeed occurs after clinical immunotherapy. However, whether there is a specific pattern in responders compared to serial biopsies of tumour tissue can only study non-responders and controls immunotherapy.

As reported previously, there were no signs of inflammation or oedema in the tumour tissue or the surrounding brain as judged by magnetic resonance tomography (MRT) after immunotherapy [22] which has been reported after treatment of high-grade gliomas with oncolytic viruses. This could be explained by inappropriate methods to detect an inflammatory reaction or by the minimal tumour volumes during immunizations in most patients. An alternative explanation is that the current immunotherapy does not induce a recordable inflammatory reaction that can be demonstrated with MRT. Immunotherapy has a potential risk of inducing autoimmune reactions that could damage normal tissue. In the CNS, these reactions could be deleterious and possibly life-threatening due to cerebral inflammation and oedema induction.

We have not recorded any such adverse reactions during immunizations. This agrees with additional immunotherapy trials of CNS tumours and is somewhat surprising as strong immune responses are evoked against antigens that might be shared with normal CNS resident cells. The reasons for this are unknown but could depend on the immune privilege of the normal CNS or the absence of shared antigens. GBM is, with anecdotal exceptions, an incurable disease in adults. Therapies that aim to cure the disease will realistically first prolong survival with gradual improvements in treating other tumours. It is now generally accepted that treatments that aim to lengthen survival should also strive to maintain or improve the quality of life. The treated patients in this study did not experience a diminished QOL during the immunizations, but further studies will have to confirm this. Neither do we know whether maintained QOL was related to the direct nor indirect effects of the immunizations.

The treated group had a statistically increased overall survival compared to both a matched control group and another control group encompassing all patients with GBM over 50 years of age, treated in our institution during the same period. There was no difference in survival between the matched control group and the non-matched control group. Furthermore, when considering RTOG-RPA classes (both treated and control patients belong to class IV-V) the expected overall survival in these groups (8.9 and 11.1 months) matches that of the overall survival of both control groups [41, 42].

5. Conclusion

In conclusion, this is the first study to show a significant prolongation of survival after immunotherapy of patients with GBM in the age group over 50 years. Taken into account that age is a predictor for survival of patients with glioblastoma multiforme; treatment of younger patients might result in longer periods of survival with unchanged or improved quality of life.

Acknowledgements

Dedicated to Hans and Märit Rausing who during 1996–2010 generously supported the research project "BRIGTT" (Brain Immuno Gene Tumour Therapy) which was performed at the Rausing Laboratory during 1996–2010.

We thank professor Hans-Olov Sjögren for his fruitful advice and discussions. We also thank research nurses Anna Evaldsson, Anita Nilsson and Charlotte Orre for coordination of pre and post-operative examinations.

The Hedvig Foundation, the Hans and Märit Rausing Charitable Foundation, the Hans and Märit Rausing Charitable Trust UK, the Swedish Cancer Foundation, the Lund University Hospital Funds, the Lund University funds and the County Council (ALF and Region Skåne) funds supported this project.

Author details

Leif G. Salford[1,2*], Peter Siesjö[1,2], Gunnar Skagerberg[1,2], Anna Rydelius[2,3], Catharina Blennow[1,2], Åsa Lilja[1,4,5], Bertil Rolf Ragnar Persson[2,4,5], Susanne Strömblad[1,2], Edward Visse[1,2] and Bengt Widegren[2,6]

1 Department of Neurosurgery, Lund University, Lund, Sweden

2 Department of Genetics, The Rausing Laboratory, Lund University, Lund, Sweden

3 Department of Neurology, Lund University, Lund, Sweden

4 Department of Psychology, Lund University, Lund, Sweden

5 Medical Radiation Physics, Lund University, Lund, Sweden

6 Medical Radiation Genetics, Lund University, Lund, Sweden

*Address all correspondence to: leif.salford@med.lu.se

References

[1] Kleihues P, Louis DN, Scheithauer BW, Rorke LB, Reifenberger G, Burger PC, et al. The WHO classification of tumors of the nervous system. Journal of Neuropathology and Experimental Neurology. 2002;**61**(3):215-225. DOI: 10.1093/jnen/61.3.215

[2] Salford LG, Brun A, Nirfalk S. Ten-year survival among patients with supratentorial astrocytomas grade-III and grade-IV. Journal of Neurosurgery. 1988;**69**(4):506-509. DOI: 10.3171/jns.1988.69.4.0506

[3] Stupp R, Mason WP, van den Bent MJ, Weller M, Fisher B, Taphoorn MJB, et al. Radiotherapy plus concomitant and adjuvant temozolomide for glioblastoma. The New England Journal of Medicine. 2005;**352**(10):987-996. DOI: 10.1056/NEJMoa043330

[4] Sandberg-Wollheim M, Malmstrom P, Stromblad LG, Anderson H, Borgstrom S, Brun A, et al. A randomized study of chemotherapy with procarbazine, vincristine, andlomustine with and without radiation therapy for astrocytoma grades 3 and/or 4. Cancer. 1991;**68**(1):22-29

[5] Stupp R, Hegi ME, Mason WP, van den Bent MJ, Taphoorn MJB, Janzer RC, et al. Effects of radiotherapy with concomitant and adjuvant temozolomide versus radiotherapy alone on survival in glioblastoma in a randomised phase III study: 5-year analysis of the EORTC-NCIC trial. The Lancet Oncology. 2009;**10**(5):459-466

[6] Wheeler CJ, Black KL, Liu G, Ying H, Yu JS, Zhang W, et al. Thymic CD8+ T cell production strongly influences tumor antigen recognition and age-dependent glioma mortality. Journal of Immunology. 2003;**171**(9):4927-4933

[7] Hakin-Smith V, Jellinek DA, Levy D, Carroll T, Teo M, Timperley WR, et al. Alternative lengthening of telomeres and survival in patients with glioblastoma multiforme. The Lancet Oncology. 2003;**361**(9360):836-838. DOI: 10.1016/S0140-6736(03)12681-5

[8] Schumacher K, Haensch W, Roefzaad C, Schlag PM. Prognostic significance of activated CD8(+) T cell infiltrations within esophageal carcinomas. Cancer Research. 2001;**61**(10):3932-3936

[9] Katsaros D, Massobrio M, Makrigiannakis A, Zhang L, Conejo-Garcia JR, Gimotty PA, et al. Intratumoral T cells, recurrence, and survival in epithelial ovarian cancer. New England Journal of Medicine. 2003;**348**(3):203-213

[10] Mattila S, Tuominen H, Koivukangas J, Stenback F. The terminal prostaglandin synthases mPGES-1, mPGES-2, and cPGES are all overexpressed in human gliomas. Neuropathology. 2009;**29**(2):156-165

[11] Hishii M, Nitta T, Ishida H, Ebato M, Kurosu A, Yagita H, et al. Human glioma-derived interleukin-10 inhibits antitumor immune responses in vitro. discussion. Neurosurgery. 1995;**37**(6):1160-1167. DOI: 10.1227/00006123-199512000-00016

[12] Parsa AT, Waldron JS, Panner A, Crane CA, Parney IF, Barry JJ, et al. Loss of tumor suppressor PTEN function increases B7-H1 expression and immunoresistance in glioma. Nature Medicine. 2007;**13**(1):84-88. DOI: 10.1038/nm1517

[13] Grauer OM, Nierkens S, Bennink E, Toonen LW, Boon L, Wesseling P, et al.

CD4+FoxP3+regulatory T cells gradually accumulate in gliomas during tumor growth and efficiently suppress antiglioma immune responses in vivo. International Journal of Cancer. 2007;**121**(1):95-105. DOI: 10.1002/ijc.22607

[14] Badn W, Visse E, Darabi A, Smith KE, Salford LG, Siesjö P. Postimmunization with IFN-gamma-secreting glioma cells combined with the inducible nitric oxide synthase inhibitor mercaptoethylguanidine prolongs survival of rats with intracerebral tumors. Journal of Immunology. 2007;**179**(6):4231-4238. DOI: 10.4049/jimmunol.179.6.4231

[15] Okada H, Pollack IF. Cytokine gene therapy for malignant glioma. Expert Opinion on Biological Therapy. 2004;**4**(10):1609-1620. DOI: 10.1517/14712598.4.10.1609

[16] Okada H, Kalinski P, Ueda R, Hoji A, Kohanbash G, Donegan TE, et al. Induction of CD8+ Tcell responses against novel glioma-associated antigen peptides and clinical activity by vaccinations with {alpha}-type 1 polarized dendritic cells and polyinosinicpolycytidylic acid stabilized by lysine and rboxymethylcellulose in patients with recurrent malignant glioma. Journal of Clinical Oncology. 2011;**29**(3):330-336. DOI: 10.1200/JCO.2010.30.7744

[17] De Vleeschouwer S, Fieuws S, Rutkowski S, Van Calenbergh F, Van Loon J, Goffin J, et al. Postoperative adjuvant dendritic cell-based immunotherapy in patients with relapsed glioblastoma multiforme. Clinical Cancer Research. 2008;**14**(10):3098-3104

[18] Steiner HH, Bonsanto MM, Beckhove P, Brysch M, Geletneky K, Ahmadi R, et al. Antitumor vaccination of patients with glioblastoma multiforme: A pilot study to assess feasibility, safety, and clinical benefit. Journal of Clinical Oncology. 2004;**22**(21):4272-4281

[19] Smith KE, Fritzell S, Badn W, Eberstal S, Janelidze S, Visse E, et al. Cure of established GL261 mouse gliomas after combined immunotherapy with GM-CSF and IFNgamma is mediated by both CD8+ and CD4+ T-cells. International Journal of Cancer. 2009;**124**(3):630-637. DOI: 10.1002/ijc.23986

[20] Visse E, Siesjo P, Widegren B, Sjogren HO. Regression of intracerebral rat glioma isografts by therapeutic subcutaneous immunization with interferon-gamma, interleukin-7, or B7-1-transfected tumor cells. Cancer Gene Therapy. 1999;**6**(1):37-44. DOI: 10.1038/sj.cgt.7700023

[21] Visse E, Johansson AC, Widegren B, Sjogren HO, Siesjo P. immune histochemical analysis of glioma-infiltrating leucocytes after peripheral therapeutic immunization with interferon-gamma-transfected glioma cells. Cancer Immunology, Immunotherapy. 2000;**49**(3):142-151. DOI: 10.1007/s002620050613

[22] Stenberg L, Englund E, Wirestam R, Siesjo P, Salford LG, Larsson E-M. Dynamic susceptibility contrast-enhanced perfusion magnetic resonance (MR) imaging combined with contrast-enhanced MR imaging in the follow-up of immunogene-treated glioblastoma multiforme. Acta Radiologica. 2006;**47**(8):852-861. DOI: 10.1080/02841850600815341

[23] Baureus-Koch C, Nyberg G, Widegren B, Salford LG, Persson BR. Radiation sterilisation of cultured human brain tumour cells for clinical immune tumour therapy. British Journal of Cancer. 2004;**90**(1):48-54. DOI: 10.1038/sj.bjc.6601467

[24] Widegren B, Baureus-Koch C, Rydelius A, Nyberg G, Järnum S, Salford LG, et al. Cultivation of human glioma cells and the use of tumour cells for immune gene therapy. Man. 2005

[25] Persson A, Skagerberg G, Salford LG, Englund E. Immunotreatment in patients with glioblastoma multiforme--a histopathological evaluation of reactive and inflammatory changes. Clinical Neuropathology. 2005;**24**(5):201-208

[26] Salford L, Ask E, Siesjo P, Skagerberg G, Baureus-Koch C, Blennow C, et al. Brain immuno gene tumour therapy. In: WFNO-II/EANO-VI Conference Secretariat Federation of European Cancer Societies, Brussels. 2005

[27] Salford L, Ask E, Siesjo P, Skagerberg G, Baureus-Koch C, Blennow C, et al. Immunization with autologous glioma cells transfected with IFN-γ gene significantly prolongs survival in GBM-patients older than 50 years. Neuro-Oncology. 2005;7(3):370-370. DOI: 10.1215/S1152851705200388

[28] Carpentier AF, Meng Y. Recent advances in immunotherapy for human glioma. Current Opinion in Oncology. 2006;**18**(6):631-636. DOI: 10.1097/01.cco.0000245321.34658.f4

[29] Ommaya AK. Immunotherapy of gliomas: A review. Advances in Neurology. 1976;**15**:337-359

[30] Sampson JH, Archer G, Mitchell DA, Heimberge AB, Herndon JE, Lally-Goss D, et al. An epidermal growth factor receptor variant III-targeted vaccine is safe and immunogenic in patients with glioblastoma multiforme. Molecular Cancer Therapeutics. 2009;**8**(10):2773-2779. DOI: 10.1158/1535-7163.MCT-09-0124

[31] Liau LM, Prins RM, Kiertscher SM, Odesa SK, Kremen TJ, Giovannone AJ, et al. Dendritic cell vaccination in glioblastoma patients induces systemic and intracranial T-cell responses modulated by the local central nervous system tumor microenvironment. Clinical Cancer Research. 2005;**11**(15):5515-5525. DOI: 10.1158/1078-0432.CCR-05-0464

[32] Yu JS, Liu G, Ying H, Yong WH, Black K, Wheeler CJ. Vaccination with tumor lysatepulsed dendritic cells elicits antigen-specific, cytotoxic T-cells in patients with malignant glioma. Cancer Research. 2004;**64**(14):4973-4979. DOI: 10.1158/0008-5472.CAN-03-3505

[33] Fakhrai H, Mantil JC, Liu L, Nicholson GL, Murphy-Satter CS, Ruppert J, et al. Phase I clinical trial of a TGF-beta antisense-modified tumor cell vaccine in patients with advanced glioma. Cancer Gene Therapy. 2006;**13**(12):1052-1060. DOI: 10.1038/sj.cgt.7700975

[34] Wang L, Wei Q, Wang LE, Aldape KD, Cao Y, Okcu MF, et al. Survival prediction in patients with glioblastoma multiforme by human telomerase genetic variation. Journal of Clinical Oncology. 2006;**24**(10):1627-1632. DOI: 10.1200/JCO.2005.04.0402

[35] Saikali S, Avril T, Collet B, Hamlat A, Bansard J-Y, Drenou B, et al. Expression of nine tumour antigens in a series of human glioblastoma multiforme: Interest of EGFRvIII, IL-13Ralpha2, gp100 and TRP-2 for immunotherapy. Journal of Neuro-Oncology. 2007;**81**(2):139-148. DOI: 10.1007/s11060-006-9220-3

[36] Mineo J-F, Bordron A, Baroncini M, Ramirez C, Maurage CA, et al. Prognosis factors of survival time in patients with glioblastoma multiforme: A multivariate analysis of 340 patients. Acta Neurochirurgica. 2007;**149**(3):245-253. DOI: 10.1007/s00701-006-1092-y

[37] Phillips HS, Kharbanda S, Chen R, Forrest WF, Soriano RH, Wu TD, et al. Molecularsubclasses of high-grade glioma predict prognosis, delineate a pattern of disease progression, and resemble stages in neurogenesis. Cancer Cell. 2006;**9**(3):157-173. DOI: 10.1016/j.ccr.2006.02.019

[38] Yu JS, Wheeler CJ, Zeltzer PM, Ying H, Finger DN, Lee PK, et al. Vaccination of malignantglioma patients with peptide-pulsed dendritic cells elicits systemic cytotoxicity and intracranial T-cell infiltration. Cancer Research. 2001;**61**(3):842-847

[39] Heimberger AB, Sun W, Hussain SF, Dey M, Crutcher L, Aldape K, et al. Immunologicalresponses in a patient with glioblastoma multiforme treated with sequential courses of temozolomide and immunotherapy: Case study. Neuro-Oncology. 2008;**10**(1):98-103. DOI: 10.1215/15228517-2007-046

[40] Wingren C, Ingvarsson J, Dexlin L, Szul D, Borrebaeck CA. Design of recombinant antibody microarrays for complex proteome analysis: Choice of sample labeling-tag and solid support. Proteomics. 2007;7(17):3055-3065. DOI: 10.1002/pmic.200700025Citations

[41] Carlsson A, Persson O, Ingvarsson J, Widegren B, Salford L, Borrebaeck CAK, et al. Plasma proteome profiling reveals biomarker patterns associated with prognosis and therapy selection in glioblastoma multiforme patients. Proteomics Clinical Applications. 2010;**4**(6-7):591-602. DOI: 10.1002/prca.200900173Citations

[42] Curran WJJ, Scott CB, Horton J, Nelson JS, Weinstein AS, Fischbach AJ, et al. Recursive partitioning analysis of prognostic factors in three Radiation Therapy Oncology Group malignant glioma trials. Journal of the National Cancer Institute. 1993;**85**(9):704-710

Chapter 11

Potential of Lipid Based Nanodrug Carriers for Targeted Treatment of Glioblastoma: Recent Progress and Challenges Ahead

Bhabani Sankar Satpathy, Binapani Barik, Ladi Alik Kumar and Sangram Biswal

Abstract

Malignant brain tumor at its fourth stage (glioblastoma) is the most dangerous and an unsolved medical challenge till today. Present therapeutic strategies including chemo treatment, radiation along with surgery all together have not succeeded to control the progression of glioblastoma. Challenges in the early detection, unavailability of specific therapeutic strategy and severe cytotoxicity of available chemotherapeutics are the some of the prime causes of treatment failure. Especially presence of blood-brain barrier (BBB) highly limits pharmacological effect of conventional chemotherapy. In lieu of this, lipid based nanodrug carriers (LNCs) have now been evolved with great potential in improving the drug efficacy for the treatment of glioma. Further, LNCs engineered with specific targeting ligand might significantly reduce the dosage regimen, increase specificity, improve bioavailability and reduce off-target distribution. Such modified LNCs possess sufficient ability to cross BBB to deliver the loaded cargo(s) at target location inside the brain; thereby ensuring improved treatment outcome with less side effects than conventional treatment. This review primarily focuses on recent advancements in various engineered LNCs for the treatment of brain cancer. Also, the existing impediments for nanomedicines associated with their effective large scale synthesis or sufficient clinical application have also been highlighted.

Keywords: lipid based nanodrug carriers, glioblastoma, advancements, challenges

1. Introduction

Brain tumor at its malignant stage is the toughest challenge to treat. Glioma is the commonest form of malignant brain tumors and silently progresses to its fourth and most aggressive stage; called giobalstoma. In fact, modern medical science in spite of cutting age technological advancements is yet to find specific answers for advanced malignant brain tumor.

An uncontrolled growth of cells beyond the cellular regulation inside the brain environment eventually leads to benign and/or malignant cancers [1]. The most common site for the development of tumor inside the brain is glial cells. Further, tumors as per their growth and location inside the brain are further classified from grade I (low grade) to grade IV (highly metastatic) type tumors [2]. Grade I stage of tumor (mostly goes unnoticed) can progress to the malignant stage more often and throws a tough challenge for treatment. Also, secondary metastatic brain tumors can be developed in adults from primary lungs/breast cancer [3]. Among the various grades of brain tumor, grade IV glioma, also called glioblastoma multiforme has been recognized as the severest and highly metastatic type brain tumor [4]. A vast majority of patients across the globe diagnoses with de novo or primary glioblastoma in recent years. Progression of brain tumors are often associated with typical increase in intracranial pressure, altered consciousness, occasional seizures along with severe headaches, vomiting, fever, gastric disturbances etc. [5]. However, these problems are highly variable from patient to patient and thus cannot be generalized prognosis parameters. Thus, primary stage of glioma often goes unnoticed. Aetiological causes related to the development of brain cancer are yet to be unravelled, which further makes the treatment extremely challenging. Classical subtype of glioma is assumed to be associated with amplification of chromosome 7 along with loss of chromosome 10. Coupled with these, over-expression of epidermal growth factor (EGFR) receptor and mutations are other proposed aetiologies of glioblastoma [6]. Mesenchymal glioblastoma has been shown to maintain a higher expression of CH13L1, MET, and genes associated with tumour necrosis factor, nuclear factor-κB, along with deletions of NF1. Mutations in IDH1, TP53 and modification of platelet-derived growth factor receptor A are also associated with secondary glioblastoma or lower-grade gliomas [7]. Though, neural glioblastomas at initial diagnosis shows similar characteristics to normal brain tissue; however, there is overexpression EGFR to several folds than normal.

At present, glioblastoma has been identified as the most complex, metastatic and treatment-resistant type of cancers with alarming prevalence around the globe. In 2020, more than 13,000 Americans have been diagnosed with GBM, which accounts for more than 48 percent of all malignant brain tumor cases [8]. Till now, average length of survival for patients with glioblastoma has been estimated to be only 1 to 1.5 years while the five-year survival rate has been roughly estimated as 6–7% only [9]. Over the past decade, mortality and survival rate of glioblastoma patients has not been improved as such in the developed nations. Even, uncontrollable prevalence of the disease is being witnessed in developing and under-developed countries. India has now become the new epi-centre for all cancer related deaths in recent years among which glioblastoma-related death cases occupies second lead position after breast cancer.

Along with extremely poor prognosis associated with glioblastoma, there is too serious dearth of promising therapeutic options. Much of the available treatment strategies alone or in combinations have been failed measurably over the past years to meet the treatment expectations. Usually, combination of various strategies like surgery, radiation, chemotherapy, non-chemodrug therapy etc. are employed to control the progression of tumor cells to other parts of the brain or to be metastatic [10, 11]. Surgery followed by radiation therapy is applied as the first line of treatment in the initial phases of glioma. Surgery is employed to remove maximum possible mass of tumor tissue from the brain, while radiation therapy is employed to circumvent tumor mass *via* precise, focused high energy beams [12]. However, in many cases, effective application of surgery and radiation are extremely constrained as majority of brain tumors are usually detected at the advanced stages, i.e., at stage III or at stage IV. Additionally, highly sensitive nature of brain tissue and presence of delicate nervous network across the brain hemispheres with all major control systems of perception, mood, behaviour, cognition etc. further limits surgical procedures and effective radiation therapy [13, 14]. Hence, chemotherapy remains as the inevitable option to check the progression of tumor cells through cytotoxic anticancer drugs. Non-chemotherapeutic drugs are also used during treatment period to control tumor-associated headache/pain and epileptic seizures [15]. However, conventional chemo-drug treatment faces the usual problem just likes other conventional dosage forms such as failure to discriminate in between cancerous tissue and normal healthy tissue or lack of targetability. As a result, off-target biodistribution of cytotoxic anticancer drugs across all vital organs inside the body occurs, which in turn aggravates a wide range of adverse drug effects including alopecia, gastric disturbances, bone marrow depression, heart problems, kidney damage, immunity suppression and many other associated complications in cancer patients [16]. It has now been an accepted fact that the presently available clinical options all together have neither succeeded in extending cancer patient lives just beyond a few extra months nor been able to improve their quality of life after chemo-treatment cycles. In a nutshell, extremely poor prognosis, highly sensitive micro-environment of brain coupled with failure of conventional treatment options has made glioblastoma as a life-threatening disease. At present, it is too one of the most expensive cancers to treat, often leaving patients and families with major financial hardship during the treatments and in turn deteriorates socio-economic burden of the society as well [17]. In the lieu of which, advanced treatment options are being investigated heavily over the past years to improve the treatment outcomes and simultaneously to minimize the dose-related toxic effects on the body.

Moving from the initial treatment options like surgery and radiation, which have their inherent limitations; anti-cancer drug therapy through modified nanocarriers with improved targeting features is being explored as alternative option to improve overall treatment outcomes in cancer patients. In view of the presence of BBB as the major obstacle in brain-drug targeting, especially, lipid based nanocarrier based delivery systems have been recognized as hopeful options in glioblastoma owing to their highly lipophilic, ultra-small size, tuneable surface features. The cytotoxic anti-cancer drugs can be loaded into such nanocarrier vehicles and thus can be effectively surpass the BBB to get into the brain. Additionally, such carriers are now being manipulated at their surface with specific targeting ligands like antibodies, aptamers, small molecules, peptides etc. to enhance their targetability and reduce off-target distribution [18]. These engineered LNCs have been emerged as the prime research area in nanomedicine mediated brain cancer therapy now-a-days.

LNCs have the capability to bypass the BBB without disrupting its normal functionalization [19, 20]. Furthermore, LNCs in lieu of their architectural uniqueness provide requisite criteria of lipophilicity and sustained release of drug from their core/matrix. Attachment of tumor-specific ligands further makes them more specific and helps to mitigate peripheral toxicities [21]. After crossing the BBB, LNCs are endocytosed by endothelial cells and release the drug inside the cell [22]. There is too a growing interest to improve the *in vivo* performance of nanocarriers *via* conjugating them with thiolated and preactivated polymers to efficiently inhibit the P-glycoprotein (P-gp) efflux at brain luminal side [22, 23]. Glioblastoma possesses a leaky vasculature, and thus may be amenable to LNC-based drug delivery systems that lead to enhanced drug deposition while limiting systemic drug exposure. Various types of LNCs have been investigated over the last decade to enhance therapeutic efficacy of anticancer drugs for the treatment of advanced stage glioma. In the present topic, we want to cover recent advancements in LNCs based drug targeting strategies for glioma. Specifically, we will restrict our discussion mostly on nanoliposomal vesicles and solid-lipid nanocarriers, which have been reported over the recent years for glioma/glioblastoma treatment. Side by side, some lights have been thrown on the challenges faced by such targeted LNCs for their successful clinical translation, regulatory hurdles along with scale-up issues for industrial production.

2. Blood-brain barrier: the prime culprit against effective drug therapy in glioblastoma

Brain, the controlling system of the whole body is undoubtedly the most complex, mysterious structure, which controls a multitude of crucial functions of the body including cognition, information processing, homeostasis, perception, motor control, mood, as well as learning and behaviour [24]. Such important functions are mediated by uncountable nervous networks which are present across the cerebellum. BBB is the main check-gate, which actively protects brain neural tissues from the influx of toxins and other compounds, including therapeutic molecules [25]. In fact, presence of BBB strictly restricts the success of chemotherapy as majority of anticancer drugs fails to permeate sufficiently across BBB, thus results in a sub-therapeutic concentration associated with low clinical outcome.

BBB is characterized by the presence of tight intercellular junctions along with lack of fenestrations. Main components of BBB are tightly placed brain endothelial cells, basal membranes, pericytes embedded in the basal membrane, along with astrocytic end feet [25]. All these structures are so uniquely placed close to each other that they collectively form a strong barrier on the way of every component having higher molecular weight or large size to pass from blood to brain. Only essential components like glucose and essential amino acids can get access inside the brain. Exogenous compounds including drugs having nano-size range or lipophilic property may cross the BBB by passive diffusion. Alternatively, some therapeutics can also cross the BBB through carrier-mediated active transport. Along with the strong barrier system like BBB, the efflux transporter systems present at the luminal side of brain also play crucial role in preventing therapeutic molecules to attain their pharmacological concentration [25, 26].

Similarly, in terms of molecule permeability, it has been found that molecules larger than 400 Da are very unlikely to cross the BBB (especially if highly water soluble) unless a suitable specific transporter is present. However, as mentioned earlier, highly lipophilic molecules tend to have better permeability than neutral or hydrophilic molecules owing to the high lipophilicity of the BBB. Temozolomide is an example of the poorly water-soluble drug with a molecular weight of 194.154 g/mol, which can readily cross the BBB. Similarly drugs like carmustine, lomustine etc. also have reasonable BBB permeation ability owing to their molecular cut-off range and lipophilic nature and have already been recommended for glioma therapy. These, along with few other drugs *viz*. capecitabine, paclitaxel etc. are presently some of the widely used chemotherapy drugs recommended in glioblastoma [27]. However, many lipophilic drugs in their native form/conventional formulation too fail to achieve required therapeutic concentration at the brain tissue owing to their molecular size, in vivo stability issue, low half-life or affected by efflux transporter systems across BBB. Drugs bound to plasma proteins are also unavailable for crossing the BBB, since most of the proteins require specific transporters for BBB permeation. This phenomenon was demonstrated using Evans blue (an albumin-binding dye), which is completely unable to permeate across the intact BBB [28].

Dose-related adverse reactions are also obvious phenomena with conventional drugs, which further limit their chemo treatment cycle [29, 30]. Hence, it must be taken into account that merely a high degree of lipophilicity or delivery in conventional dosage forms does not either guarantee sufficient availability of drug inside the brain nor ensures its decreased off-target distribution throughout the healthy tissues.

In this context, there always felt an age-old need for an ideal delivery system that has to transport a drug with high efficiency to target brain cells, with minimal healthy tissue toxicity or off-target distribution. To achieve this, delivery of drugs/chemotherapeutics through the LNC based platforms has been attempted over the past few years by the pharma researchers and formulation scientists across the globe.

2.1 Lipid based nanocarriers: effective drug targeting platforms to brain

LCNs have been heavily investigated in recent years to improve the drug delivery at brain tissues owing to their lipophilic nature and ultra-small size. The key features of LNCs primarily involve their desirable size range, surface properties, and also ease of surface manipulation with targeting ligands [31]. The development of a broad range of LCNs with varying size, composition, and functionality has provided a significant resource for nanomedicine based glioblastoma therapy.

However, requirements for LCNs fabrication for effective glioma therapy also depend on tumor characteristics, its location and complicacy. Although LCNs avoid renal clearance preferably within the range of 10–50 nm, but they tend to accumulate heavily in the reticulo-endothelial system (RES), which is also another major setback for their sufficient brain bioavailability. Further, LCNs like other nanodrug carriers below the size of 10 nm possess the risk of higher glomerular filtration followed by renal clearance [32, 33]. All such problems are now being addressed successfully by the advanced formulation technologies, adaptation of cutting age research instruments and effective surface manipulation and employment of novel polymers (natural/synthetic). For example, problem associated with higher RES uptake can be subsided by surface coating/shielding of the LNCs with specific hydrophilic polymers like polyethylene glycol (PEG). Presence of PEG over the surface of LNCs renders hydrophilicity with subsequent reduction in RES uptake and enhancement in plasma half-life [34]. Similarly, by optimizing critical in-process parameters during formulation development such as polymer:drug ratio, amount of drug, sonication time, speed of centrifugation, filtration/separation technique, surface conjugation etc., desired size range of LCNs can be attained (preferably within 10–50 nm) for effective BBB permeation.

Likewise, the off-target bio distribution of the nanodrug carriers can be effectively reduced by surface conjugation with tumor-specific ligands. Several ligands like aptamers, antibodies, small molecules, peptides, sugar moiety etc., can be attached to LCNs to make them more specific with enhanced brain targetability [35]. Such engineered LCNs can effectively reduce healthy tissue toxicity along with chemoresistance of cancer cells, since they promote higher brain uptake of cytotoxic drugs around the tumor area with considerable decrease in drug efflux, thereby enhancing therapeutic outcome as well as (**Figure 1**).

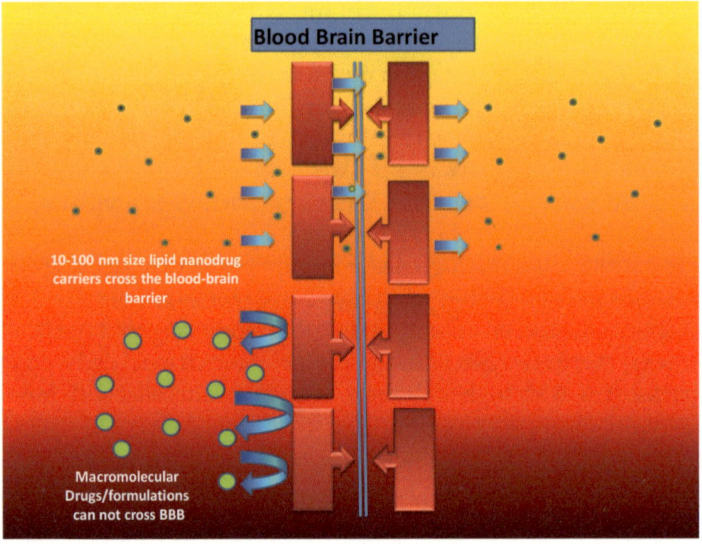

Figure 1.
A representative diagram of blood-brain barrier showing permeation of ultra-small size lipophilic drug carriers, whereas inability of macromolecular drug/ carriers to cross the barrier.

2.2 Types of lipid nanocarriers employed for drug targeting to brain

Lipid based nanocarriers are categorized into mainly three types, *viz*. nanoliposomes, solid-lipid nanoparticles, nanostructured lipid carriers. In our study, we would mostly restrict the discussion on these lipid based nanodrug carriers for glioblastoma therapy, excluding other organic/inorganic nanoparticles or other novel carriers.

2.2.1 Nanoliposomes

This is the first generation of novel drug delivery system, developed in 1960. It is prepared to resemble to the cell membrane compositions mainly by using fats, phospholipids, and cholesterol [36]. Due to its high flexibility, low toxicity, better stability, and biocompatibility, specifically targeting character with highly versatile nature, it has got immense attention in glioblastoma therapy [37, 38].

Liposomes are colloidal nano carriers, comprised in a vesicle. It can be uni-lamellar or multi lamellar i.e. comprising of more than one number of lipid bilayers encapsulating hydrophilic core or aqueous core. Due to unique structural features, both hydrophilic and lipophilic drugs can be delivered through nanoliposomes. By applying various in vitro techniques, the surface of liposomes can be easily modified with surfactants (e.g. tween 80, tween 20) bile salts, or tumor-specific targeting ligands [39, 40]. However, one of the major limitations related to liposome is their earlier uptake by phagocytic cells leading to shorter in circulation half-life. To avoid this PEG is functionalized over the conventional liposomes to keep it safe from the eyes of macrophages and to extend blood circulation profile [41].

2.2.2 Solid lipid nano carrier (SLNs)

This the first generation of solid-lipid based nano carrier was developed in 1991. It is usually spherical in shape having the diameter about 50–100 nm, dispersed in water or in an aqueous surfactant phase [42]. SLNs have advantages like better stability, low melting point, nontoxic, ease to preparation, higher plasma pharmacokinetics, better bioavailability across BBB, good biocompatibility, bio degradability, very low cytotoxicity along with cost effective method of production [43]. It is an oil in water (o/w) system, in which the oil phase/liquid-lipid is replaced with the solid lipid to make it solid in both room and body temperature. The main ingredients used for the production of SLNs includes monostearates, stearyl alcohol, stearic acid, glycerol, cetyl palmitate etc. including stabilizers like tween 80, poloxamer 188, and dimethyl dioctadecyl ammonium bromine. The variation of ratio occurs in between the range of solid lipid (4:1) to the liquid lipid (1:4), surfactant concentration (0.25 to 6% w/v) to the total lipid concentration (1–30% w/v) [44]. However, it has also got few limitations like moderately drug loading capacity and expulsion of drug due to crystallization during under long-term storage condition.

2.3 Targeting strategies adopted by lipid nanodrug carriers for brain delivery

LNCs with their loaded cargo can be directly targeted to the brain owing to their ultra-small size and lipophilicity, as discussed previously. Since, most of the LNCs constitute phospholipid, sphingo lipid, cholesterol-based structures, they usually possess a cell-mimicking property, for which once get inside the cell, they tend to retain there with subsequent release of loaded cargo. In such cases, no artificial surface manipulation is done, and thus it does not guarantee glioma cell-specific drug targeting also.

Tumor vasculature usually shows abnormal architecture with highly permeable capillaries. Along with that the tumor mass too possesses a poor lymphatic drainage system, which thus allows accumulation of micromolecules having molecular cut-off size ≤40 kDa. LCNs mediated drug targeting actually utilizes this unique feature along with its lipophilic nature to invade inside the tumor tissue. The phenomenon popularly known as the enhanced permeability and retention (EPR) effect is taken as the prime mechanism in passive targeting of nanodrug carriers [45, 46]. Passive method of targeting the chemotherapeutics does not involve targeting to any specific receptor/protein expressed over tumor cell surface. It, thus primarily depends on the size and physicochemical properties of the nanocarriers. The ideal size range to benefit from the EPR effect is usually between 10 and 100 nm. But for successful BBB permeation of LNCs, an average hydrodynamic diameter around 10–50 is now preferably investigated. Outside this range, smaller particles usually clear by the kidney, preventing accumulation within the tumor site, while larger size particles fail to adequately penetrate through the glioma vasculature [46, 47].

In lieu of problems associated with passive targeting, surface engineering of nanocarriers with tumor cell-specific ligands have been investigated widely in past few years. The development of a broad range of LCNs with varying size, composition, and functionality has actually provided a significant revolution in glioblastoma therapy. While, passive targeting utilizes unique internal architecture of tumor tissue to target nano size delivery vehicles, active targeting is primarily based on surface engineering of nanodrug carriers with specific targeting ligands to make them more precise. Though, the leaky tumor vasculature coupled with weak lymphatic drainage of tumor provides a golden opportunity for direct targeting of nanosize drug carriers even without any surface manipulation [48], however, the chances of healthy tissue accumulation still remain there. Thus, surface engineering of LNCs has been emerged as hopeful alternative to decrease drug uptake in normal tissue and to increase accumulation in glioma to elicit better therapeutic outcome.

Active targeting in glioblastoma involves targeting surface membrane proteins that are upregulated in cancer cells [49]. Targeting molecules can be monoclonal antibodies or their fragments, aptamers, small molecules, oligopeptides etc. LNCs attached with surface ligands can be preferably localized to tumor tissue, expressing the associated receptors or antigens and can deliver the loaded drug *via* ligand-receptor interaction [50]. Some ligand receptor interactions also facilitate receptor-mediated endocytosis, which in turn enhances payload delivery inside the tumor cell.

2.4 Major types of targeting ligands in glioblastoma

2.4.1 Monoclonal antibodies (mAb)

Biocompatible mAb has been utilized from a decade as the first line of targeting ligand owing to their highly specific nature in various cancer treatments including malignant brain tumors. Many tumors up-regulate growth factor receptors, such as HER2/ neu in certain breast cancers, which can be targeted with anti-HER2/ neu surface antibodies [51]. Similar mAb mediated targeting strategy has now been investigated for glioblastoma. Though, unlike breast or prostate cancer, the specific receptors/ proteins having higher expression in case of brain tumor are very limited, but some of the recently reported research has provided evidence of improved treatment efficacy with mAb-engineered LNCs in malignant brain tumor as compared to conventional chemo-treatment. One recent example of such mAb is CD 133. This pentaspan transmembrane glycoprotein family member is also known as prominin-1 and has been found closely associated with glioblastoma. Research finding has identified CD133 as a major hallmark of glioblastoma stem cells [52]. Recent reports have further shown that CD133 antigen has elevated expression in glioblastoma, medulloblastomas, along with other brain cancers [53]. Thus, it could serve as a prognostic indicator of tumor recurrence or malignant progression.

2.4.2 Aptamers

Aptamers have recently emerged as effective ligands for their higher specificity, safer in vivo application with lesser chances of immunogenicity. They are basically folded single stranded oligonucleotides (25–100 nucleotides) that bind to specific molecular targets [54]. Aptamer-conjugated nanoparticles *in vitro* have displayed increased cytotoxicity and decreased volume of xenografts compared with non-targeted nanoparticles [55]. Aptamers possess many unique characteristics which make them an ideal imaging and targeting agent for the treatment of glioblastoma. Owing to their higher sensitivity, selective nature, ease of fabrication aptamers are presently lucrative drug-delivery platforms in glioblastoma [56, 57]. Although mAbs have been long history of use as potent therapeutic tool, however, their therapeutic application for glioblastoma including other neurodegenerative diseases has been limited, thanks to the presence of BBB, which checks effective entry of traditional antibodies. As compared to conventional mAbs, aptamers are more stable, smaller size and also easily accessible to chemical modifications. Adverse effects associated with aptamers are also rare. They can be physically/ chemically conjugated to a wide range of probes and therapeutic agents, which make them promising entity for imaging and detection in brain cancer. Successful application of aptamers for the diagnosis or treatment of glioblastoma has been reported in many recent researches. Recent research identified A40s, a novel aptamer that was internalized effectively in GBM stem cells and successfully delivered miR-34c and anti-miR10b to the stem cell population. The data demonstrated that A40s crossed the BBB to reach the tumor location and selectively attached with the EphA2 receptor, which in turn led to inhibition in tumor growth and reduction in tumor relapse [58].

2.4.3 Folic acid (FA)

FA is essential for DNA synthesis, DNA repair, and methylation of DNA and is therefore necessary for cell survival and proliferation. The human folate receptor (FR), a glycosyl phosphatidyl inositol anchored membrane protein of 38 kDa, which shows high affinity for FA. At present, FR is considered an essential marker component in most of the cancers including glioblastoma. FR expression is very low or almost undetectable in most of the normal cells/tissues, but its expression is much higher in ovarian, breast, brain, lung, colorectal cancers [59]. FR-mediated liposomal delivery has been shown to enhance the antitumor efficacy of doxorubicin both in vitro and in vivo, and to overcome P-glycoprotein-mediated multi-drug resistance. Using folate as a targeting ligand, FR-targeting nanodrug delivery systems have been developed to target in situ glioma tumors [60].

2.4.4 Transferrin (Tf)

Tf receptor has been evolved as another important target for receptor-mediated transcytosis across the BBB. Owing to its higher expression on BBB endothelium, Tf-conjugation to the LNCs could be used as an effective active targeting strategy to enhance therapeutic outcomes in glioblastoma. Tf is basically a single chain iron-transporting glycoprotein that supplies iron into cells via receptor-mediated endocytosis [61]. Though, expression of Tf receptor remains very low in most of the normal tissues but its expression increases drastically in case of brain cancer. The binding affinity of Tf to its receptors on the external surface of tumor endothelial cells has been found 10 to 100 times more than in normal endothelial cells [62]. LNCs can take advantage of this feature through surface conjugation with Tf, which will be then actively transported into the tumor cells. Tf modified liposomes, nanoparticles and dendrimers have been widely investigated in recent years.

2.4.5 Oligopeptides

Oligopeptides are another class of emerging targeting ligands, which are now heavily investigated for glioma-specific drug targeting [63, 64]. The Arg-Gly-Asp (RGD) oligopeptide is a component of the extracellular matrix protein fibronectin, which is involved in the cell adhesion, migration and proliferation [64]. RGD is known to serve as a recognition motif in multiple ligands for several different integrin receptors. RGD-containing peptide can be internalized into cells by integrin-mediated endocytosis.

3. Advancements in lipid nanocarrier based drug delivery research in glioblastoma

LNCs in view of their architectural uniqueness and preferable in vitro characteristics have become leading choice of delivery vehicle in glioblastoma research [33].

Many recent studies have depicted superiority of the LNCs in successful drug targeting to brain as compared to conventional formulations. S D. Hettiarachchi and his co-researchers developed a nano drug formulation of triple conjugated delivery system which included conjugation of two drugs to achieve synergistic effect in glioma. The triple conjugated delivery system comprised of transferrin, epirubicin and temozolomide. The in vitro results showed higher anticancer effect for transferrin conjugated samples. MTT assay depicted dramatically reduced cell viability in case of targeted nanocarriers as compared to non-transferrin conjugated carriers. The triple system of transferrin conjugated samples was significantly more cytotoxic to glioblastoma cell lines and was more effective than their equivalent single agents [65].

Another new strategy reported potentiality of aptamer-based immunoliposomes in modifying PD-1-silencing T cells. PD-1 gene was knocked out from CD8+ T cells using CRISPR/Cas9 system to liberate T cell activity from immunosuppression. The work involved stimulation of PD-1– T cells followed by functional modification of tumor-specific nanoliposomes (hEnd-Apt/CD3-Lipo) to generate FC/PD-1– CTLs. The activation and proliferation of the modified FC/PD-1– CTLs were then measured [66]. The anticancer potential of experimental CTLs against HepG2-tumors was evaluated in xenograft mice. Results indicated that the modification of hEnd-Apt/CD3-Lipo nanocomposites on the FC/PD-1– CTLs had a more substantial synergetic effect in inhibiting tumor growth and prolonging animal survival, rather than other control liposomes [66]. Though, the study was not directed towards glioblastoma therapy, but the active targeting of immunoliposomes towards PD-1 receptor could be taken an attractive strategy for futuristic potential application in glioblastoma. Seeing the over-expression of PD-1 in many brain/CNS disorders including glioma, the outcome of the study could be used as an important input for further research of LNCs based PD-1 targeting to glioblastoma.

The therapeutic potential of hyaluronic acid (HA) as a targeting ligand for glioblastoma was investigated in a study by Stephen L et al. Anticancer effect of HA-conjugated doxorubicin loaded LNCs was reported in cortical astrocytes, MG, and A172 cells. In the study, three different glioblastoma cell lines were employed *viz.* invasive/non-tumorigenic (A172 cells), non-invasive/slightly tumorigenic (U251), and invasive/ highly tumorigenic (U87MG). A 24-hour potency assay demonstrated that the LC_{50} of experimental LNCs on A172 cells was nearly 5 folds lower than the corresponding LC_{50} for the cortical astrocytes and nearly 3 folds lower than that for MG cells [67]. The study thus highlighted potential application of HA in promoting preferential tumor cell uptake, with significant enhancement in chemotherapeutic potency in glioblastoma cells as compared to astrocytes.

Application of monoclonal antibodies as glioma-specific ligands through nano-liposomal vesicular carriers has already been reported. A recent liposomal delivery study has suggested conjugation of CD133 antibodies as a suitable method for targeting glioblastoma [52]. The study reported brain targeted delivery of gemcitabine, a widely used anticancer drug for cancers. However, being a BCS class III category of drug, it has higher water solubility with low permeability. Hence, to meet the challenge of sufficient brain uptake, gemcitabine was loaded in nanoliposome and the surface of the gemcitabine loaded liposome was functionalized with CD 133. The experimental CD 133 modified nanolipsomes was then tested for their in vitro and in vivo performance in glioblastoma cells. The in vitro study showed that conjugation of CD133 significantly enhanced the cytotoxicity of gemcitabine through endocytosis of CD133 surface markers overexpressed on glioblastoma cells [52]. The anti-tumor effect of CD133-modified nanoliposome was 15 times higher than that of free drug.

The formulation also showed enhanced in vivo stability and cytotoxicity through in glioma bearing xenograft models. Moreover, monitoring of body weight changes showed that the use of targeted nanoliposomes significantly reduced the toxicity of gemicitabine.

Compared to single anticancer drug based chemotherapy, a combination of gene and drug therapy is being investigated in recent studies to achieve breakthrough in glioma treatment. It was expected that therapeutic genes and chemical drugs could act on different targeting sites with different mechanisms and could achieve synergistic therapeutic efficacy. The study explored the potential application of angiopep-2 through paclitaxel loaded cationic nanoliposomes. Angiopep-2 possesses the ability to target the low-density lipoprotein receptor-related protein, which is over-expressed on the BBB and glioma cells [68]. In a study, angiopep-2 modified cationic liposome was developed (ANG-CLP) for effective co-delivery of a therapeutic gene and an anticancer drug. The gene encoding the human tumour necrosis factor-related apoptosis-inducing ligand (pEGFP-hTRAIL) was used along with paclitaxel as the drug of choice for targeted delivery to glioma through LNCs. The dual targeting co-delivery system improved cellular uptake and gene expression in U87 MG human glioblastoma cells and also in the infiltrating margin of intracranial U87 MG glioma-bearing models [69]. The dual targeting LNCs selectively induced apoptosis in U87 MG cells while reducing toxicity to BCECs. Results of the pharmacodynamics studies showed that the apoptosis of glioma cells in *in vitro* BBB models and in U87 MG glioma-bearing mice treated by the experimental LNCs was more apparent and widespread than that treated by single medication systems and unmodified co-delivery system. Along with that, the median survival time of brain tumour-bearing mice group treated with angiopep-2-targetd LNCs was 69.5 days, which was significantly longer than that of conventional nanolipsome and standard drug treated groups. The treatment groups received commercial temozolomide showed median survival time of 47 days only [69].

Receptor-mediated endocytosis is one of the major mechanisms which can be effectively employed as active targeting approach to deliver the conventional chemotherapeutic agents to permeate across BBB. The receptors for insulin, transferrin, endothelial growth factors, amino acids, follic acid along with various metabolic nutrients are expressed on BBB, which thus can be taken as an opportunity to modify the surface of nanocarriers with relevant targeting moiety to make them brain specific. Dual-targeting doxorubicin encapsulated nanoliposomes were produced by conjugating the experimental liposomes with both folate and Tf, which were then tested for their effectiveness in glioma model [70]. The nanoliposomes were characterized by particle size, drug entrapment efficiency, and in vitro drug release profile. Drug accumulation, P-gp expression, and drug transport across the BBB in the dual-targeting nanoliposomes were examined by using bEnd3 BBB models. In vivo studies demonstrated that the dual-targeted nanoliposomes could successfully transport doxorubicin across the BBB and mainly distributed in the brain glioma. The anti-tumor effect of the dual-targeting liposome was also found significantly higher as compared to plain liposomes and free drug in terms of increased survival time and decreased tumor volume [70].

From our laboratory, we also carried out few works related to the brain delivery or BBB permeation ability of anticancer drugs through LNCs based strategy. Though our works were mostly based on passive targeting approach where we have mostly utilized the lipophilic nature and nanosize property of our developed liposomal vesicles to target the anticancer drug to brain, but the outcomes of the work was quite impressive, which has compelled us for their further clinical translational studies. One of the recent studies from our laboratory reported the successful delivery of lomustine in glioma cells via lipid nanovesicular constructs [71]. Experimental LNCs were developed by modified lipid layer hydration technique and evaluated for different *in vitro* characteristics. Anticancer potential of selected lomustine loaded LNCs was tested on C6 glioma cell line *in vitro*. The experimental LNCs were within a size of less than 50 nm along with 8.8% drug loading capacity. Confocal microscopy revealed reasonable internalization of the selected LNCs in C6 cells. Experimental formulations were found more cytotoxic than free lomustine and blank LNCs as depicted from MTT assay. A clear improvement in pharmacokinetic profile both in blood and brain in the experimental mice models was observed for drug loaded LNCs than free drug. The formulations showed negligible haemolysis in mice blood cells, which further justified their safer in vivo applications.

Another similar study by Satapathy et al., reported delivery of docetaxel successfully to the rat brain through DSPE-modified nanoliposomes. In the work, the researchers simply aggravated the passive targeting strategy by utilizing DSPE, a sphingolipid, which has abundant presence the in brain and CNS. In the work, they developed a DSPE incorporated LNCs encapsulating docetaxel and investigated its BBB crossing potential, both qualitatively and quantitatively, in vivo [72]. Pharmacokinetic and biodistribution data showed an enhanced residence time of the docetaxel in the blood and efficient permeation of the drug from the docetaxel loaded LNCs through the BBB, as compared to free drug. The technetium-99 m labeled experimental LNCs effectively crossed the BBB and accumulated in the brain tissue in a time dependant manner as depicted from single photon emission tomography data [72]. At 4 h experimental time period, radiolabelled-LNCs were clearly tracked in the rat brain, whereas the same signal was absent in case of radiolabelled-free drug, which thus clearly confirmed that the sphingolipid modified LNCs possessed the necessary potential for BBB permeation and could be effective for the treatment of glioblastoma. Similar study from another research group in same department revealed successful delivery of docetaxel to rat brain through experimental nanoliposomes. Anti-proliferative effect of the experimental docetaxel loaded LNCs was conducted on C6 rat glioma cells. MTT assay showed that IC_{50} values of docetaxel from experimental nanoliposomes (9.5 ± 0.8 nM) was significantly less in comparison to free-drug (IC_{50} value, 70.8 ± 0.1 nM) and marketed Taxotere (IC_{50} value, 86.5 ± 0.3 nM) [73]. Flow cytometric analysis of C6 glioma cells incubated with fluorescein isothiocyanate (FITC)-labelled docetaxel loaded LNCs indicated about 18 and 23% enhancement of cellular uptake at 0.5 h at 0.5 h and 6 h of treatments in comparison to untreated cells.

Triggered drug delivery now-a-days has been merged as an interesting active targeting option for improved delivery of drugs through nanocarriers for the treatment of glioblastoma. A recent study showed that repeated pulsed high-intensity focused ultrasound can be used to improve the delivery of doxorubicin loaded nanocarriers to brain [74]. Atherosclerotic plaque-specific peptide-1 (AP-1) was used as the targeting ligand over the surface of doxorubicin loaded LNCs to selectively target glioblastoma cells. Compared with the control group, the animals treated with AP-1-conjugated nanoliposomes (5 mg/kg) showed significantly enhanced accumulation of drug at the sonicated tumor site and also a significantly elevated tumor-to-normal brain drug ratio ($p = 0.001$) (**Table 1**).

4. Challenges ahead

It is a fact that nanomedicine has revolutionized the field of medical diagnostics and treatment and significantly improved the therapeutic and pharmacokinetic profile of conventional chemotherapy for effective targeting at brain. However, in spite of all eye-catching progress in nanocarrier based drug targeting, lots of challenges still remain, which in fact need serious insight analysis. Common obstacles with the use of LNCs for successful treatment of glioblastoma yet remain unaddressed largely in the form of the RES uptake, opsonisation, *in vivo* stability etc. [85].

Another issue is the cell/tissue accumulation and toxicity concern of engineered LNCs. Ultra-small size and brain specific delivery through targeting ligands though helpful for increased cellular uptake and diminished off-target toxicity, but accumulation of such engineered nanodrug systems in healthy organ cannot be fully ruled out. Such *in vivo* studies related to the toxicological concern of engineered nanodrug carriers are too highly lacking. Since, the toxic effects upon long-term accumulation of nanodrug carriers largely depend on various physico-chemical factors including shape, size, composition, biocompatibility, route of administration, degradation mechanism, drug-tissue interaction, protein binding etc., these factors thus need to be vividly analysed from case to case basis. The safety and pharmacological effect of engineered LNCs can be influenced by minor variations in multiple parameters and need to be carefully examined in preclinical and clinical studies. Systematic impact analysis of the possible acute/chronic toxicity effects of novel LNCs on humans and environment is the need of the hour.

Oral administration of LNCs is still not a feasible strategy due to stability and liver metabolism issues. Even, after intravenous administration, it is still unclear, how the properties of engineered LNCs change in brain microenvironments, or their effect on complement activation, blood coagulation, etc. Thus, many such important factors related to the *in vivo* behaviour engineered LNCs and their post treatment effect on normal brain cells need thorough investigation.

There is still dearth of ample pre-clinical research outcome of engineered LNCs on glioblastoma. Most of the studies related to glioblastoma are confined to *in vitro* cell line studies. Though experiments on *in vivo* efficacy of LNCs in brain tumor bearing xenograft model is there, but results of such research are highly variable with lack *of in vitro-in vivo* correlation data. Due to reliable *in vitro-in vivo* correlation related studies with variable research outcomes, such engineered LNCs face serious hurdle in clearing requisite regulatory approval for clinical trials [85]. The insufficiency of specific regulatory guidelines for the development, evaluation, *in vivo* testing of engineered LNCs is also another crucial factor in clinical translation. The leading pharma houses or pharma-research and development laboratories are still in confusion, whether to rely on the clinical efficacy of engineered nanodrug carriers for the treatment of glioblastoma on large scale basis. To find a sponsor for clinical trial of engineered nanodrug carriers still remains a tough task.

For anticancer drug loaded LNCs, dose ranges need to be correctly defined along with sufficient blood and brain pharmacokinetics data. Since, clinical testing of nanodrug carriers intended for the treatment of glioblastoma starts from phase II stage, i.e. subsiding phase I clinical trial on healthy volunteers, therefore establishment of proper in vivo safety, pharmacokinetic and dose-range data are highly crucial. In case of in vivo experiments, concerns are also being raised by some formulation scientists and medical experts on the rationality of *in vivo* experiments using xenograft

Lipid nanocarrier based delivery system	Drug/ therapeutic agent	Targeting strategy/ targeting ligand	Research findings	Reference
H-ferritin siRNA conjugated nanoliposome	siRNA	Active targeting/ H-ferritin	H-ferritin siRNA decreased protein expression by 80% within 48 hours. Increased apoptosis in glioma cells *in vitro*	[75]
FTH1 loaded nanoliposome	FTH1 siRNA	Passive targeting	FTH1 down-regulation demonstrated by decreased cell viability, impaired DNA repair and reduced colony formation	[76]
Glutathione PEGylated liposomal Doxorubicin	Doxorubicin	Active targeting/ Glutathione	4.8 fold increase in brain-to-blood ratio of doxorubicin as compared to generic Caelyx® ($p = 0.0016$)	[77]
Dual-functioned nanoliposome	Doxorubicin	Active targeting/ Transferrin and cell-penetrating peptide	Tf/TAT-modified nanoliposomes showed higher anti-proliferative activity against U87 cells and also in orthotropic glioma model *in vivo*.	[78]
OX26/CTX-conjugated liposome	Plasmid DNA	Active targeting/ OX26 and chlorotoxin	The targeted nanoliposome exhibited enhanced therapeutic effects on C6 cells.Dual-targeting effect diminished tumor volumes (18.81 ± 6.15 mm3) and extended median survival time (46 days) in C6 glioma-bearing rats.	[79]
Dual-targeting nanoliposme	Doxorubincin	Active targeting/ folate and transferrin	Dual-targeting liposome demonstrated increased survival time, decreased tumor volume in glioblastoma model	[80]
Folic acid modified nanoliposome	Lidocaine	Active targeting/ Follic acid	Higher uptake of targeted nanoliposomes by U87 cells. Suppressed the motility of U87 glioma cells and stimulated apoptosis.	[81]
Dual-targeting liposome	Paclitaxel	Active targeting/ Transferrin and arginine-glycine-aspartic acid	In vivo imaging demonstrated RGD peptide and transferrin provided the highest brain distribution. Targeted liposomes showed preferential anti-proliferative activity against C6 glioma cells	[82]

Lipid nanocarrier based delivery system	Drug/ therapeutic agent	Targeting strategy/ targeting ligand	Research findings	Reference
Theranostic liposomes	Docetaxel	Active targeting / folate	Higher cellular uptake lower IC_{50} showed for folate-targeted nanoliposomes than non-targeted liposomes and marketed formulation	[83]
Ligand modified nanoliposme	Doxorubicin	Active targeting/ c(RGDfK) and Peptide-22	c(RGDfK) and Peptide-22-modified nanoliposomes increased the internalization in U87 cells. In vivo imaging verified higher brain tumor distribution for targeted nanoliposmes than un-modified liposomes.	[84]

Table 1.
Research outcomes on lipid nanocarrier based drug delivery systems, targeting strategy adopted in metastatic glioma.

mice/rat model bearing brain tumor. As such animal systems are usually athymic or immune-compromised; data derived out of these animal experiments cannot be fully relied on to carry out direct clinical testing on human subjects. In view of the significant anatomical/ physiological differences between immune-compromised laboratory animal model and human subjects in the development and progression of glioblastoma, it has been a point of long argument that whether these animal models could really mimic the human brain micro environment or whether such pre-clinical safety/ dose-range data can be reciprocated in clinical settings. It is a fact that laboratory rodents employed for the study do not suffer from glioblastoma or any other brain/ CNS cancers frequently as normal humans. Furthermore, immune response, cellular reaction, metabolism profile between laboratory animals and human subjects vary significantly differently. In a lay man language the material, which behave nontoxic to animals may show severe toxicity to humans or vice versa. Again till now, exact mechanism behind development/progression of glioblastoma in humans is largely unclear just as other cancer types. We seriously lack sufficient knowledge or well characterized data on specific biochemical factors, diseased conditions or antigens/ proteins responsible for development of glioblastoma. Thus, how much it will be rational to trust on the animal experiment data involving artificial/forcefully develop glioblastoma in nude/athymic animal models. Whether the use of such genetically modified animal models could really serve the purpose of successful clinical translation of LNCs? The budding scientists and medical/pharmacy/clinical professionals have to find specific answer for these unsolved questions in order to convince the manufacturers/sponsors to go ahead for large scale production.

Moving from the regulatory or clinical application problems towards large scale production at industrial scale, there is too lots of challenges remain unaddressed. Many pharmaceutical companies are still hesitant to invest directly in the large scale production of LNCs based delivery platforms. Batch to batch variation, problems with scale up, high cost of raw materials, availability of standardized unique protocol for manufacturing and testing, stability issues, low drug carrying capacity are some of the major issues associated with LNCs. As a result, maximum research outcomes are confined in academic or small scale research laboratories and cannot able to reach from bench to bed side. To simplify the approval process for LNC based drug delivery system, a closer cooperation among various regulatory agencies is also warranted. Government of various countries too have ample responsibility with regard to develop advanced/simplified protocols that must be genuine, less tedious, yet sufficiently rigorous to address any safety concerns in a timely manner.

5. Conclusion

Glioblastoma still remains an area of unmet medical challenge despite remarkable progress in understanding its genesis and propagation. With advancements in molecular biology, biotechnology and interdisciplinary research horizon covering nanotechnology, computational biology, genetic engineering etc., successful treatment strategies are highly expected in near future. Continuous research by formulation scientists have led to development of novel lipid nanocarrier based formulations, which are showing promise in glioblastoma both *in vitro* and *in vivo* rodent models of the disease. Few of the nanodrug carriers have already seen day light with successful clinical applications in brain cancer patients. However, number of such advanced engineered nanocarrier system at clinical trial stage is still very limited. Stringent regulatory procedure coupled with lack of sponsors/industrial collaborators are being the major hurdles in successful clinical translation of the nanodrug carriers from laboratory to bed side. Active targeting strategies with tumor-specific ligands though emerged as hopeful approach in elevating treatment outcomes and to reduce chemo-induced side effects in glioblastoma, but in reality, lots of challenges are need to be focused. Recent studies have introduced MRI and near infrared imaging to the administration of dual-targeted nanodrug carriers, enabling targeting to be imaged with these new theranostics. Although the engineered LNCs could be plausible option for treating glioblastoma, detailed in depth analysis is highly essential to bring out desired outcomes in patients. In vivo performances of engineered LNCs are yet highly variable and *in vitro-in vivo* correlation data is seriously lacking. Till now, the leading pharma manufactures in India hesitate to go ahead for the large-scale production of targeted nanodrug carriers. Data are also scarce and dissatisfactory for targeted nanomedicnes to show improved clinical outcomes or improved quality of life post treatment in glioblastoma. Despite these daunting facts there is still hope. Personalized cancer planning, advance diagnosis, ample pre-clinical research, continuous research idea exchange between industry and academia are some of the highly focused area, which could finally make this goal a reality. With the growing global trend, the future of modern multimodal, multi-centered treatment approach of LNCs for regular clinical application in glioblastoma looks feasible.

Author details

Bhabani Sankar Satpathy[1]*, Binapani Barik[2], Ladi Alik Kumar[2] and Sangram Biswal[1]

1 School of Pharmaceutical Sciences, Siksha 'O' Anusandhan (Deemed to be University), Bhubaneswar, Odisha, India

2 Centurion University of Technology and Management, R. Sitapur, Odisha, India

*Address all correspondence to: bhabanisatapathy@soa.ac.in; bbhabanisatapathy@yahoo.com

References

[1] Aldape K, Brindle KM, Chesler L, Chopra R, Gajjar A, Gilbert MR, et al. Challenges to curing primary brain tumours. Nature Reviews Clinical oncology. 2019;**16**(8):509-520. DOI: 10.1038/s41571-019-0177-5

[2] Gilbert MR, Dignam JJ, Armstrong TS, Wefel JS, Blumenthal DT, Vogelbaum MA, et al. A randomized trial of bevacizumab for newly diagnosed glioblastoma. New England Journal of Medicine. 2014;**370**(8):699-708. DOI: 10.1056/nejmoa1308573

[3] Nimmervoll BV, Boulos N, Bianski B, Dapper J, DeCuypere M, Shelat A, et al. Establishing a preclinical multidisciplinary board for brain tumors: A preclinical multidisciplinary brain tumor board. Clinical Cancer Research. 2018;**24**(7):1654-1666. DOI: 10.1158/1078-0432.ccr-17-2168

[4] Mackay A, Burford A, Carvalho D, Izquierdo E, Fazal-Salom J, Taylor KR, et al. Integrated molecular meta-analysis of 1000 pediatric high-grade and diffuse intrinsic pontine glioma. Cancer Cell. 2017;**32**(4):520-537. DOI: 10.1016/j.ccell.2017.08.017

[5] Zacharakis N, Chinnasamy H, Black M, Xu H, Lu YC, Zheng Z, et al. Immune recognition of somatic mutations leading to complete durable regression in metastatic breast cancer. Nature Medicine. 2018;**24**(6):724-730. DOI: 10.1038/s41591-018-0040-8

[6] Szopa W, Burley TA, Kramer-Marek G, Kaspera W. Diagnostic and therapeutic biomarkers in glioblastoma: Current status and future perspectives. BioMed Research International. 2017;**8013575**:1-14. DOI: 10.1155/2017/8013575

[7] Ohgaki H, Kleihues P. The definition of primary and secondary glioblastoma. Clinical Cancer Research. 2013;**19**:764-772. DOI: 10.1158/1078-0432

[8] National Brain Tumor Society. Glioblastoma Facts & Figures. 2019. Available from: https://braintumor.org/events/glioblastoma-awareness-day/about-glioblastoma

[9] Hanif F, Muzaffar K, Perveen K, Malhi SM, Simjee SU. Glioblastoma multiforme: A review of its epidemiology and pathogenesis through clinical presentation and treatment. Asian Pacific Journal of Cancer Prevention. 2017;**18**(1):3-9. DOI: 10.22034/APJCP.2017.18.1.3

[10] Leone JP, Leone BA. Breast cancer brain metastases: The last frontier. Experimental Hematology & Oncology. 2015;**4**(33):1-10. DOI: 10.1186/s40164-015-0028-8

[11] Urbańska K, Sokołowska J, Szmidt M, Sysa P. Glioblastoma multiforme—An overview. Contemporary Oncology. 2014;**5**:307-312. DOI: 10.5114/wo.2014.40559

[12] Davis ME. Glioblastoma: Overview of disease and treatment. Clinical Journal of Oncology Nursing. 2016;**20**(5):1-8. DOI: 10.1188/16.cjon.s1.2-8

[13] Tamimi AF, Juweid M. Epidemiology and Outcome of Glioblastoma. Brisbane (AU): Codon Publications; 2017. pp. 143-153. DOI: 10.15586/codon.glioblastoma.2017.ch8

[14] Franchino F, Rudà R, Soffietti R. Mechanisms and therapy for cancer metastasis to the brain. Frontiers in Oncology. 2018;**8**:161. DOI: 10.3389/fonc.2018.00161

[15] Fernandes C, Costa A, Osório L, Lago RC, Linhares P, Carvalho B, et al. Current Standards of Care in Glioblastoma Therapy. Exon Publications; 2017. pp. 197-241. DOI: 10.15586/codon.glioblastoma.2017.ch11

[16] Baskar R, Dai J, Wenlong N, Yeo R, Yeoh KW. Biological response of cancer cells to radiation treatment. Frontiers in Molecular Biosciences. 2014;**1**:24. DOI: 10.3389/fmolb.2014.00024

[17] Makale MT, McDonald CR, Hattangadi-Gluth J, Kesari S. Brain irradiation and long-term cognitive disability: Current concepts. Nature reviews. Neurology. 2017;**13**(1):52-64. DOI: 10.1038/nrneurol.2016.185

[18] Zhou J, Rossi JJ. Cell-specific aptamer-mediated targeted drug delivery. Oligonucleotides. 2011;**21**(1): 1-10. DOI: 10.1089/oli.2010.0264

[19] Su S, Kang P. Recent advances in nanocarrier-assisted therapeutics delivery systems. Pharmaceutics. 2020;**12**(9):837. DOI: 10.3390/pharmaceutics12090837

[20] Yingchoncharoen P, Kalinowski DS, Richardson DR. Lipid-based drug delivery systems in cancer therapy: What is available and what is yet to come. Pharmacological Reviews. 2016;**68**(3):701-787. DOI: 10.1124/pr.115.012070

[21] Wen H, Jung H, Li X. Drug delivery approaches in addressing clinical pharmacology-related issues: Opportunities and challenges. The AAPS Journal. 2015;**17**(6):1327-1340. DOI: 10.1208/s12248-015-9814-9

[22] Alavijeh MS, Chishty M, Qaiser MZ, Palmer AM. Drug metabolism and pharmacokinetics, the blood-brain barrier, and central nervous system drug discovery. NeuroRx. 2005;**2**(4):554-571. DOI: 10.1602/neurorx.2.4.554

[23] Ventola CL. The nanomedicine revolution: Part 1: Emerging concepts. Pharmacy and Therapeutics. 2012;**9**:512

[24] Zheng M, Tao W, Zou Y, Farokhzad OC, Shi B. Nanotechnology-based strategies for siRNA brain delivery for disease therapy. Trends in Biotechnology. 2018;**36**(5):562-575. DOI: 10.1016/j.tibtech.2018.01.006

[25] Dong X. Current strategies for brain drug delivery. Theranostics. 2018;**8**(6):1481-1493. DOI: 10.7150/thno.21254

[26] Daniëlle ME, Mark L, Ronald B, Robert CS, Albert DW, Philip S, et al. P-Glycoprotein function at the blood–brain barrier: Effects of age and gender. Molecular Imaging and Biology. 2012;**14**(6):771-776. DOI: 10.1007/s11307-012-0556-0

[27] Narvekar M, Xue HY, Eoh JY, Wong HL. Nanocarrier for poorly water-soluble anticancer drugs-barriers of translation and solutions. AAPS PharmSciTech. 2014;**15**(4):822-833. DOI: 10.1208/s12249-014-0107-x

[28] Meng-Chih W, Jye-Lin H, Ted WL. Evans blue dye as an indicator of albumin permeability across a brain endothelial cell monolayer in vitro. Neuroreport. 2021;**32**(11):957-964. DOI: 10.1097/WNR.0000000000001690

[29] Din F, Aman W, Ullah I, Qureshi OS, Mustapha O, Shafique S, et al. Effective use of nanocarriers as drug delivery systems for the treatment of selected tumors. International Journal of Nanomedicine. 2017;**12**:7291-7309. DOI: 10.2147/IJN.S146315

[30] Blanco E, Shen H, Ferrari M. Principles of nanoparticle design for

overcoming biological barriers to drug delivery. Nature Biotechnology. 2015;**33**(9):941-951. DOI: 10.1038/nbt.3330

[31] Manasa MH, Suma P, Srinivas M, Abhishek C, Jayant SG, Satish Rao BS. Multifunctional lipidic nanocarriers for effective therapy of glioblastoma: Recent advances in stimuli-responsive, receptor and subcellular targeted approaches. Journal of Pharmaceutical Investigation. 2022;**52**:49-74. DOI: 10.1007/s40005-021-00548-6

[32] Tu L, Luo Z, Wu YL, Huo S, Liang XJ. Gold-based nanomaterials for the treatment of brain cancer. Cancer Biology & Medicine. 2021;**18**(2):372-387. DOI: 10.20892/j.issn.2095-3941.2020.0524

[33] Patra JK, Das G, Fraceto LF, Campos EV, Rodriguez-Torres MD, Acosta-Torres LS, et al. Nano based drug delivery systems: Recent developments and future prospects. Journal of Nanobiotechnology. 2018;**16**(1):1-33. DOI: 10.1186/s12951-018-0392-8

[34] Jung SS, Qingguo X, Namho K, Justin H, Laura ME. PEGylation as a strategy for improving nanoparticle-based drug and gene delivery. Advanced Drug Delivery Reviews. 2016;**99**(Pt A):28-51. DOI: 10.1016/j.addr.2015.09.012

[35] Rizvi SA, Saleh AM. Applications of nanoparticle systems in drug delivery technology. Saudi Pharmaceutical Journal. 2018;**26**(1):64-70. DOI: 10.1016/j.jsps.2017.10.012

[36] Bozzuto G, Molinari A. Liposomes as nanomedical devices. International Journal of Nanomedicine. 2015;**10**:975. DOI: 10.2147/ijn.s68861

[37] Guimarães D, Cavaco-Paulo A, Nogueira E. Design of liposomes as drug delivery system for therapeutic applications. International Journal of Pharmaceutics. 2021;**601**:120571. DOI: 10.1016/j.ijpharm.2021.120571

[38] Daraee H, Etemadi A, Kouhi M, Alimirzalu S, Akbarzadeh A. Application of liposomes in medicine and drug delivery. Artificial Cells, Nanomedicine, and Biotechnology. 2016;**44**(1):381-391. DOI: 10.3109/21691401.2014.953633

[39] Ahmed KS, Hussein SA, Ali AH, Korma SA, Lipeng Q, Jinghua C. 2019. Liposome: Composition, characterisation, preparation, and recent innovation in clinical applications. Journal of Drug Targeting. 2019;**27**(7):742-761. DOI: 10.1080/1061186x.2018.1527337

[40] Large DE, Abdelmessih RG, Fink EA, Auguste DT. Liposome composition in drug delivery design, synthesis, characterization, and clinical application. Advanced Drug Delivery Reviews. 2021;**176**:113851. DOI: 10.1016/j.addr.2021.113851

[41] Pasut G, Paolino D, Celia C, Mero A, Joseph AS, Wolfram J, et al. Polyethylene glycol (PEG)-dendron phospholipids as innovative constructs for the preparation of super stealth liposomes for anticancer therapy. Journal of Controlled Release. 2015;**199**:106-113. DOI: 10.1016/j.jconrel.2014.12.008

[42] Lingayat VJ, Zarekar NS, Shendge RS. Solid lipid nanoparticles: A review. Nanoscience and Nanotechnology Research. 2017;**2**:67-72

[43] Mu H, Holm R. Solid lipid nanocarriers in drug delivery: Characterization and design. Expert Opinion on Drug Delivery. 2018;**15**(8):771-785. DOI: 10.1080/17425247.2018.1504018

[44] Geszke-Moritz M, Moritz M. Solid lipid nanoparticles as attractive drug vehicles: Composition, properties and therapeutic strategies. Materials Science and Engineering. 2016;**68**:982-994. DOI: 10.1016/j.msec.2016.05.119

[45] Senapati S, Mahanta AK, Kumar S, Maiti P. Controlled drug delivery vehicles for cancer treatment and their performance. Signal Transduction and Targeted Therapy. 2018;**3**(1):1-9. DOI: 10.1038/s41392-017-0004-3

[46] Hoshyar N, Gray S, Han H, Bao G. The effect of nanoparticle size on in vivo pharmacokinetics and cellular interaction. Nanomedicine. 2016;**11**(6):673-692. DOI: 10.2217/nnm.16.5

[47] Longmire M, Choyke PL, Kobayashi H. Clearance properties of nano-sized particles and molecules as imaging agents: considerations and caveats. Nanomedicine (Lond). 2005;**3**(5):703-717. DOI: 10.2217/17435889.3.5.703

[48] Bazak R, Houri M, El Achy S, Hussein W, Refaat T. Passive targeting of nanoparticles to cancer: A comprehensive review of the literature. Molecular and Clinical Oncology. 2014;**2**(6):904-908. DOI: 10.3892/mco.2014.356

[49] Yao Y, Zhou Y, Liu L, Xu Y, Chen Q, Wang Y, et al. Nanoparticle-based drug delivery in cancer therapy and its role in overcoming drug resistance. Frontiers in Molecular Biosciences. 2020;**7**:193. DOI: 10.3389/fmolb.2020.00193

[50] Hirsjarvi S, Passirani C, Benoit JP. Passive and active tumour targeting with nanocarriers. Current Drug Discovery Technologies. 2011;**8**(3):188-196. DOI: 10.2174/157016311796798991

[51] Mukherjee B, Satapathy BS, Mondal M, Dey NS, Maji R. Potentials and challenges of active targeting at the tumor cells by engineered polymeric nanoparticles. Current Pharmaceutical Biotechnology. 2013;**14**(15):1250-1263. DOI: 10.2174/138920101566614060814 3235

[52] Shin DH, Xuan S, Kim W-Y, Bae G-U, Kim J-S. CD133 antibody-conjugated immunoliposomes encapsulating gemcitabine for targeting glioblastoma stem cells. Journal of Materials Chemistry B. 2014;**2**:3771-3781. DOI: 10.1039/c4tb00185k

[53] Zeppernick F, Ahmadi R, Campos B, Dictus C, Helmke BM, Becker N, et al. Clinical Cancer Research. 2008;**14**:123-129. DOI: 10.1158/1078-0432.ccr-07-0932

[54] Zhou J, Rossi J. Aptamers as targeted therapeutics: Current potential and challenges. Nature Reviews Drug Discovery. 2017;**16**(3):181-202. DOI: 10.1038/nrd.2016.199

[55] Keefe AD, Pai S, Ellington A. Aptamers as therapeutics. Nature Reviews Drug Discovery. 2010;**9**(7):537-550. DOI: 10.1038/nrd3141

[56] Emma MH, Wei D, Sarah S. Aptamers and glioblastoma: Their potential use for imaging and therapeutic applications. International Journal of Molecular Sciences. 2017;**18**:1-17. DOI: 10.3390/ijms18122576

[57] Ni X, Castanares M, Mukherjee A, Lupold SE. Nucleic acid aptamers: Clinical applications and promising new horizons. Current Medicinal Chemistry. 2011;**18**(27):4206-4214. DOI: 10.2174/092986711797189600

[58] Affinito A, Quintavalle C, Esposito CL, Roscigno G, Vilardo C, Nuzzo S, et al. The discovery of RNA aptamers that selectively bind glioblastoma stem cells. Molecular

Therapy-Nucleic Acids. 2019;**18**:99-109. DOI: 10.1016/j.omtn.2019.08.015

[59] Fernández M, Javaid F, Chudasama V. Advances in targeting the folate receptor in the treatment/imaging of cancers. Chemical Science. 2018;**9**(4):790-810

[60] Chen YC, Chiang CF, Wu SK, et al. Targeting microbubbles-carrying TGFβ1 inhibitor combined with ultrasound sonication induce BBB/BTB disruption to enhance nanomedicine treatment for brain tumors. Journal of Controlled Release. 2015;**11**:53-62. DOI: 10.1016/j.jconrel.2015.05.288

[61] Ediriwickrema A, Saltzman WM. Nanotherapy for cancer: Targeting and multifunctionality in the future of cancer therapies. ACS Biomaterials Science & Engineering. 2015;**1**(2):64-78. DOI: 10.1021/ab500084g

[62] Yu MK, Park J, Jon S. Targeting strategies for multifunctional nanoparticles in cancer imaging and therapy. Theranostics. 2012;**2**(1):3-44. DOI: 10.7150/thno.3463

[63] Lajoie JM, Shusta EV. Targeting receptor-mediated transport for delivery of biologics across the blood-brain barrier. Annual Review of Pharmacology and Toxicology. 2015;**55**:613. DOI: 10.1146/annurev-pharmtox-010814-124852

[64] Pulgar VM. Transcytosis to cross the blood-brain barrier, new advancements and challenges. Frontiers in Neuroscience. 2019;**12**:1019. DOI: 10.3389/fnins.2018.01019

[65] Hettiarachchi SD, Graham RM, Mintz KJ, Zhou Y, Vanni S, Peng Z, et al. Triple conjugated carbon dots as a nano-drug delivery model for glioblastoma brain tumors. Nanoscale. 2019;**11**(13):6192-6205. DOI: 10.1039/c8nr08970a

[66] Xie S, Hou X, Yang W, Shi W, Yang X, Duan S, et al. Endoglin-aptamer-functionalized liposome-equipped PD-1-silenced T cells enhance Antitumoral immunotherapeutic effects. International Journal of Nanomedicine. 2021;**16**:6017-6034. DOI: 10.2147/ijn.s317220

[67] Hayward SL, Wilson CL, Kidamb S. Hyaluronic acid-conjugated liposome nanoparticles for targeted delivery to CD44 overexpressing glioblastoma cells. Oncotarget. 2016;7:34158-34171. DOI: 10.18632/oncotarget.8926

[68] Ke W, Shao K, Huang R, Han L, Liu Y, Li J, et al. Gene delivery targeted to the brain using an Angiopep-conjugated polyethyleneglycol-modified polyamidoamine dendrimer. Biomaterials. 2009;**30**(36):697. DOI: 10.1016/j.biomaterials.2009.08.049

[69] Sun X, Pang Z, Ye H, Qiu B, et al. Co-delivery of pEGFP-hTRAIL and paclitaxel to brain glioma mediated by an angiopep-conjugated liposome. Biomaterials. 2011;**33**:916-926. DOI: 10.1016/j.biomaterials.2011.10.035

[70] Gao J-Q, Lv Q, Li L-M, Tang X-J, Li F-Z, Yu-Lan H, et al. Glioma targeting and bloodebrain barrier penetration by dual-targeting doxorubincin liposomes. Biomaterials. 2013;**14**:5628-5639. DOI: 10.1016/j.biomaterials.2013.03.097

[71] Satapathy BS, Kumar LA, Pattnaik G, Barik B. Lomustine incorporated lipid nanostructures demonstrated preferential anticancer properties in C6 glioma cell lines with enhanced pharmacokinetic profile in mice. Acta Chimica Slovenica. 2021;**68**:970-982. DOI: 10.17344/acsi.2021.6977

[72] Satapathy BS, Mukherjee B, Baishya R, Debnath MC, Dey NS, Maji R.

Lipid nanocarrier-based transport of docetaxel across the blood brain barrier. RSC Advances. 2016;**6**:85261-85274. DOI: 10.1039/c6ra16426a

[73] Shaw TK, Mandal D, Dey G, Pal MM. Successful delivery of docetaxel to rat brain using experimentally developed nanoliposome: a treatment strategy for brain tumor. Drug Delivery. 2017;**24**(1):346-357. DOI: 10.1080/10717544.2016.1253798

[74] Yang FY, Teng MC, Lu M, Liang HF, Lee YR, Yen CC, et al. Treating glioblastoma multiforme with selective high-dose liposomal doxorubicin chemotherapy induced by repeated focused ultrasound. International Journal of Nanomedicine. 2012;7:965-974. DOI: 10.2147/IJN.S29229

[75] Liu X, Madhankumar AB, Slagle-Webb B, Sheehan JM, Surguladze N, Connor JR. Heavy chain ferritin siRNA delivered by cationic liposomes increases sensitivity of cancer cells to chemotherapeutic agents. Cancer Research. 2011;**71**(6):2240-2249. DOI: 10.1158/0008-5472.CAN-10-1375

[76] Vagisha R, Achuthamangalam BM, Thomas A, Becky SW, James RC. Liposomal delivery of ferritin heavy chain 1 (FTH1) siRNA in patient xenograft derived glioblastoma initiating cells suggests different sensitivities to radiation and distinct survival mechanisms. PLoS One. 2019;**14**(9):e0221952. DOI: 10.1371/journal. pone.0221952

[77] Thomas B, Reingard R, Werner G, Christina G, Edgar G, Arijit G, et al. Enhanced doxorubicin delivery to the brain administered through glutathione PEGylated liposomal doxorubicin (2B3-101) as compared with generic Caelyx,(®)/Doxil(®)—A cerebral open flow microperfusion pilot study. Journal of Pharmaceutical Sciences. 2014;**103**(7):1945-1948. DOI: 10.1002/jps.23994

[78] Chuanyi Z, Chunyang M, Enqi B, Kun Y, Ruxiang X. Transferrin and cell-penetrating peptide dual-functioned liposome for targeted drug delivery to glioma. International Journal of Clinical and Experimental Medicine. 2015;**8**(2):1658-1668. DOI: 10.3892/ol.2014.2449

[79] Yue PJ, He L, Qiu SW, Li Y, Liao YJ, Li XP, et al. OX26/CTX-conjugated PEGylated liposome as a dual-targeting gene delivery system for brain glioma. Molecular Cancer. 2014;**13**:191. DOI: 10.1186/1476-4598-13-191

[80] Gao JQ, Qing L, Li-Ming L, Jiang T, Fan-Zhu L, Yu-Lan H, et al. Glioma targeting and bloodebrain barrier penetration by dual-targeting doxorubincin liposomes. Biomaterials. 2013;**34**:5628-5639. DOI: 10.1016/j.biomaterials.2013.03.097

[81] Li D, Yang X, Li B, Yang C, Sun J, Yu M, et al. Lidocaine liposome modified with folic acid suppresses the proliferation and motility of glioma cells via targeting the PI3K/AKT pathway. Experimental and Therapeutic Medicine. 2021;**22**(3):1-10. DOI: 10.3892/etm.2021.10457

[82] Qin L, Wang CZ, Fan HJ, Zhang CJ, Zhang HW, Lv MH, et al. A dual-targeting liposome conjugated with transferrin and arginine-glycine-aspartic acid peptide for glioma-targeting therapy. Oncology Letters. 2014;**8**(5):2000-2006. DOI: 10.3892/ol.2014.2449

[83] Muthu MS, Kulkarni SA, Raju A, Feng S-S. Theranostic liposomes of TPGS coating for targeted co-delivery of docetaxel and quantum dots.

Biomaterials. 2012;**33**:3494-3501. DOI: 10.1016/j.biomaterials.2012.01.036

[84] Chen C, Duan Z, Yuan Y, Li R, Pang L, Liang J, et al. Peptide-22 and cyclic RGD functionalized liposomes for glioma targeting drug delivery overcoming BBB and BBTB. ACS Applied Materials & Interfaces. 2017;**9**(7):5864-5873. DOI: 10.1021/acsami.6b15831

[85] Kumar LA, Pattnaik G, Satapathy BS, Swapna S, Mohanty D. Targeting to brain tumor: Nanocarrier-based drug delivery platforms, opportunities, and challenges. Journal of Pharmacy & Bioallied Sciences. 2021;**13**:172-177. DOI: 10.4103/jpbs.JPBS_239_20

Chapter 12

Glycan and Glycosylation as a Target for Treatment of Glioblastoma

Atit Silsirivanit

Abstract

Glycosylation is an important post-translational modification regulating many cellular processes. In cancer, aberrant glycosylation leads to the expression of tumor-associated glycans that are possibly used as therapeutic targets or biomarkers for diagnosis, monitoring, and prognostic prediction. The cumulative evidence suggested the significance of alteration of glycosylation in glioblastoma (GBM). Aberrant glycosylation presents truncated or uncommon glycans on glycoproteins, glycolipids, and other glycoconjugates. These aberrant glycans consequently promote the tumor development, metastasis, and therapeutic resistance. The glycosylation changes occurred in either cancer cells or the tumor microenvironment. GBM-associated glycans and their corresponding enzymes are proposed to be a target for GBM treatment. Several tools, such as lectin and inhibitors, are possibly applied to target the tumor-associated glycans and glycosylation for the treatment of GBM. This chapter provides information insight into glycosylation changes and their roles in the development and progression of GBM. The perspectives on targeting glycans and glycosylation for the treatment of GBM are enclosed.

Keywords: glioma, glioblastoma, glycosylation, glycan, lectin

1. Introduction

Glycosylation is a critical process to maturate the glycoproteins and glycolipids. Many factors were demonstrated to regulate this process, including 1) nucleotide sugar donors, 2) glycosyltransferase enzymes, and 3) glycosidase enzymes. The activated nucleotide sugars, synthesized through the hexosamine biosynthesis pathway, are served as sugar donors for the glycosylation process. More than 200 glycosyltransferase (GT) and glycosidase (GA) enzymes, residing in the endoplasmic reticulum (ER) or Golgi apparatus, are responsible for the addition and removal of sugar onto the glycoconjugates [1]. There are two major types of protein core-glycosylation, including N-linked and O-linked glycosylation (**Figure 1**). Both N-linked and O-linked glycans are generally terminal-modified with sialic acid and fucose *via* sialylation and fucosylation, respectively. Glycosylation is a sensitive process that could be influenced by several stimulants and cellular stresses. Many studies

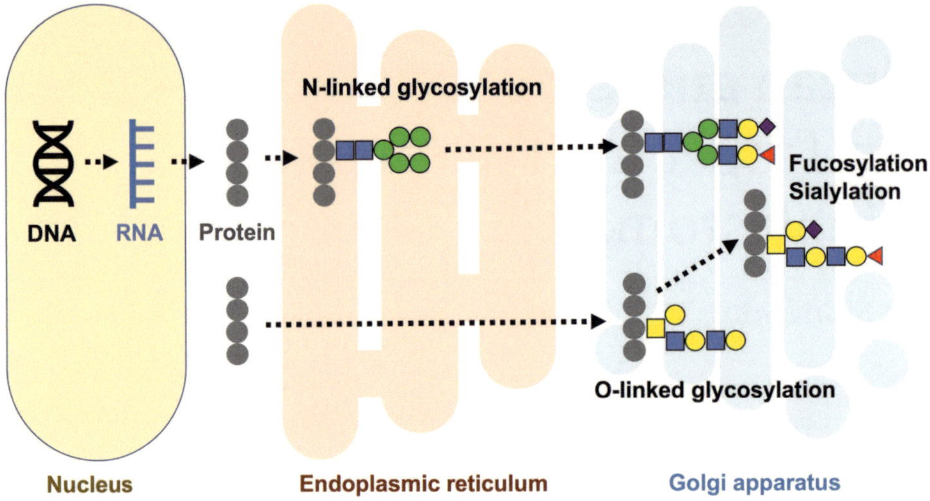

Figure 1.
Protein glycosylation. After transcription and translation, the proteins undergo N-linked glycosylation in endoplasmic reticulum or O-linked glycosylation in Golgi apparatus. Both N-linked glycans and O-linked glycans undergo peripheral modifications, fucosylation, and sialylation in the Golgi apparatus.

showed that altered glycosylation is associated with the carcinogenesis and progression of cancers [2, 3]. Defects in glycosylation are possibly caused by the alteration of nucleotide sugar synthesis or the imbalanced expression of glycosyltransferases or glycosidases [4]. Aberrant glycosylation in cancer cells causes the glycan truncation or the expression of uncommon glycans. These aberrantly expressed glycans are possibly used as a biomarker or a target for the treatment of cancers. Many tumor-associated glycans were demonstrated to play essential roles in tumor development, progression, and therapeutic resistance [2, 5].

Recent evidence suggests the alteration of glycosylation in glioblastoma (GBM) [3, 4, 6, 7]. GBM-associated glycans and glycoconjugates, such as the cluster of differentiation 44 (CD44), CD133, and ephrin-A1, were discovered to play important roles in tumor progression, leading to the poor prognosis of patients [8, 9]. Defects of glycosylation in GBM tumors were found in glycoproteins, glycolipids, glycosaminoglycans, or proteoglycans. The alteration of protein glycosylation occurred in both N-linked and O-linked glycosylation. Besides, aberrant terminal glycan modification of sialylation or fucosylation was also observed in GBM [3]. Moreover, the glycans and glycosylation also exhibited the functional significance in glioma stem-like cells (GSC) by regulating the stem cell-related phenotypes [10, 11].

Not only in cancer cells, the tumor microenvironment (TME) was also presented with aberrant glycosylation [12, 13]. Glycosylation changes in TME were found to promote tumor progression, immunosuppression, and therapeutic resistance [14]. Therefore, it is proposed that glycosylation changes of TME might be an alternative target for the treatment of GBM.

This chapter collectively summarizes the recent information on glycan and glycosylation changes and their roles in GBM progression and therapeutic resistance. The information provided here may fulfill our understanding of the roles of glycosylation and its potential to be a target for the treatment of GBM.

2. N-linked glycosylation

The N-linked glycosylation transfers the oligosaccharide chain to the target polypeptide by forming the linkage between the *N*-acetyl glucosamine (GlcNAc) residue and the amide side chain of the asparagine residue. The process starts in ER; an oligosaccharide is firstly synthesized on the dolichol phosphate carrier and transferred to the protein acceptor by the oligosaccharyltransferase enzyme. The premature glycan chain of N-linked glycoprotein is subsequently modified by the sequential reactions of sugar addition or removal, controlled by several GTs and GAs. The final steps, sialylation and fucosylation, are accomplished in the Golgi apparatus. Many studies demonstrated the alteration of *N*-linked glycosylation and its related enzymes in GBM (**Table 1**).

Enzymes	Glycan products	Related functions	References
N-linked glycosylation			
MGAT-1	Hybrid N-linked oligosaccharide	• Proliferation • Migration	[15]
MGAT-5	Biantennary or β1,6-GlcNAc-containing *N*-linked oligosaccharide	• Invasion • Radioresistance	[16–18]
B4GalT-5	Highly branched N-glycans	• Drug resistance • Self-renewal • Tumorigenicity	[19–21]
B3GnT-8	Polylactosamine on branched N-glycans	• Proliferation • Migration	[22]
O-linked glycosylation			
GALNT-2	O-GalNAc glycan	• Migration • Invasion	[23]
GALNT-12	O-GalNAc glycan	• Proliferation • Migration	[24]
Fucosylation			
FUT-8	α1,6-fucosylated N-glycan	• Proliferation • Migration • Invasion • Drug resistance	[25]
Sialylation			
ST3Gal-3	α2,3-sialylated glycan	• Invasion	[18]

β1,3-N-acetylglucosaminyltransferase-8, B3GnT8; β1,4-Galactosyltransferase 5, B4GalT5; mannosylglycoprotein β-N-acetylglucosaminyltransferase-1, MGAT1; mannosylglycoprotein β-N-acetylglucosaminyltransferase-5, MGAT5; polypeptide GalNAc transferase-2, GALNT-2; polypeptide GalNAc transferase-12, GALNT-12; Fucosyltransferase-8, FUT-8; α2,3-sialyltransferase-3, ST3Gal-3.

Table 1.
Glycosyltransferases involved in the progression of GBM.

An increase of bi-, tri-, and tetra-anternary N-linked glycans was found to be associated with the progression of GBM [15–17, 26]. The α1,6-mannosylglycoprotein-β-*N*-acetylglucosaminyltransferase-5 (MGAT), an enzyme responsible for the synthesis of biantennary *N*-linked oligosaccharide, was found to promote the invasiveness of GSC [16]. N-linked glycosylation of the receptor protein tyrosine phosphatase type mu (RPTPmu) controlled by MGAT5 was demonstrated to suppress its function and consequently enhance the migration ability of GBM cells through phospholipase C (PLC)/protein kinase C (PKC) pathway [17]. In addition, the MGAT1 (a member of the N-linked associated *N*-acetylglucosaminyltransferase group) was highly detected in GBM and plays an essential role in promoting the proliferation and invasion of cancer cells [15, 17].

A new subclass of *N*-glycosylation called-Paucimannosylation, producing a truncated N-glycan ($Man_3GlcNAc_2Fuc$), was found to elevate in GBM compared with non-tumor tissues [27, 28]. The glycan was found to be involved in the proliferation, migration, and invasion of cancer cells [27].

Another N-link-associated enzyme, a β1,3-*N*-acetylglucosaminyltransferase-8 (B3GnT8), an enzyme that controls the formation of polylactosamine on β1–6 branched N-glycans, was found to regulate the proliferation and metastatic ability of cancer cells [22]. The β1,4-galactosyltransferase-5 (B4Gal-5) producing highly branched N-glycans was found to regulate the sensitivity of cancer cells to anticancer drugs-etoposide and arsenic trioxide. Suppression of B4GalT-5 could enhance the apoptosis induction effects of these drugs in cancer cells, suggesting its potential to improve the therapeutic efficiency for malignant glioma [19, 20]. Moreover, the B4GalT-5 was also found to regulate self-renewal and tumorigenicity of glioma stem-like cells [20].

Inhibition of N-glycan synthesis by the specific siRNA or inhibitors significantly suppresses tumor growth, metastasis, and radioresistance of GBM [15–18, 29–31]. This information suggested the potential of N-glycosylation to be a target for the treatment of GBM.

3. O-linked glycosylation

Golgi-resident glycosyltransferases are responsible for the synthesis of O-glycans *via* O-linked glycosylation. A particular serine (Ser) and threonine (Thr) residues can be O-glycosidic linked with various kinds of oligosaccharides. This chapter focuses on the mucin-type O-glycosylation or O-GalNAcylation, an O-linked modification of Ser/Thr by *N*-acetylgalactosamine (GalNAc), followed by the formation of complex oligosaccharide structure. There are 20 isoforms of polypeptide GalNAc transferase (ppGalNAcT or GALNT) identified in humans; the enzymes catalyze the transferring of GalNAc from activated nucleotide sugar donor to initially modify the Ser or Thr residues of a specific glycoprotein [32]. Alteration of O-linked, especially O-GalNAc, glycosylation was observed in many types of cancer [1, 5, 32]. Truncated O-glycans and their associated mucin glycoproteins were applicable as a marker for diagnosis, monitoring, and prognostic prediction of cancer [1].

In GBM, the alteration of O-linked glycosylation played a significant role in the tumor progression and therapeutic resistance [23, 24]. The significance of GALNT enzymes in the progression of GBM has been revealed, suggesting their possibility of being a new target for GBM treatment (**Table 1**). GALNT-2 was demonstrated to promote the migration and invasion of cancer cells [23]. Expression of GALNT-12 was associated with poor prognosis of GBM patients as it promotes cancer cell proliferation, migration, and invasion *via* PI3K/Akt/mTOR cascade [24]. The tumor-associated truncated O-linked glycan and its receptor, macrophage galactose-type lectins, were found to modulate the function of tumor-associated macrophages and microglia in GBM [33]. Using lectin from *Dolichos biflorus*, the GalNAc-associated glycan was highly detected in GSC compared with its differentiated form, suggesting its potential to be a GSC marker (**Table 2**) [11]. This information suggested the possibility of using GALNTs as a biomarker and a therapeutic target for GBM.

4. Fucosylation

The terminal glycan modification by fucose, called "Fucosylation," is controlled by the fucosyltransferase (FUT) enzymes. In human, 13 FUTs are classified according to their activities into 1) α1,2-FUTs (FUT-1 and FUT-2), 2) α1,3-FUTs (FUT-3, FUT-4, FUT-5, FUT-6, FUT-7, FUT-9, FUT-10, and FUT-11), 3) α1,4-FUTs (FUT-3 and FUT-5), 4) α1,6-FUTs (FUT-8), and 5) O-FUTs (Pofut-1 and Pofut-2) [34]. Altered expression of FUTs and the fucosylated-glycans were found to associate with tumor development and progression [5, 35]. In GBM, the aggressiveness and malignant phenotypes GBM were associated with fucosylated Lewis antigens' expression [36]. The enzyme FUT-8, responsible for α-1,6-fucosylation of N-glycans, was discovered to promote the growth, migration, and invasion of GBM cells [25]. Inhibition of fucosylation by the inhibitor-2F-peracetyl-fucose could sensitize the effect of temozolomide (TMZ), suggesting the potential of FUT-8 to be a target for GBM treatment [25].

5. Sialylation

Sialylation is a modification of glycoproteins and glycolipids by sialic acid (Sia). There are 20 sialyltransferase enzymes (STs) responsible for three types of sialylations: 1) α2,3-sialylation, 2) α2,6-sialylation, and 3) α2,8-sialylation (**Table 2**) [37, 38].

Sialylations	Enzymes	Glycan structure
α2,3-sialylation	ST3Gal-1, ST3Gal-2, ST3Gal-3, ST3Gal-4, ST3Gal-5, ST3Gal-6	Sia-α2,3-Gal
α2,6-sialylation	ST6Gal-1 and ST6Gal-2	Sia-α2,6-Gal
	ST6GalNAc-1, ST6GalNAc-2, ST6GalNAc-3, ST6GalNAc-4, ST6GalNAc-5, and ST6GalNAc-6	Sia-α2,6-GalNAc
α2,8-sialylation	ST8Sia1, ST8Sia2, ST8Sia3, ST8Sia4, ST8Sia5, and ST8Sia6	Sia-α2,8-Sia

Sialyltransferase, ST; Galactose, Gal; N-acetylgalactosamine, GalNAc; Sialic acid, Sia.

Table 2.
Sialylation and the associated enzymes and glycan structures.

Sialylation was demonstrated to involve in the stemness maintenance of GSC and tumor progression, suggesting its possibility to be a promising target for the treatment of GBM [39, 40]. An α-2,3 sialylation was found to promote the progression, while α-2,6 sialylation suppresses the GBM. Inhibition of α-2,3 or enhancement of α-2,6 sialylation significantly suppresses the metastatic ability of GBM cells [41–43]. Using lectin from *Maackia amurensis*, α-2,3 sialylation was found to be enhanced in GSC and play an essential role in stemness maintenance [39]. Suppression of sialylation using ST inhibitor or sialidase leads to the apoptosis of GSC [39]. The mechanism by which α-2,3 sialylation regulates stemness of GSC is probably explained by its role in the stabilization of surface CD133, an important functional GSC marker [43]. Moreover, the lectin *M. amurensis* lectin-II (MAL-II) could significantly induce the apoptosis of GSC, suggesting its potential for GBM treatment [39]. In addition, suppression of sialylation by a specific inhibitor was found to enhance the sensitivity of GBM cells to the general chemo-drugs—cisplatin and 5-fluorouracil [39]. This collective evidence suggested the potential of α-2,3 sialylation as a target for the treatment of GBM.

In addition, sialidases or neuraminidases (NEU), the enzymes that remove terminal Sia from the oligosaccharide chain of glycoproteins and glycolipids, were also altered in GBM. The overexpression of NEU3 significantly suppresses cancer cells' migration and invasion ability by promoting focal adhesions through calpain-dependent proteolysis [44]. NEU4 was found to be upregulated in GSC, and suppression of NEU4 significantly reduces cell survival and stemness properties of the cells [45].

6. Gangliosides, glycosaminoglycans, and proteoglycans

Altered syntheses of gangliosides, glycosaminoglycans, and proteoglycans were observed to play significant roles in GBM [46–52]. The GD3-gangliosides, heparan sulfate (HS) glycosaminoglycans, and their responsible enzymes were found to be altered in GBM and proposed as a potential GBM marker [46–48]. Glycosaminoglycans played essential roles in the communication between GBM cells and their TME. Alteration of HS synthesis by ablation of heparanase (HPSE) results in the significant reduction of tumor cell adhesion and invasion [48]. This information implied that HS is an important factor in promoting GBM invasion; it is therefore possibly proposed as a therapeutic target for GBM.

Alteration of proteoglycan synthesis was found to associate with the development and progression of GBM [49–52]. Expression of tumor-associated proteoglycans and their related enzymes were found to facilitate the tyrosine kinase signaling pathway, which benefits the progression of GBM, suggesting their potential as a promising prognostic marker and target for GBM treatment [49]. The elevation of neuro-glial proteoglycan-NG2 was associated with the invasiveness of GBM [50]. NG2 was found to control the vascular morphology and functions, suggesting its role in facilitating metastasis *via* tumor vascularization of GBM [51]. Targeting NG2, in combination with GD3A (a GBM-associated ganglioside), could significantly reduce the viability of GBM cells [53]. This information suggested the significance of NG2 in the progression of GBM and its possibility of being a target for treatment. Moreover, chondroitin sulfate proteoglycans (CSPGs) play important roles in organizing the tumor microenvironment to prevent tumor invasion. CSPGs were drastically decreased in a diffusely infiltrating tumor of GBM [52].

7. Conclusion and perspectives

Alteration of glycosylation was predominantly observed in either cancer cells or TME in GBM. Both core-glycosylation and peripheral glycan modifications were important factors in regulating the tumor development, progression, and therapeutic resistance. Several strategies have been proposed to target glycans and glycosylation for the treatment of GBM.

Suppression of glycosylation using specific interferences or inhibitors is a potential strategy to target glycosylation [54, 55]. However, there is a limitation to using the broad-spectrum glycosylation inhibitors for cancer treatment as they also affect the neighboring non-tumor cells. Targeting glycosylation of a particular glycoprotein or glycoconjugate is a possible strategy for cancer treatment. In GBM, interference of hyaluronic acid synthesis by methylumbelliferone (4-MU), an inhibitor of hyaluronic acid synthase capable of crossing the blood-brain barrier (BBB), was found to significantly inhibit the proliferation of GBM [56].

The short peptide is recently applicable for targeting or suppressing the specific glycoform of a particular glycoprotein in cancer cells. The deglycosylated form of brevican (dg-Bcan), an ECM-associated glycoprotein upregulated in GBM, was explicitly bound by a small 8-amino acid dg-Bcan-Targeting Peptide (BTP). The radiolabeled-BTP could be internalized into the cancer cell, suggesting its potential to be used as an imaging agent to detect GBM [57]. Further studies to apply this peptide for the treatment of GBM by conjugating it with chemo-drugs or other substances are noteworthy.

Based on the sugar preferential of lectins, the plant lectins were widely used to determine the expression of GBM-associated glycans as well as the functional analyses either *in vitro* or *in vivo* model (**Table 3**) [11, 18, 19, 21, 26, 59, 60]. Using the lectin as a therapeutic agent for GBM is another approach, either combined with other chemo-drugs or as a single agent.

The *Phaseolus vulgaris* erythroagglutinin (PHA-E) was used to detect the β1,4-GlcNAc-containing N-glycans. It strongly inhibits the migration ability of GBM cells, suggesting its potential to be used for the treatment of GBM [18]. In addition, PHA-E was also found to inhibit the functions of the epidermal growth factor receptor (EGF-R) and a drug efflux pump-P-glycoprotein on GBM [59, 61]. This information suggested the involvement of β1,4-GlcNAc in cancer cells' growth and drug resistance. Moreover, the potential of PHA-E as a chemosensitizing agent for GBM was also reported [61]. MAL-II is another lectin that can suppress the stemness maintenance and induce apoptosis of GSCs, suggesting its application as a therapeutic agent for GBM [39]. Lectin from *Griffonia simplicifolia* I (GSL-I) was used to identify the GBM-specific cell surface glycobiomarkers compared with the low-grade glioma. The identified markers may be applicable for diagnosis and possibly used as a target for the treatment of GBM [58]. With another type of brain tumor, the lectin from *Canavalia brasiliensis* seeds (ConBr) was found to suppress the ERK1/2 and Akt signaling pathways, consequently inhibiting the migration ability of rat neuroblastoma cells [62]. Besides the lectins, monoclonal antibodies against the specific glycans have been established and used to detect cancer-associated glycans. The antibodies can also suppress or activate the functions of glycans in cancer cells; this information suggests the possibility of using a glycan-specific antibody to treat the GBM patients [63, 64].

In conclusion, glycans and glycosylation have been identified to play significant roles in GBM progression and therapeutic resistance. Targeting glycans and glycosylation is possibly an alternative strategy for the treatment of GBM; however, further studies to target specific glycosylation of a particular glycoconjugate are still needed. In addition,

Lectins		Preferred glycan structure	Applications	References
Dolichos biflorus **agglutinin**	**DBA**	**GalNAc-modified glycan**	• Detection of GSC	**[11]**
Griffonia simplicifolia lectin-I	GSL-I	βGal/GalNAc	• Detection of GBM	[58]
Lens culinaris agglutinin	LCA	Core-fucosylated biantennary N-glycans	• Proliferation inhibition and apoptosis induction	[26]
Maackia amurensis lectin-II	MAL-II	α-2,3 sialylated glycans	• Detection of GSC • Apoptosis induction of GSC	[39]
Phaseolus vulgaris erythro-agglutinin	E-PHA	Bisecting β1,4-GlcNAc N-glycans	• Suppression of cell migration • Suppression of EGF-induced proliferation	[18, 59, 60]
Ricinus communis agglutinin-I	RCA-I	Highly branched N-glycans	• Enhancement of etoposide-induced apoptosis	[19, 21]

Table 3.
Lectins used in GBM studies.

the clinical studies or trials on the potential of using glycans and glycosylation as a target for GBM treatment are still a large gap that needs to be further evaluated.

Acknowledgements

The author would like to thank the supports from the National Research Council of Thailand and Khon Kaen University, Thailand.

Conflict of interest

The author declares no conflict of interest.

Author details

Atit Silsirivanit
Faculty of Medicine, Department of Biochemistry, Khon Kaen University, Khon Kaen, Thailand

*Address all correspondence to: atitsil@kku.ac.th

References

[1] Silsirivanit A. Glycosylation markers in cancer. Advances in Clinical Chemistry. 2019;**89**:189-213

[2] Vajaria BN, Patel PS. Glycosylation: A hallmark of cancer? Glycoconjugate Journal. 2017;**34**(2):147-156

[3] Veillon L, Fakih C, Abou-El-Hassan H, Kobeissy F, Mechref Y. Glycosylation changes in brain cancer. ACS Chemical Neuroscience. 2018;**9**(1):51-72

[4] Ashkani J, Naidoo KJ. Glycosyltransferase gene expression profiles classify cancer types and propose prognostic subtypes. Scientific Reports. 2016;**6**:26451

[5] Silsirivanit A. Glycans: Potential therapeutic targets for cholangiocarcinoma and their therapeutic and diagnostic implications. Expert Opinion on Therapeutic Targets. 2021;**25**(1):1-4

[6] Lemjabbar-Alaoui H, McKinney A, Yang YW, Tran VM, Phillips JJ. Glycosylation alterations in lung and brain cancer. Advances in Cancer Research. 2015;**126**:305-344

[7] Furukawa J, Tsuda M, Okada K, Kimura T, Piao J, Tanaka S, et al. Comprehensive glycomics of a multistep human brain tumor model reveals specific glycosylation patterns related to malignancy. PLoS One. 2015;**10**(7):e0128300

[8] Lehnus KS, Donovan LK, Huang X, Zhao N, Warr TJ, Pilkington GJ, et al. CD133 glycosylation is enhanced by hypoxia in cultured glioma stem cells. International Journal of Oncology. 2013;**42**(3):1011-1017

[9] Ferluga S, Hantgan R, Goldgur Y, Himanen JP, Nikolov DB, Debinski W. Biological and structural characterization of glycosylation on ephrin-A1, a preferred ligand for EphA2 receptor tyrosine kinase. The Journal of Biological Chemistry. 2013;**288**(25):18448-18457

[10] Cheray M, Petit D, Forestier L, Karayan-Tapon L, Maftah A, Jauberteau MO, et al. Glycosylation-related gene expression is linked to differentiation status in glioblastomas undifferentiated cells. Cancer Letters. 2011;**312**(1):24-32

[11] Tucker-Burden C, Chappa P, Krishnamoorthy M, Gerwe BA, Scharer CD, Heimburg-Molinaro J, et al. Lectins identify glycan biomarkers on glioblastoma-derived cancer stem cells. Stem Cells and Development. 2012;**21**(13):2374-2386

[12] Sethi MK, Downs M, Shao C, Hackett WE, Phillips JJ, Zaia J. In-depth matrisome and glycoproteomic analysis of human brain glioblastoma versus control tissue. Molecular & Cellular Proteomics. 2022;**21**(4):100216

[13] Quirico-Santos T, Fonseca CO, Lagrota-Candido J. Brain sweet brain: Importance of sugars for the cerebral microenvironment and tumor development. Arquivos de Neuro-Psiquiatria. 2010;**68**(5):799-803

[14] Tondepu C, Karumbaiah L. Glycomaterials to investigate the functional role of aberrant glycosylation in glioblastoma. Advanced Healthcare Materials. 2022;**11**(4):e2101956

[15] Li Y, Liu Y, Zhu H, Chen X, Tian M, Wei Y, et al. N-acetylglucosaminyltransferase I promotes glioma cell proliferation and migration through increasing

the stability of the glucose transporter GLUT1. FEBS Letters. 2020;**594**(2):358-366

[16] Marhuenda E, Fabre C, Zhang C, Martin-Fernandez M, Iskratsch T, Saleh A, et al. Glioma stem cells invasive phenotype at optimal stiffness is driven by MGAT5 dependent mechanosensing. Journal of Experimental & Clinical Cancer Research. 2021;**40**(1):139

[17] Gao Y, Yang F, Su Z, He Z, Xiao J, Xu Y, et al. beta1,6 GlcNAc branches-modified protein tyrosine phosphatase Mu attenuates its tyrosine phosphatase activity and promotes glioma cell migration through PLCgamma-PKC pathways. Biochemical and Biophysical Research Communications. 2018;**505**(2):569-577

[18] Yamamoto H, Swoger J, Greene S, Saito T, Hurh J, Sweeley C, et al. Beta1,6-N-acetylglucosamine-bearing N-glycans in human gliomas: Implications for a role in regulating invasivity. Cancer Research. 2000;**60**(1):134-142

[19] Jiang J, Shen J, Wu T, Wei Y, Chen X, Zong H, et al. Down-regulation of beta1,4-galactosyltransferase V is a critical part of etoposide-induced apoptotic process and could be mediated by decreasing Sp1 levels in human glioma cells. Glycobiology. 2006;**16**(11):1045-1051

[20] Wei Y, Zhou F, Ge Y, Chen H, Cui C, Li Q, et al. Beta1,4-galactosyltransferase V regulates self-renewal of glioma-initiating cell. Biochemical and Biophysical Research Communications. 2010;**396**(3):602-607

[21] Wei Y, Liu D, Ge Y, Zhou F, Xu J, Chen H, et al. Down-regulation of beta1,4GalT V at protein level contributes to arsenic trioxide-induced glioma cell apoptosis. Cancer Letters. 2008;**267**(1):96-105

[22] Liu J, Shen L, Yang L, Hu S, Xu L, Wu S. High expression of beta3GnT8 is associated with the metastatic potential of human glioma. International Journal of Molecular Medicine. 2014;**33**(6):1459-1468

[23] Liu J, Yang L, Jin M, Xu L, Wu S. Regulation of the invasion and metastasis of human glioma cells by polypeptide N-acetylgalactosaminyltransferase 2. Molecular Medicine Reports. 2011;**4**(6):1299-1305

[24] Zheng Y, Liang M, Wang B, Kang L, Yuan Y, Mao Y, et al. GALNT12 is associated with the malignancy of glioma and promotes glioblastoma multiforme *in vitro* by activating Akt signaling. Biochemical and Biophysical Research Communications. 2022;**610**:99-106

[25] Wei KC, Lin YC, Chen CH, Chu YH, Huang CY, Liao WC, et al. Fucosyltransferase 8 modulates receptor tyrosine kinase activation and temozolomide resistance in glioblastoma cells. American Journal of Cancer Research. 2021;**11**(11):5472-5484

[26] Tsuchiya N, Yamanaka R, Yajima N, Homma J, Sano M, Komata T, et al. Isolation and characterization of an N-linked oligosaccharide that is increased in glioblastoma tissue and cell lines. International Journal of Oncology. 2005;**27**(5):1231-1239

[27] Becker Y, Forster S, Gielen GH, Loke I, Thaysen-Andersen M, Laurini C, et al. Paucimannosidic glycoepitopes inhibit tumorigenic processes in glioblastoma multiforme. Oncotarget. 2019;**10**(43):4449-4465

[28] Chatterjee S, Lee LY, Kawahara R, Abrahams JL, Adamczyk B,

Anugraham M, et al. Protein Paucimannosylation is an enriched N-glycosylation signature of human cancers. Proteomics. 2019;**19**(21-22):e1900010

[29] Contessa JN, Bhojani MS, Freeze HH, Ross BD, Rehemtulla A, Lawrence TS. Molecular imaging of N-linked glycosylation suggests glycan biosynthesis is a novel target for cancer therapy. Clinical Cancer Research. 2010;**16**(12):3205-3214

[30] Shen L, Dong XX, Wu JB, Qiu L, Duan QW, Luo ZG. Radiosensitisation of human glioma cells by inhibition of beta1,6-GlcNAc branched N-glycans. Tumour Biology. 2016;**37**(4):4909-4918

[31] Wahl DR, Lawrence TS. No sugar added: A new strategy to inhibit glioblastoma receptor tyrosine kinases. Clinical Cancer Research. 2019;**25**(2):455-456

[32] Bennett EP, Mandel U, Clausen H, Gerken TA, Fritz TA, Tabak LA. Control of mucin-type O-glycosylation: A classification of the polypeptide GalNAc-transferase gene family. Glycobiology. 2012;**22**(6):736-756

[33] Dusoswa SA, Verhoeff J, Abels E, Mendez-Huergo SP, Croci DO, Kuijper LH, et al. Glioblastomas exploit truncated O-linked glycans for local and distant immune modulation via the macrophage galactose-type lectin. Proceedings of the National Academy of Sciences of the United States of America. 2020;**117**(7):3693-3703

[34] Shan M, Yang D, Dou H, Zhang L. Fucosylation in cancer biology and its clinical applications. Progress in Molecular Biology and Translational Science. 2019;**162**:93-119

[35] Indramanee S, Sawanyawisuth K, Silsirivanit A, Dana P, Phoomak C, Kariya R, et al. Terminal fucose mediates progression of human cholangiocarcinoma through EGF/EGFR activation and the Akt/Erk signaling pathway. Scientific Reports. 2019;**9**(1):17266

[36] Cuello HA, Ferreira GM, Gulino CA, Toledo AG, Segatori VI, Gabri MR. Terminally sialylated and fucosylated complex N-glycans are involved in the malignant behavior of high-grade glioma. Oncotarget. 2020;**11**(52):4822-4835

[37] Wang L, Liu Y, Wu L, Sun XL. Sialyltransferase inhibition and recent advances. Biochimica et Biophysica Acta. 2016;**1864**(1):143-153

[38] Harduin-Lepers A, Vallejo-Ruiz V, Krzewinski-Recchi MA, Samyn-Petit B, Julien S, Delannoy P. The human sialyltransferase family. Biochimie. 2001;**83**(8):727-737

[39] Putthisen S, Silsirivanit A, Panawan O, Niibori-Nambu A, Nishiyama-Ikeda Y, Ma-In P, et al. Targeting alpha2,3-sialylated glycan in glioma stem-like cells by Maackia amurensis lectin-II: A promising strategy for glioma treatment. Experimental Cell Research. 2022;**410**(1):112949

[40] Wielgat P, Niemirowicz-Laskowska K, Wilczewska AZ, Car H. Sialic acid-modified nanoparticles-new approaches in the glioma management-perspective review. International Journal of Molecular Sciences. 2021;**22**(14):7494

[41] Dawson G, Moskal JR, Dawson SA. Transfection of 2,6 and 2,3-sialyltransferase genes and GlcNAc-transferase genes into human glioma cell line U-373 MG affects glycoconjugate expression and enhances cell death. Journal of Neurochemistry. 2004;**89**(6):1436-1444

[42] Yamamoto H, Oviedo A, Sweeley C, Saito T, Moskal JR. Alpha2,6-sialylation of cell-surface N-glycans inhibits glioma formation *in vivo*. Cancer Research. 2001;**61**(18):6822-6829

[43] Zhou F, Cui C, Ge Y, Chen H, Li Q, Yang Z, et al. Alpha2,3-sialylation regulates the stability of stem cell marker CD133. Journal of Biochemistry. 2010;**148**(3):273-280

[44] Takahashi K, Proshin S, Yamaguchi K, Yamashita Y, Katakura R, Yamamoto K, et al. Sialidase NEU3 defines invasive potential of human glioblastoma cells by regulating calpain-mediated proteolysis of focal adhesion proteins. Biochimica et Biophysica Acta (BBA) - General Subjects. 2017;**1861** (11 Pt A):2778-2788

[45] Silvestri I, Testa F, Zappasodi R, Cairo CW, Zhang Y, Lupo B, et al. Sialidase NEU4 is involved in glioblastoma stem cell survival. Cell Death & Disease. 2014;**5**:e1381

[46] Sarbu M, Petrica L, Clemmer DE, Vukelic Z, Zamfir AD. Gangliosides of human glioblastoma multiforme: A comprehensive mapping and structural analysis by ion mobility tandem mass spectrometry. Journal of the American Society for Mass Spectrometry. 2021;**32**(5):1249-1257

[47] Fabris D, Rozman M, Sajko T, Vukelic Z. Aberrant ganglioside composition in glioblastoma multiforme and peritumoral tissue: A mass spectrometry characterization. Biochimie. 2017;**137**:56-68

[48] Tran VM, Wade A, McKinney A, Chen K, Lindberg OR, Engler JR, et al. Heparan sulfate glycosaminoglycans in glioblastoma promote tumor invasion. Molecular Cancer Research. 2017;**15**(11):1623-1633

[49] Wade A, Robinson AE, Engler JR, Petritsch C, James CD, Phillips JJ. Proteoglycans and their roles in brain cancer. The FEBS Journal. 2013;**280**(10):2399-2417

[50] Wiranowska M, Ladd S, Smith SR, Gottschall PE. CD44 adhesion molecule and neuro-glial proteoglycan NG2 as invasive markers of glioma. Brain Cell Biology. 2006;**35**(2-3):159-172

[51] Brekke C, Lundervold A, Enger PO, Brekken C, Stalsett E, Pedersen TB, et al. NG2 expression regulates vascular morphology and function in human brain tumours. NeuroImage. 2006;**29**(3):965-976

[52] Silver DJ, Siebzehnrubl FA, Schildts MJ, Yachnis AT, Smith GM, Smith AA, et al. Chondroitin sulfate proteoglycans potently inhibit invasion and serve as a central organizer of the brain tumor microenvironment. The Journal of Neuroscience. 2013;**33**(39):15603-15617

[53] Higgins SC, Fillmore HL, Ashkan K, Butt AM, Pilkington GJ. Dual targeting NG2 and GD3A using Mab-Zap immunotoxin results in reduced glioma cell viability in vitro. Anticancer Research. 2015;**35**(1):77-84

[54] Costa AF, Campos D, Reis CA, Gomes C. Targeting glycosylation: A new road for cancer drug discovery. Trends in Cancer. 2020;**6**(9):757-766

[55] Bowles WHD, Gloster TM. Sialidase and Sialyltransferase inhibitors: Targeting pathogenicity and disease. Frontiers in Molecular Biosciences. 2021;**8**:705133

[56] Yan T, Chen X, Zhan H, Yao P, Wang N, Yang H, et al. Interfering with hyaluronic acid metabolism suppresses glioma cell proliferation by regulating

autophagy. Cell Death & Disease. 2021;**12**(5):486

[57] von Spreckelsen N, Fadzen CM, Hartrampf N, Ghotmi Y, Wolfe JM, Dubey S, et al. Targeting glioblastoma using a novel peptide specific to a deglycosylated isoform of brevican. Advanced Therapeutics. 2021;**4**(4):2000244

[58] Park YE, Yeom J, Kim Y, Lee HJ, Han KC, Lee ST, et al. Identification of plasma membrane glycoproteins specific to human glioblastoma multiforme cells using lectin arrays and LC-MS/MS. Proteomics. 2018;**18**(1)

[59] Rebbaa A, Yamamoto H, Moskal JR, Bremer EG. Binding of erythroagglutinating phytohemagglutinin lectin from Phaseolus vulgaris to the epidermal growth factor receptor inhibits receptor function in the human glioma cell line, U373 MG. Journal of Neurochemistry. 1996;**67**(6):2265-2272

[60] Aoyanagi E, Sasai K, Nodagashira M, Wang L, Nishihara H, Ihara H, et al. Clinicopathologic application of lectin histochemistry: Bisecting GlcNAc in glioblastoma. Applied Immunohistochemistry & Molecular Morphology. 2010;**18**(6):518-525

[61] Rebbaa A, Chou PM, Vucic I, Mirkin BL, Tomita T, Bremer EG. Expression of bisecting GlcNAc in pediatric brain tumors and its association with tumor cell response to vinblastine. Clinical Cancer Research. 1999;**5**(11):3661-3668

[62] Wolin IAV, Heinrich IA, Nascimento APM, Welter PG, Sosa LDV, De Paul AL, et al. ConBr lectin modulates MAPKs and Akt pathways and triggers autophagic glioma cell death by a mechanism dependent upon caspase-8 activation. Biochimie. 2021;**180**:186-204

[63] Silsirivanit A, Araki N, Wongkham C, Vaeteewoottacharn K, Pairojkul C, Kuwahara K, et al. CA-S27: A novel Lewis a associated carbohydrate epitope is diagnostic and prognostic for cholangiocarcinoma. Cancer Science. 2013;**104**(10):1278-1284

[64] Kato Y, Kaneko MK. A cancer-specific monoclonal antibody recognizes the aberrantly glycosylated podoplanin. Scientific Reports. 2014;**4**:5924